2011
YEAR BOOK OF
OTOLARYNGOLOGY–
HEAD AND NECK SURGERY®

The 2011 Year Book Series

Year Book of Anesthesiology and Pain Management™: Drs Chestnut, Abram, Black, Gravlee, Lien, Mathru, and Roizen

Year Book of Cardiology®: Drs Gersh, Cheitlin, Elliott, Gold, Graham, and Thourani

Year Book of Critical Care Medicine®: Drs Dellinger, Parrillo, Balk, Dorman, Dries, and Zanotti-Cavazzoni

Year Book of Dermatology and Dermatologic Surgery™: Dr Del Rosso

Year Book of Diagnostic Radiology®: Drs Osborn, Abbara, Elster, Manaster, Oestreich, Offiah, Rosado de Christenson, Stephens, and Walker

Year Book of Emergency Medicine®: Drs Hamilton, Bruno, Handly, Mullin, Quintana, and Ramoska

Year Book of Endocrinology®: Drs Schott, Apovian, Clarke, Eugster, Ludlam, Meikle, Ovalle, Schinner, Schteingart, and Toth

Year Book of Gastroenterology™: Drs Talley, DeVault, Harnois, Pearson, Picco, Scolapio, Smith, and Vege

Year Book of Hand and Upper Limb Surgery®: Drs Yao and Steinmann

Year Book of Medicine®: Drs Barker, Garrick, Gersh, Khardori, LeRoith, Seo, Talley, and Thigpen

Year Book of Neonatal and Perinatal Medicine®: Drs Fanaroff, Benitz, Donn, Neu, Papile, Polin, and van Marter

Year Book of Neurology and Neurosurgery®: Drs Klimo and Rabinstein

Year Book of Obstetrics, Gynecology, and Women's Health®: Drs Dungan and Shulman

Year Book of Oncology®: Drs Arceci, Bauer, Gordon, Lawton, and Thigpen

Year Book of Ophthalmology®: Drs Rapuano, Cohen, Flanders, Hammersmith, Milman, Myers, Nelson, Penne, Pyfer, Sergott, Shields, and Vander

Year Book of Orthopedics®: Drs Morrey, Beauchamp, Huddleston, Swiontkowski, and Trigg

Year Book of Otolaryngology-Head and Neck Surgery®: Drs Sindwani, Balough, Franco, Gapany, and Mitchell

Year Book of Pathology and Laboratory Medicine®: Drs Raab, Parwani, Bejarano, and Bissell

Year Book of Pediatrics®: Dr Stockman

Year Book of Plastic and Aesthetic Surgery™: Drs Miller, Gosain, Gurtner, Gutowski, Ruberg, Salisbury, and Smith

Year Book of Psychiatry and Applied Mental Health®: Drs Talbott, Ballenger, Buckley, Frances, Krupnick, and Mack

Year Book of Pulmonary Disease®: Drs Barker, Jones, Maurer, Raza, Tanoue, and Willsie

Year Book of Sports Medicine®: Drs Shephard, Cantu, Feldman, Jankowski, Khan, Lebrun, Nieman, Pierrynowski, and Rowland

Year Book of Surgery®: Drs Copeland, Behrns, Daly, Eberlein, Fahey, Huber, Klodell, Mozingo, and Pruett

Year Book of Urology®: Drs Andriole and Coplen

Year Book of Vascular Surgery®: Drs Moneta, Gillespie, Starnes, and Watkins

2011

The Year Book of
OTOLARYNGOLOGY–
HEAD AND NECK
SURGERY®

Editor-in-Chief
Raj Sindwani, MD, FACS, FRCS(C)

Associate Editors
Ben J. Balough, CAPT, MC, USN
Ramon A. Franco, Jr, MD
Markus Gapany, MD, FACS
Ron B. Mitchell, MD

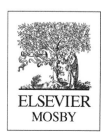

ELSEVIER
MOSBY

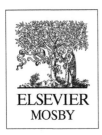

ELSEVIER
MOSBY

Vice President, Continuity: Kimberly Murphy
Editor: Jessica Demetriou
Production Supervisor, Electronic Year Books: Donna M. Skelton
Electronic Article Manager: Emily Ogle
Illustrations and Permissions Coordinator: Dawn Vohsen

2011 EDITION

Composition by TNQ Books and Journals Pvt Ltd, India
Printed and bound by CPI Group (UK) Ltd, Croydon, CR0 4YY
Transferred to Digital Print 2011

Editorial Office:
Elsevier
Suite 1800
1600 John F. Kennedy Blvd.
Philadelphia, PA 19103-2899

International Standard Serial Number: 1041-892X
International Standard Book Number: 978-0-323-08423-9

Editorial Board

Editor-in-Chief
Raj Sindwani, MD, FACS, FRCS(C)
Section Head, Rhinology, Sinus and Skull Base Surgery, Head and Neck Institute, Cleveland Clinic Foundation, Cleveland, Ohio

Associate Editors
Ben J. Balough, CAPT, MC, USN
Captain, Medical Corps, United States Navy; Deputy Director, Clinical Research, Navy Medical Research and Developmental Center, Navy Medicine Institute, Bureau of Medicine and Surgery, Washington, D.C.

Ramon A. Franco, Jr, MD
Assistant Professor, Department of Otology and Laryngology, Harvard Medical School; Director, Division of Laryngology, Medical Director of the Voice and Speech Laboratory, Massachusetts Eye and Ear Infirmary, Boston, Massachusetts

Markus Gapany, MD, FACS
Associate Professor of Otolaryngology, University of Minnesota; Chief of Otolaryngology, Minneapolis VA Medical Center; Paparella Ear, Head, and Neck Institute, Minneapolis, Minnesota

Ron B. Mitchell, MD
Professor and Chief, Division of Pediatric Otolaryngology, Saint Louis University School of Medicine, Cardinal Glennon Children's Hospital, St. Louis, Missouri

Table of Contents

Journals Represented

Journals represented in this YEAR BOOK are listed below.
Acta Otolaryngol
American Journal of Medicine
American Journal of Otolaryngology
American Journal of Respiratory and Critical Care Medicine
American Surgeon
Anesthesia & Analgesia
Annals of Neurology
Annals of Otology Rhinology & Laryngology
Annals of Surgical Oncology
Annals of Thoracic Surgery
Archives of Disease in Childhood
Archives of Otolaryngology Head & Neck Surgery
Archives of Surgery
British Journal of Cancer
Burns
Cancer Research
Clinical Journal of Pain
Dermatologic Surgery
Digestive Diseases and Sciences
European Journal of Nuclear Medicine and Molecular Imaging
Head & Neck
Headache
International Journal of Oral and Maxillofacial Surgery
International Journal of Radiation Oncology Biology Physics
Journal of Allergy and Clinical Immunology
Journal of Clinical Endocrinology & Metabolism
Journal of Dental Research
Journal of Laryngology and Otology
Journal of Oral and Maxillofacial Surgery
Journal of Otolaryngology: Head and Neck Surgery
Journal of Plastic, Reconstructive & Aesthetic Surgery
Journal of Trauma
Laryngoscope
Neurosurgery
New England Journal of Medicine
Oral Oncology
Otolaryngology-Head and Neck Surgery
Otology & Neurotology
Pediatric Dermatology
Pediatrics
Respiratory Medicine
Thyroid
World Journal of Surgery

STANDARD ABBREVIATIONS

The following terms are abbreviated in this edition: acquired immunodeficiency syndrome (AIDS), cardiopulmonary resuscitation (CPR), central nervous system (CNS), cerebrospinal fluid (CSF), computed tomography (CT), deoxyribonucleic acid (DNA), electrocardiography (ECG), health maintenance organization (HMO), human immunodeficiency virus (HIV), intensive care unit (ICU), intramuscular (IM), intravenous (IV), magnetic resonance (MR) imaging (MRI), ribonucleic acid (RNA), and ultrasound (US).

NOTE

The YEAR BOOK OF OTOLARYNGOLOGY–HEAD AND NECK SURGERY is a literature survey service providing abstracts of articles published in the professional literature. Every effort is made to assure the accuracy of the information presented in these pages. Neither the editors nor the publisher of the YEAR BOOK OF OTOLARYNGOLOGY–HEAD AND NECK SURGERY can be responsible for errors in the original materials. The editors' comments are their own opinions. Mention of specific products within this publication does not constitute endorsement.

To facilitate the use of the YEAR BOOK OF OTOLARYNGOLOGY–HEAD AND NECK SURGERY as a reference tool, all illustrations and tables included in this publication are now identified as they appear in the original article. This change is meant to help the reader recognize that any illustration or table appearing in the YEAR BOOK OF OTOLARYNGOLOGY–HEAD AND NECK SURGERY may be only one of many in the original article. For this reason, figure and table numbers will often appear to be out of sequence within the YEAR BOOK OF OTOLARYNGOLOGY–HEAD AND NECK SURGERY.

Introduction

Welcome to the 2011 edition of the YEAR BOOK OF OTOLARYNGOLOGY–HEAD AND NECK SURGERY.

As amazing as it may seem, the history and steep lineage of this unique publication dates back more than 110 years. The first edition of the YEAR BOOK OF OTOLARYNGOLOGY–HEAD AND NECK SURGERY was published in the year 1900 by Gustavus P. Head, MD, Professor of Laryngology and Rhinology at the Chicago Postgraduate Medical School. Dr Head's forward-thinking idea was to create "an epitome of much of the best literature of the year" in a volume convenient for reference. The first title of this publication was the YEAR BOOK OF THE NOSE, THROAT AND EAR, and it contained 274 pages. This book became the first ever in a series of YEAR BOOKS, which now have volumes representing 26 specialties.

From these humble beginnings, the sentiment of hand-selecting and then commenting upon and framing some of the seminal articles within our specialty has continued consecutively—and without pause—for more than a century. In addition to being a written repository of the most intriguing and landmark articles, the YEAR BOOK has evolved with the times and now offers streaming online publication of abstracts and editor commentaries as well. The endeavor has grown to include a large audience of hundreds of individuals and institutions, including more than 57 foreign institutions, which subscribe annually. This issue also boasts a truly international flavor, and a variety of papers from investigators around the globe are showcased herein.

As always, I am indebted to my tireless associate editors for their insightful reviews and cutting-edge commentaries, and they continue to make it a true pleasure to be involved with this project.

Raj Sindwani, MD, FACS, FRCS(C)

1 Allergy and Immunology

General

Allergy and Immunotherapy: Are They Related to Migraine Headache?
Martin VT, Taylor F, Gebhardt B, et al (Univ of Cincinnati College of Medicine, OH; Park Nicollet Clinic, Minneapolis, MN; Saint Vincent Hosp, Erie, PA; et al)
Headache 51:8-20, 2011

Introduction.—Several studies have reported that migraine headaches are more common in patients with allergic rhinitis and that immunotherapy decreases the frequency of headache in atopic headache sufferers.

Objective.—To determine if the degree of allergic sensitization and the administration of immunotherapy are associated with the prevalence, frequency, and disability of migraine headache in patients with allergic rhinitis.

Methods.—Consecutive patients between the ages of 18-65 presenting to an allergy practice that received a diagnosis of an allergic rhinitis subtype (eg, allergic or mixed rhinitis) were enrolled in this study. All participants underwent allergy testing as well as a structured verbal headache diagnostic interview to ascertain the clinical characteristics of each headache type. Those reporting headaches were later assigned a headache diagnosis by a headache specialist blinded to the rhinitis diagnosis based on 2004 International Classification Headache Disorders-2 (ICHD-2) diagnostic criteria. Migraine prevalence was defined as the percentage of patients with a diagnosis of migraine headache (ICHD-2 diagnoses 1.1-1.5). Migraine frequency represented the number of days per month with migraine headache self-reported during the headache interview and migraine disability was the number of days with disability obtained from the Migraine Disability Assessment questionnaire. Generalized linear models were used to analyze the migraine prevalence, frequency, and disability with the degree of allergic sensitization (percentage of positive allergy tests) and administration of immunotherapy as covariates. Patients were categorized into high (> 45% positive allergy tests) and low (≤45% positive allergy tests) atopic groups based on the number of allergy tests that were positive for the frequency and disability analyses.

Results.—A total of 536 patients (60% female, mean age 40.9 years) participated in the study. The prevalence of migraine was not associated with the degree of allergic sensitization, but there was a significant age/immunotherapy interaction ($P < .02$). Migraine headaches were less prevalent in the immunotherapy group than the nonimmunotherapy at ages <40 years and more prevalent in the immunotherapy group at ages ≥40 years of age. In subjects ≤45 years of age, increasing percentages of allergic sensitization were associated with a decreased frequency and disability of migraine headache in the low atopic group (risk ratios [RRs] of 0.80 [95% CI; 0.65, 0.99] and 0.81[95% CI; 0.68, 0.97]) while increasing percentages were associated with an increased frequency (not disability) in the high atopic group (RR = 1.60; [95% CI; 1.11, 2.29]). In subjects ≤45 years of age, immunotherapy was associated with decreased migraine frequency and disability (RRs of 0.48 [95% CI; 0.28, 0.83] and 0.55 [95% CI; 0.35, 0.87]). In those >45 years of age, there was no effect of degree of allergic sensitization or immunotherapy on the frequency and disability of migraine headache.

Conclusions.—Our study suggests that the association of allergy with migraine headaches depends upon age, degree of allergic sensitization, administration of immunotherapy, and the type of headache outcome measure that are studied. Lower "degrees of atopy" are associated with less frequent and disabling migraine headaches in younger subjects while higher degrees were associated with more frequent migraines. The administration of immunotherapy is associated with a decreased prevalence, frequency, and disability of migraine headache in younger subjects.

▶ The interplay between migraine headache and nasal conditions such as allergic rhinitis (AR) is poorly understood and sharply contested by some. Both conditions are of course very common and a daily part of an otolaryngologist's practice. Previous studies have reported an increased prevalence of migraine headache in patients with a diagnosis of AR. Some studies have also reported that migraine headaches are more common in patients with AR and that immunotherapy decreases the frequency of headache in atopic headache sufferers. This well-performed study examined these very important questions. Over 500 adult AR patients (60% female; mean age, 40.9 years) underwent allergy testing and immunotherapy as well as a structured verbal headache diagnostic interview with completion of the Migraine Disability Assessment questionnaire. Patients were categorized into high and low atopic groups based on the number of allergy tests that were positive. The study found that the prevalence of migraine was not associated with the degree of allergic sensitization, but there was a significant age/immunotherapy interaction. Migraine headaches were less prevalent in the immunotherapy group than in the nonimmunotherapy group for younger patients. In younger subjects (≤45 years of age), immunotherapy was associated with decreased migraine frequency and disability, while in older patients there was no effect of degree of allergic sensitization or immunotherapy on the frequency and disability of migraine headache. The study suggested that the association of allergy with migraine headaches depends on age, degree of allergic sensitization, administration of immunotherapy, and the type of headache outcome measure. Lower levels of atopy are associated with less frequent and disabling migraine headaches in younger subjects, while higher degrees were associated with more frequent migraines. Immunotherapy decreased prevalence, frequency, and disability of migraines in this same group of patients. The administration of immunotherapy and its relationship to the prevalence of migraine headache is one of the more interesting findings of this article. Younger migraineurs receiving immunotherapy had lower prevalence rates of migraine headache than those not receiving immunotherapy. Conversely, older subjects receiving immunotherapy had higher prevalence rates than those not receiving this therapy. This could suggest that age modulates the effect of immunotherapy on the prevalence of migraine headache, with immunotherapy decreasing prevalence at younger ages and increasing it at older ages. Further work is needed, but this and other articles do suggest that there is more going on in relation to headaches and nasal conditions than we currently appreciate.

R. Sindwani, MD

Efficacy of Leukotriene Antagonists as Concomitant Therapy in Allergic Rhinitis

Cingi C, Gunhan K, Gage-White L, et al (Osmangazi Univ, Eskisehir, Turkey; Celal Bayar Univ, Manisa, Turkey; Louisiana State Univ, Shreveport)
Laryngoscope 120:1718-1723, 2010

Objectives/Hypothesis.—The symptoms of allergic rhinitis result from an immunoglobulin E-dependent mast cell activation cascade, marked by the release of inflammatory mediators, including histamine. Patients with perennial allergic rhinitis also have elevated levels of cysteinyl leukotrienes (CysLTs) in nasal lavage fluid. Histamine and CysLTs produce different responses in the pathogenesis of allergic rhinitis, and this study tested the hypothesis that the effects of combined antihistamine and leukotriene antagonist therapy would be more effective than antihistamine alone.

Study Design.—Multicentered, prospective, randomized, placebo-controlled, parallel-group.

Methods.—Three groups totaling 275 patients using: 1) fexofenadine alone, 2) fexofenadine with montelukast, or 3) fexofenadine with placebo, participated in a 21-day trial conducted during the spring pollen season. Objective analysis included pre- and poststudy physical examination findings and nasal resistance measurements. Subjective data gathered included a daily patient diary and pre- and poststudy patient satisfaction measurements.

Results.—The group using both fexofenadine and montelukast showed significantly better control of nasal congestion both subjectively, using patient diary and visual analog scale evaluations, and objectively, using rhinomanometry and physical examination, compared to groups using antihistamine alone or with placebo.

Conclusions.—Our data provided both objective and subjective evidence that leukotriene receptor antagonist- antihistamine combination therapy is more effective than antihistamine alone in the control of allergic rhinitis symptoms.

▶ Histamine and cysteinyl leukotrienes (CysLTs) have different roles in the pathogenesis of allergic rhinitis, and it certainly seems logical to expect that the effects of combined antihistamine and antileukotriene therapy would be more effective than either treatment alone. Although several publications report the mostly subjective effectiveness of LTRA in the treatment of allergic rhinitis, the results are inconsistent. The objective of this well-designed well-conducted trial was to measure any synergistic effect of LTRA medication when combined with antihistamine in treating patients with seasonal allergic rhinitis, as measured by objective and subjective parameters. Specifically, the authors hypothesized that the key symptom of congestion would be reduced with the combined therapy. This was a multicentered, prospective, randomized, placebo-controlled, parallel-group study in which 275 patients were divided into 3 groups using (1) fexofenadine alone, (2) fexofenadine with montelukast, or (3) fexofenadine with placebo. They participated in a 21-day trial conducted during the spring pollen season; the data gathered included prestudy and post-study physical examination findings and nasal resistance measurements and subjective results of a daily patient diary and prestudy and poststudy patient satisfaction scores. The group using both fexofenadine and montelukast showed significantly better control of nasal congestion both subjectively and objectively compared with groups using antihistamine alone or with placebo. Interestingly, the subjective patient satisfaction in all groups was similar until the 10th day of medication use, and the difference in efficacy became significant only after the 10th day. This confirms prior studies showing leukotriene receptor antagonist (LTRA) alone or with antihistamine combination medication was not found very effective for the first week in some of the earlier reported studies. This study provides a solid basis for the use of LTRA-antihistamine combination therapy in the control of allergic rhinitis. The effect is likely because of the additional anti-inflammatory activity provided by the reduction of inflammatory infiltrate and cytokine levels. Lastly, it is worth mentioning that unlike some studies, this one contains no conflicts of interest with respect to its authors and there was no funding or other input from any pharmaceutical company.

R. Sindwani, MD

Fluticasone Reverses Oxymetazoline-induced Tachyphylaxis of Response and Rebound Congestion

Vaidyanathan S, Williamson P, Clearie K, et al (Univ of Dundee, Scotland, UK)
Am J Respir Crit Care Med 182:19-24, 2010

Rationale.—Chronic use of intranasal decongestants, such as oxymetazoline, leads to tachyphylaxis of response and rebound congestion, caused by α-adrenoceptor mediated down-regulation and desensitization of response.

Objectives.—We evaluated if tachyphylaxis can be reversed by intranasal fluticasone propionate, and the relative α_1- and α_2-adrenoceptor components of tachyphylaxis using the α_1-antagonist prazosin.

Methods.—In a randomized, double-blind, placebo-controlled, crossover design, 19 healthy subjects received intranasal oxymetazoline, 200 μg three times a day for 14 days, followed by the addition of fluticasone, 200 μg twice a day for a further 3 days. At Days 1, 14, and 17, participants received a single dose of oral prazosin, 1 mg, or placebo with measurements made before and 2 hours later.

Measurements and Main Results.—Outcomes evaluated were peak nasal inspiratory flow, nasal resistance, blood flow, and oxymetazoline dose–response curve (DRC). On Day 14 versus Day 1, inspiratory flow decreased (mean difference, 95% confidence interval) $(-47.9\,\text{L·min}^{-1}; -63.9$ to $-31.9; P < 0.001)$ and the DRC shifted downward $(24.8\,\text{L·min}^{-1}; 20.3–29.3; P < 0.001)$. On Day 17 versus Day 14, after fluticasone, inspiratory flow increased $(45\,\text{L·min}^{-1}; 30–61; P < 0.001)$ and the DRC shifted upward $(26.2\,\text{L·min}^{-1}; 21.7–30.7; P < 0.001)$. On Day 1, prazosin reduced inspiratory flow $(-52.6\,\text{L·min}^{-1}; -19.2$ to $-86)$ compared with baseline. This effect was abolished on Day 14 $(7.9\,\text{L·min}^{-1}; -41.3$ to $25.5)$.

Conclusions.—Oxymetazoline-induced tachyphylaxis and rebound congestion are reversed by intranasal fluticasone. Further studies are indicated to evaluate if combination nasal sprays of decongestant and corticosteroid are an effective strategy to obviate tachyphylaxis and rebound in rhinitis.

Clinical trial registered with www.clinicaltrials.gov (NCT 00487032).

▶ Intranasal decongestants, such as oxymetazoline (an α-adrenoceptor agonist), are highly efficacious in treating nasal congestion in rhinitis for short time periods. It is held that prolonged use is heralded by a reduction in efficacy (tachyphylaxis) and a rebound increase in nasal airway congestion and nonspecific nasal hyperreactivity, which together have been given the term rhinitis medicamentosa. This effect is thought to be caused by α-adrenoceptor-mediated down-regulation and desensitization of response. This clever study explored if tachyphylaxis can be reversed by intranasal fluticasone propionate and the relative α_1- and α_2-adrenoceptor components of tachyphylaxis using the α_1-antagonist prazosin. In a randomized, double-blind, placebo-controlled, crossover design, 19 healthy subjects received intranasal oxymetazoline, 200 μg 3 times a day for 14 days, followed by the addition of fluticasone, 200 μg twice a day for a further 3 days. At days 1, 14, and 17, participants received a single dose of oral prazosin (1 mg) or placebo, and outcomes of peak nasal inspiratory flow, nasal resistance, blood flow, and oxymetazoline dose-response curve (DRC) were measured. On day 14 versus day 1, inspiratory flow significantly decreased (mean difference, 95% confidence interval) and the DRC shifted downward. On day 17 versus day 14, after the addition of fluticasone, inspiratory flow increased significantly and the DRC shifted upward. On day 1, prazosin reduced inspiratory flow compared with baseline, and this effect was not present by day 14, suggesting a predominantly α_1-mediated response. The group concluded that oxymetazoline-induced tachyphylaxis and rebound congestion are reversed by intranasal fluticasone and suggested that further studies are indicated to evaluate if combination nasal sprays of decongestant and corticosteroid are an effective strategy to obviate tachyphylaxis and rebound in rhinitis. The positive impact of corticosteroid spray and this interesting interplay between these 2 agents is indeed suggested by their findings, based on objective measurements, but the subjective patient experience was not adequately explored by this study. Even if fluticasone helps to mitigate against the tachyphylaxis and rebound congestion characteristic of long-term oxymetazoline use, the addiction that usually accompanies these physical manifestations may not be altered with this medication. This is a potentially important angle that also deserves further study. The onset, mechanism, and modulation of α-adrenoceptor tolerance in the nose are poorly understood.

R. Sindwani, MD

Long-lasting effects of sublingual immunotherapy according to its duration: A 15-year prospective study

Marogna M, Spadolini I, Massolo A, et al (Macchi Hosp Foundation, Varese, Italy; Med Dept, Anallergo, Florence, Italy; Univ of Calgary, Alberta, Canada; et al)

J Allergy Clin Immunol 126:969-975, 2010

Background.—Data on the long-term effects of sublingual immunotherapy (SLIT) are sparse, and the optimal duration of treatment is a matter of debate.

Objective.—We sought to prospectively evaluate the long-term effect of SLIT given for 3, 4, or 5 years and to compare the effect of those different durations.

Methods.—In this prospective open controlled study we followed up patients with respiratory allergy who were monosensitized to mites for 15 years. The subjects were divided in 4 groups receiving drug therapy alone or SLIT for 3, 4, or 5 years. Clinical scores, skin sensitizations, methacholine reactivity, and nasal eosinophil counts were evaluated every year during the winter months. The clinical effect was considered to persist until clinical scores remained at less than 50% of the baseline value, and then patients underwent another course of SLIT.

Results.—Seventy-eight patients were enrolled, and 59 completed the study. In the 12 control subjects no relevant change in clinical scores was seen throughout the study. In the patients receiving SLIT for 3 years, the clinical benefit persisted for 7 years. In those receiving immunotherapy for 4 or 5 years, the clinical benefit persisted for 8 years. New sensitizations occurred in all the control subjects over 15 years and in less than a quarter of the patients receiving SLIT (21%, 12%, and 11%, respectively). The second course of vaccination induced a benefit more rapidly than the first course. The behavior of bronchial hyperreactivity and nasal eosinophils paralleled the clinical score.

Conclusion.—Under the present conditions, it can be suggested that a 4-year duration of SLIT is the optimal choice because it induces a long-lasting clinical improvement similar to that seen with a 5-year course and greater than that of a 3-year vaccination.

▶ Over the past few years, management of allergic rhinitis using sublingual immunotherapy (SLIT) as opposed to subcutaneous immunotherapy has gained popularity, despite robust data on the long-term efficacy of this treatment. This study prospectively evaluated the long-term effect of SLIT given for 3, 4, or 5 years for dust mite allergy and compared the effect of those different durations to examine the optimal duration of treatment. Patients were monosensitized to mites for 15 years and were divided into 4 groups, receiving drug therapy alone or SLIT for 3, 4, or 5 years. A variety of outcomes, including clinical scores, skin sensitizations, methacholine reactivity, and nasal eosinophil counts, were followed annually. The clinical effect was considered to persist until clinical scores remained at less than 50% of the baseline value, and then patients underwent another course of SLIT. Fifty-nine patients completed this study, which found that in patients receiving SLIT for 3 years, the clinical benefit persisted for 7 years; in those receiving immunotherapy for 4 or 5 years, the clinical benefit persisted for 8 years. The second course of vaccination induced a benefit more rapidly than the first course. The authors concluded that a 4-year duration of SLIT was the optimal choice for immunotherapy duration. The results from this study are fascinating, and the long-term follow-up of 15 years is indeed impressive. Its weaknesses, however, include the lack of an initial randomization (eg, patients receiving SLIT vs control subjects), lack of placebo group, and the high rate of subject drop-outs. Continued efforts to examine the efficacy of SLIT compared with traditional immunotherapy techniques are warranted.

R. Sindwani, MD

2 Head and Neck Surgery and Tumors

Basic and Clinical Research

18F-FDG-PET/CT versus panendoscopy for the detection of synchronous second primary tumors in patients with head and neck squamous cell carcinoma

Haerle SK, Strobel K, Hany TF, et al (Univ Hosp Zurich, Switzerland; et al)
Head Neck 32:319-325, 2010

Background.—This study assesses the additional value of ^{18}F-fluoro-2-deoxy-D-glucose positron emission tomography/CT (^{18}F-FDG-PET/CT) with respect to synchronous primaries in patients undergoing panendoscopy for staging of head and neck squamous cell carcinoma.

Methods.—In all, 311 patients underwent both modalities. Cytology, histology, and/or clinical/imaging follow-up served as reference standard.

Results.—The prevalence of second primary tumors detected by panendoscopy was 4.5%, compared with 6.1% detected by ^{18}F-FDG-PET/CT. The sensitivity for panendoscopy was 74%, the specificity was 99.7%, the positive predictive value (PPV) was 93%, and the negative predictive value (NPV) was 98%. The sensitivity for ^{18}F-FDG-PET/CT was 100%, the specificity was 95.7%, the PPV was 59%, and the NPV was 100%.

Conclusions.—[18]F-FDG-PET/CT is superior to panendoscopy. With a negative ^{18}F-FDG-PET/CT, the extent of endoscopy can be reduced to the area of the primary tumor. Due to the costs, ^{18}F-FDG-PET/CT is recommended only in advanced disease to assess potential distant disease. In early-stage cancer, panendoscopy is accurate enough to rule out secondary tumors.

▶ Fluoro-2-deoxy-D-glucose positron emission tomography/computed tomography (FDG-PET/CT) has emerged as the most sensitive imaging modality for detection of head and neck cancer. Its very high sensitivity, however, is associated with a high rate of false-positive results (low positive predictive value), which makes this study suboptimal for initial staging of the tumor. Nevertheless, the study is ideal for detecting synchronous tumors and distant metastatic disease at the time of the initial cancer work-up. This reviewed retrospective study has compared the efficacy of FDG-PET with that of operative panendoscopy for detection of synchronous primary tumors. The results of this study confirm the superiority of FDG-PET/CT as compared with operative endoscopy in this setting (6% of second primaries detected by PET/CT as compared with 4.5% by operative endoscopy). However, routine FDG-PET/CT screening for second primaries and distant metastases in all new cases of head and neck cancer is not cost-effective. There is a trend in the modern practice of head and neck oncology to perform endoscopic evaluation of head and neck cancer for staging and biopsies in the office setting, using modern fiberoptic instruments. This practice in most cases obviates the need for operative endoscopy and significantly reduces the cost of such evaluation. FDG-PET/CT is a very useful adjunct imaging modality usually reserved for advanced head and neck tumors, where distant metastatic disease and second primary pulmonary cancers are more prevalent.

M. Gapany, MD

A Community-based RCT for Oral Cancer Screening with Toluidine Blue
Su WW-Y, Yen AM-F, Chiu SY-H, et al (Natl Taiwan Univ, Taipei; Chang Gung Univ, Tao-Yuan, Taiwan)
J Dent Res 89:933-937, 2010

Early detection of oral premalignant lesions (OPMLs) by visual inspection with toluidine blue has not been addressed. We conducted a community-based randomized controlled trial to assess whether using toluidine blue as an adjunctive tool for visual screening had a higher detection rate of OPMLs and could further reduce the incidence of oral cancer. In 2000, in Keelung, we randomly assigned a total of 7975 individuals, aged 15 years or older and with high-risk oral habits, to either the toluidine-blue-screened (TBS) group or the visual screening group. Results showed 5% more oral premalignant lesions and 79% more oral submucous fibrosis detected in the TBS group than in the control group. After a five-year follow-up ascertaining oral cancer development through linkage to the National Cancer Registry, the incidence rate in the TBS group (28.0×10^{-5}) was non-significantly 21% lower than that in the control group (35.4×10^{-5}).

▶ Early-stage (T1N0) squamous cell carcinoma of oral tongue and floor of mouth is associated with relatively high incidence of occult cervical metastases (25%-30%). Surgeons treating early oral cavity cancer are thus often confronted with the dilemma of performing a prophylactic neck dissection. While multiple retrospective studies have shown a correlation between the depth of tumor invasion and the incidence of occult neck metastases, this useful parameter can be reliably assessed only through measurements by the pathologist of the entire resected specimen and thus become available as part of the final pathology report. Frozen sections on the resected tumor are often used for intra-operative decision making regarding the indication to perform a prophylactic neck dissection but are useful only when the thickness of the sampled area exceeds 4 mm. The idea of the preoperative measurement of tumor thickness using ultrasound is therefore very attractive. This study confirms the validity of this concept, showing a significant correlation between the measurements obtained by preoperative ultrasonography and histological measurements of tumor depth. Gaining experience with this simple diagnostic modality appears to be very worthwhile.

M. Gapany, MD

Diagnostic efficacy of surgeon-performed ultrasound-guided fine needle aspiration: A randomized controlled trial
Robitschek J, Straub M, Wirtz E, et al (Tripler Army Med Ctr, Honolulu, HI)
Otolaryngol Head Neck Surg 142:306-309, 2010

Objective.—To evaluate the clinical efficacy of surgeon-performed, office-based head and neck ultrasound in facilitating diagnostic fine needle aspiration (FNA) of lesions in the head and neck.

Study Design.—A randomized controlled trial of ultrasound-guided FNA versus traditional palpation-guided technique for palpable masses in the head and neck.

Setting.—An office-based study performed in a military academic medical center.

Subjects and Methods.—Eighty-one adults older than 18 years of age with a palpable head and neck mass (less than 3 cm in largest diameter) were randomized to ultrasound-guided or traditional palpation-guided FNA of a head and neck mass. Measured variables and outcomes for the study included tissue adequacy rates, tissue type, and operator variability.

Results.—Following three passes using either palpation or ultrasound guidance, a comparative tissue adequacy rate of 84 percent for ultrasound guidance versus 58 percent for standard palpation was established ($P < 0.014$). With regard to tissue type, a statistically significant comparative diagnostic advantage for ultrasound guidance was observed in thyroid tissue while remaining statistically insignificant for lymphatic and salivary tissues. No statistical significance was found when comparing the ability of otolaryngology residents versus attending otolaryngologists to obtain ultrasound-guided diagnostic samples.

Conclusion.—Office-based surgeon-performed ultrasound-guided FNA of palpable lesions in the head and neck yields a statistically significant higher diagnostic rate compared to standard palpation technique. Our institutional experience supports the utility of surgeon-performed ultrasound as a core competency in clinical practice.

▶ Despite the efforts by the American Academy of Otolaryngology-Head and Neck Surgery to facilitate the training of otolaryngologists in office-based real-time ultrasonography (through a joint American College of Surgeons and American Academy of Otolaryngology course in ultrasonography for surgeons), this diagnostic modality has been very slow to catch on in the United States. There are multiple reasons for this reluctance by otolaryngologists in the United States to incorporate this very useful imaging modality into their daily practice. Among them, is high cost of ultrasound equipment and rapidly changing technology, creating financial difficulty to amortize the purchased equipment, problems with coding and billing for the studies, and potential conflict of interest with radiologists regarding the scopes of practice. Most importantly, however, it takes great interest and dedication for an otolaryngologist to become a skillful ultrasonographer. In a busy clinical practice, there is just not enough time and/or financial incentive to perform adequate numbers of ultrasound studies to reach the level of required proficiency. This selected article demonstrates clear advantages of office-based surgeon-performed ultrasound-guided fine needle aspiration (FNA) over standard nonultrasound-guided FNA.

M. Gapany, MD

Histopathologic Findings of HPV and p16 Positive HNSCC
Mendelsohn AH, Lai CK, Shintaku IP, et al (David Geffen School of Medicine at UCLA)
Laryngoscope 120:1788-1794, 2010

Objective.—Human papilloma virus (HPV) and p16INKa (p16) positivity in head and neck squamous cell carcinomas (HNSCCs) is currently thought to be an encouraging prognostic indicator. However, the histopathologic changes responsible for this behavior are poorly understood. It is our objective to elucidate these histopathologic characteristics to help define the clinical utility of these markers.

Design.—Retrospective cohort study.

Methods.—71 HNSCC tumors between July 1, 2008 and August 30, 2009 were examined for HPV, p16, and epidermal growth factor receptor (EGFR). Specified pathologic features were examined: perivascular invasion (PVI), perineural invasion (PNI), grade of squamous differentiation, basaloid classification.

Results.—HPV and p16 had no direct impact on perineural or perivascular invasion. However, HPV and p16 were strongly predictive of poorly differentiated tumors, as well as basaloid squamous cell carcinoma (SCCA) ($P < .001$). Additionally, upon multivariate analysis, HPV(+) and p16(+) tumors had an increased risk of nodal metastasis (HPV: odds ratio [OR] = 23.9 (2.2, 265.1) $p = .01$; p16: OR = 6.5 (1.4, 31.2) $p = .02$; PVI: OR = 6.0 (1.6, 22.8) $p < .01$). The area under the curve (AUC) of receiver operating characteristic (ROC) curves demonstrated improved predictive value for lymph node metastasis above standard H&E histopathologic features (76.7%) for both HPV (83.2%) and p16 (81.3%) individually.

Conclusions.—HPV(+) and p16(+) are highly predictive for poorly differentiated tumors and basaloid SCCA. Additionally, HPV and p16 positivity demonstrate superior predictive value for lymph node metastasis above standard H&E histopathologic features. Although exact recommendations should be tempered by considerations of primary tumor subsite, T-stage, and depth of invasion, head and neck multidisciplinary teams should strongly consider aggressive lymph node treatment for any HPV(+) or p16(+) tumor.

▶ Human papilloma virus (HPV)-positive head and neck cancer is on a dramatic rise. The individuals affected are young nonsmokers and have no history of alcohol abuse. The other striking feature of HPV-positive cancers is their propensity to metastasize to cervical lymph nodes early in the course of the disease as judged by early T stages at the primary site, usually in the oropharynx. In contrast to this propensity to metastasize is a relatively good prognostic outcome of these tumors as compared with tobacco- and alcohol-linked HPV-negative head and neck cancer. Of particular interest are most recent observations that surgery with adjuvant radiotherapy is as equally effective as radiochemotherapy in controlling HPV-positive cancer (please refer to other studies on this subject), suggesting that HPV-positive cancer will have a better prognosis regardless of the method of therapy. This study is interesting in that it provides the scientific evidence for what we have been observing empirically in clinical practice, that is, HPV-positive tumors are strongly associated with poor differentiation and basaloid histopathologic features and have a strong propensity for lymph node metastases.

M. Gapany, MD

Human Papillomavirus and Oropharynx Cancer: Biology, Detection and Clinical Implications
Allen CT, Lewis JS Jr, El-Mofty SK, et al (Washington Univ School of Medicine, St Louis, MO)
Laryngoscope 120:1756-1772, 2010

Objectives.—To review evidence for the role of human papillomavirus (HPV) in the etiology of oropharyngeal cancers, methods of viral detection, and the resulting clinical implications.

Study Design.—Contemporary review.

Methods.—Published journal articles identified through PubMed and conference proceedings were reviewed.

Results.—HPV-associated squamous cell carcinomas represent a distinct disease entity from carcinogen-associated squamous cell carcinomas. HPV oncoproteins lead to mucosal cell transformation through well-defined mechanisms. Different methods of detecting HPV exist with variable levels of sensitivity and specificity for biologically active virus. Although virus is detected in a number of head and neck subsites, studies demonstrate improved outcomes in HPV-associated carcinoma of the oropharynx only. The cell cycle regulatory protein p16 is upregulated by biologically active HPV and serves as a biomarker of improved response to therapy.

Conclusions.—HPV-associated squamous cell carcinoma of the oropharynx is a biologically distinct entity from carcinogen-associated carcinoma. Understanding the molecular mechanisms behind the improved outcomes in patients with HPV-associated oropharyngeal carcinoma may lead to novel therapeutics for patients with carcinogen-associated carcinomas.

▶ Evidence has been mounting that human papillomavirus (HPV) infection constitutes an independent etiologic factor for causing oropharyngeal cancer and that HPV-associated oropharyngeal cancer has different epidemiologic, biologic, and clinical characteristics from non-HPV cancer. Epidemiologic implications of these findings are of utmost importance because it is likely that we are witnessing a new form of sexually transmitted disease from changes in sexual behavior. Furthermore, there is ample evidence in the literature that links HPV tumor status with relatively favorable clinical course of tonsillar cancer. This is in part because of different tumor biology of HPV-positive tumors, as compared with HPV-negative, smoking-linked, and alcohol-linked cancers. In part, better outcome could also be associated with improved response to therapy. This selected contemporary review article provides a good source of information on the latest findings and developments pertaining to HPV and oropharyngeal cancer. It is definitely worth reviewing for otolaryngologists who treat head and neck cancer and general otolaryngologists who want to stay abreast with latest development in our specialty.

M. Gapany, MD

Is preoperative ultrasonography accurate in measuring tumor thickness and predicting the incidence of cervical metastasis in oral cancer?
Mark Taylor S, Drover C, MacEachern R, et al (Dalhousie Univ, Halifax, Nova Scotia, Canada)
Oral Oncol 46:38-41, 2010

The need for elective neck dissection in patients with early stage oral cancer is controversial. A preoperative predictor of the risk of subclinical nodal metastasis would be useful. Studies have shown a strong correlation between histological tumor depth and the risk of nodal metastasis.

To determine if preoperative ultrasonography is an accurate measure of tumor depth in oral carcinoma. To assess if preoperatively measured tumor depth predicts an increased risk of subclinical metastatic neck disease and thus the need for elective neck dissection.

Twenty one consecutive patients with biopsy proven squamous cell carcinoma of the tongue/floor of mouth were analyzed prospectively. Each patient received a preoperative ultrasonography to assess tumor depth which was compared to histological measures. Univariate analysis was used to correlate tumor thickness and T stage with neck metastasis.

There was a significant correlation between the preoperative ultrasonography and histological measures of tumor depth (correlation coefficient 0.981, $P < 0.001$). The overall rate of lymph node metastasis was 52%. The rate of metastasis was 33% in N0 necks. In the group with tumors <5 mm in depth, the neck metastatic rate was 0%, as compared with 65% in the group $\geq$5 mm. Using univariate analysis tumor depth and T stage were significant predictors of cervical metastasis ($P = 0.0351$ and $P = 0.0300$, respectively).

Preoperative ultrasonography is an accurate measure of tumor depth in oral carcinoma. Tumor thickness is a significant predictor of nodal metastasis and elective neck dissection should be considered when this thickness is $\geq$5 mm.

▶ Early-stage (T1N0) squamous cell carcinoma of oral tongue and floor of mouth is associated with relatively high incidence of occult cervical metastases (25%-30%). Surgeons treating early oral cavity cancer are thus often confronted with the dilemma of performing a prophylactic neck dissection. While multiple retrospective studies have shown a correlation between the depth of tumor invasion and the incidence of occult neck metastases, this useful parameter can be reliably assessed only through measurements by the pathologist of the entire resected specimen and thus become available as part of the final pathology report. Frozen sections on the resected tumor are often used for intra-operative decision making regarding the indication to perform a prophylactic neck dissection but are useful only when the thickness of the sampled area exceeds 4 mm. The idea of the preoperative measurement of tumor thickness using ultrasound is therefore very attractive. This study confirms the validity of this concept, showing a significant correlation between the measurements obtained by preoperative ultrasonography and histological measurements of tumor depth. Gaining experience with this simple diagnostic modality appears to be very worthwhile.

M. Gapany, MD

Management of Patients Treated With Chemoradiotherapy for Head and Neck Cancer Without Prophylactic Feeding Tubes: The University of Pittsburgh Experience

McLaughlin BT, Gokhale AS, Shuai Y, et al (Univ of Pittsburgh Cancer Inst Biostatistics Facility, PA; et al)
Laryngoscope 120:71-75, 2010

Objectives/Hypothesis.—Mucositis and dysphagia are common complications of chemoradiotherapy (CRT) for head and neck cancer that may necessitate nutritional support with a gastrostomy tube (G-tube).

Methods.—We reviewed records of patients who underwent and completed CRT, which included at least one traditional chemotherapeutic, for previously untreated head and neck cancer. G-tubes were placed as needed. The timing and duration of G-tube placement and treatment-related complications and risk factors for long-term G-tube use were analyzed.

Results.—A total of 91 consecutive patients who received CRT, 68 as primary and 23 as postoperative treatment, were studied. Radiation doses ranged from 59.4 to 74 Gy (median, 70 Gy). Seventy-nine percent of patients received platinum-based therapy during CRT. Severe mucositis occurred in 40% of patients. Forty percent of patients required G-tube placement (15 prior to CRT and 21 during CRT). Median duration of G-tube use was 5.8 months. Two patients who had a G-tube placed during CRT developed a G-tube-related complication. At 6 and 12 months, 15 (18%) and four (6%) patients who were disease free were using G-tubes, respectively. Patients with G-tubes placed prior to CRT or advanced T stage had longer G-tube dependence.

Conclusions.—With aggressive supportive care it is feasible to avoid G-tubes in the majority of patients undergoing CRT for head and neck cancer. G-tube placement prior to CRT due to pre-existing dysphagia and advanced T stage are associated with prolonged G-tube dependence.

▶ Recent studies have shown that nutrition is an important factor in determining the outcomes of head and neck cancer treated with radiochemotherapy. As a result, many head and neck cancer treatment centers have adopted a policy of placing prophylactic percutaneous endoscopic gastrostomies (PEGs) before initiation of radiochemotherapy. As it often happens with policy-driven therapies, some patients who get PEGs might in fact not have needed them, if given a chance to maintain oral nutrition. This article, which is a retrospective review, challenges the approach of prophylactic PEG. In patients who did not require a PEG at the time of their initial evaluation because of pre-existing critical weight loss, severe dysphagia, or high risk for aspiration, only 30% required PEG placement during the course of radiochemotherapy. The complication rates and PEG dependence rates were similar in patients who had their PEGs placed before or during the therapy. Of course, prophylactic PEG saves a lot of headaches to the managing team, such as frequent monitoring of the patient's nutritional status and logistical problems of arranging an emergency PEG in failing patients during the therapy. I do not quite agree with one of the authors' arguments for wait-and-observe approach, which pertains to the detrimental role of absent oral intake. Undoubtedly, lack of use of swallowing musculature through the course of radiochemotherapy can be detrimental, but PEG should not prevent oral intake of small amounts of pureed diet or liquids, mainly for exercise of those muscles.

M. Gapany, MD

Multivitamins, Folate, and Green Vegetables Protect against Gene Promoter Methylation in the Aerodigestive Tract of Smokers

Stidley CA, Picchi MA, Leng S, et al (Univ of New Mexico, Albuquerque; Lovelace Respiratory Res Inst, Albuquerque, NM; et al)
Cancer Res 70:568-574, 2010

One promising approach for early detection of lung cancer is by monitoring gene promoter hypermethylation events in sputum. Epidemiologic studies suggest that dietary fruits and vegetables and the micronutrients they contain may reduce risk of lung cancer. In this study, we evaluated whether diet and multivitamin use influenced the prevalence of gene promoter methylation in cells exfoliated from the aerodigestive tract of current and former smokers. Members ($N = 1,101$) of the Lovelace Smokers Cohort completed the Harvard Food Frequency Questionnaire and provided a sputum sample that was assessed for promoter methylation of eight genes commonly silenced in lung cancer and associated with risk for this disease. Methylation status was categorized as low (fewer than two genes methylated) or high (two or more genes methylated). Logistic regression models were used to identify associations between methylation status and 21 dietary variables hypothesized to affect the acquisition of gene methylation. Significant protection against methylation was observed for leafy green vegetables [odds ratio (OR) = 0.83 per 12 monthly servings; 95% confidence interval (95% CI), 0.74–0.93] and folate (OR, 0.84 per 750 μg/d; 95% CI, 0.72–0.99). Protection against gene methylation was also seen with current use of multivitamins (OR, 0.57; 95% CI, 0.40–0.83). This is the first cohort-based study to identify dietary factors associated with reduced promoter methylation in cells exfoliated from the airway epithelium of smokers. Novel interventions to prevent lung cancer should be developed based on the ability of diet and dietary supplements to affect reprogramming of the epigenome.

▶ Several recently published epidemiologic studies for the first time provided factual evidence in support of promoting a diet rich in fresh fruit, juices, vegetables, and vitamins for head and neck cancer patients and populations at risk of developing oral cavity premalignancy. This simple dietary modification may be the least expensive and most effective method of decreasing the risk of head and neck cancer (even in smokers). This selected article is the first cohort-based study to evaluate the role of leafy green vegetables, folate, and multivitamins in protection against the acquisition of gene promoter methylation in the upper aerodigestive tract epithelial cells, thus reducing the risk of lung cancer in smokers. After reviewing this new body of literature, I started to routinely recommend to all my head and neck cancer patients to alter their dietary habits and include into their diet large amounts of vitamin C-rich fruit, juices, leafy green vegetables, and multivitamins.

M. Gapany, MD

N2 Disease in Patients With Head and Neck Squamous Cell Cancer Treated With Chemoradiotherapy: Is There a Role for Posttreatment Neck Dissection?

Cho AH, Shah S, Ampil F, et al (Louisiana State Univ Health Sciences Ctr, Shreveport; et al)

Arch Otolaryngol Head Neck Surg 135:1112-1118, 2009

Objectives.—To determine whether nodal necrosis and node size of 3 cm or larger are risk factors for recurrent neck disease and whether negative computed tomography–positron emission tomography (CT-PET) results 8 weeks or more after therapy indicate complete response in the neck in patients with N2 disease.

Design.—Retrospective study.

Setting.—State university hospital.

Patients.—Fifty-six patients with head and neck squamous cell cancer and N2 disease treated with chemoradiotherapy were evaluated for persistent or recurrent neck disease. Tumor characteristics analyzed were primary site, T category, nodal size (<3 cm or ≥3 cm), nodal necrosis based on hypodensity of one-third or more of the node, and type of N2 disease (N2a, N2b, or N2c). Forty-eight of the 56 patients underwent CT-PET to determine treatment response after chemoradiotherapy. Clinical examination, imaging, and pathologic specimens were used to confirm disease recurrence.

Main Outcome Measures.—The number of recurrence events, disease-free interval, and positive posttreatment CT-PET result in the neck.

Results.—Most patients had oropharyngeal tumors (n = 37; 66%), T2 tumors (n = 21; 38%), nodes 3 cm or larger (n = 43; 77%), positive necrosis (n = 40; 71%), and N2c disease (n = 28; 50%). Multivariate analysis determined that no factors were significant predictors of recurrence, except for positive posttreatment PET results ($P < .001$). Comparison of CT-PET with nodal recurrence demonstrated a sensitivity of 82%, a specificity of 97%, a negative predictive value of 95%, and a positive predictive value of 90%.

Conclusion.—Posttreatment neck dissections may not be indicated for patients with N2 disease and a negative CTPET result, even in patients with nodal necrosis and nodes 3 cm or larger.

▶ The introduction of combined radiochemotherapy protocols for advanced head and neck cancer have improved the regional response of cervical metastases to treatment and reduced the incidence of treatment failures in the neck, bringing the rationale of planned neck dissection into question. A growing number of studies have shown that CT-positron emission tomography (PET) can be very useful in selecting patients for neck dissection after completion of radiochemotherapy for head and neck cancers with advanced neck metastases. Accumulating data in the literature show that negative CT-PET at 12 weeks after completion of radiochemotherapy has a very high predictive value for the absence of residual cancer. This retrospective study focused on advanced metastatic neck disease staged as N2 and showed a very high negative predictive value (95%) for detecting complete response in the cervical lymph nodes staged as N2. The very high specificity (97%) of PET-CT in this study can probably be attributed to delay of the study until at least 8 weeks after completion of radiochemotherapy. A consensus in the literature is emerging in favor of avoiding posttreatment neck dissections in patients with complete clinical and radiographic response as determined by negative CT-PET at 12 weeks after completion of radiochemotherapy.

M. Gapany, MD

Neck restaging with sentinel node biopsy in T1-T2N0 oral and oropharyngeal cancer: Why and how?
Burcia V, Costes V, Faillie JL, et al (Montpellier Univ Hosp Ctr, France; et al)
Otolaryngol Head Neck Surg 142:592-597, 2010

Objective.—To evaluate the lack of accuracy in neck staging with the classical technique (i.e., neck dissection and routine histopathology) with the sentinel node (SN) biopsy in oral and oropharyngeal T1-T2N0 cancer.
Study Design.—Cross-sectional study with planned data collection.
Setting.—Tertiary center care.
Subjects and Methods.—In 50 consecutive patients, the pathological stage of sentinel node (pSN) was established after analyzing SN biopsies (n = 148) using serial sectioning and immunohistochemistry. Systematic selective neck dissection was performed. The pN stage was established with routine histopathologic analysis of both the non-SN (n = 1075) and the 148 SN biopsies.
Results.—The sensitivity and negative predictive value of pSN staging were 100 percent. Conversely, if one considers pSN staging procedure as the reference test for micro- and macro-metastasis diagnosis, the sensitivity of the classical pN staging procedure was 50 percent (9/1; 95% CI 26.9-73.1) and its negative predictive value was 78 percent (95% CI 61.9-88.8). Fifteen patients (30%) were upstaged, including nine cases from pN0 to pSN $\geq$ 1 and six cases from pN1 to pSN2. Two of the pN0-pSN1 upstaged patients died with relapsed neck disease.
Conclusion.—The SN biopsy technique appeared to be the best staging method in cN0 patients and provided evidence that routinely undiagnosed lymph node invasion may have clinical significance.

▶ Sentinel node biopsy (SNB) in head and neck oncology is a minimally invasive method designed to determine the nodal involvement status of cervical lymph nodes, thus replacing the standard cervical lymphadenectomy. SNB can potentially improve the accuracy of histopatholological cervical lymph node staging, decreasing the morbidity stemming from overtreating patients with head and neck cancer. The feasibility of SNB has been shown in patients with oral and oropharyngeal cancer. It allows sampling of lymph nodes that are at the most risk of harboring metastatic disease and focusing on the pathological analysis of those nodes. This article validates this approach and demonstrates that in cN0 oral and oropharyngeal cancers, SNB and subsequent serial section immunohistochemical analysis of the removed lymph nodes allows detection of micrometastases otherwise undetectable with standard histopathological sections; it is thus much more accurate in establishing a correct pN stage. SNB is emerging as a potentially very useful method for staging cN0 oral and oropharyngeal cancers. I strongly recommend readers to review the recently published "Joint Practice Guidelines for Radionuclide Lymphoscintigraphy for Sentinel Node Localization in Oral/Oropharyngeal Squamous Cell Carcinoma."[1]

M. Gapany, MD

Reference

1. Alkureishi LW, Burak Z, Alvarez JA, et al. European Association of Nuclear Medicine Oncology Committee; European Sentinel Node Biopsy Trial Committee. Joint practice guidelines for radionuclide lymphoscintigraphy for sentinel node localization in oral/oropharyngeal squamous cell carcinoma. *Ann Surg Oncol.* 2009;16: 3190-3210.

Chemotherapy

Low-Dose Weekly Platinum-Based Chemoradiation for Advanced Head and Neck Cancer

Watkins JM, Zauls AJ, Wahlquist AH, et al (Med Univ of South Carolina, Charleston)
Laryngoscope 120:236-242, 2010

Objectives/Hypothesis.—The optimal concurrent chemoradiotherapy regimen for definitive treatment of locoregionally advanced head and neck cancer remains to be determined. The present investigation reports toxicities, disease control, patterns of failure, and survival outcomes in a large mature cohort of patients treated with low-dose weekly platinum-based concurrent chemoradiotherapy.

Study Design.—Retrospective single-institution series.

Methods.—Toxicity and outcome data for locoregionally advanced head and neck cancer patients treated with low-dose weekly platinum-based chemotherapy concurrent with standard fractionation radiotherapy were retrospectively collected and analyzed from a clinical database. Survival analysis methods, including Kaplan-Meier estimation and competing risks analysis, were used to assess locoregional disease control, freedom from failure, and overall survival.

Results.—Ninety-six patients were eligible for the present analysis. Nearly all patients had American Joint Committee on Cancer clinical stage III to IVB disease (99%). Severe acute toxicities included grade 3 mucositis (61%), grade 3/4 nausea (27%/1%), and grade 3 neutropenia (8%). Thirty-seven patients (38%) required hospitalization for a median of 7 days (range, 1–121). Ninety-two percent of patients completed the fully prescribed course of radiotherapy, and 87% completed ≥6 cycles of chemotherapy. At a median survivor follow-up of 40 months (range, 8–68), 47% of patients were without evidence of disease recurrence. The estimated 4-year freedom from failure and overall survival were 48% and 58%, respectively. Initial site(s) of disease failure were locoregional for 22 patients, locoregional and distant (five patients), and distant only (14 patients).

Conclusions.—Weekly low-dose platinum-based chemotherapy with full-dose daily radiotherapy is a tolerable alternative regimen for locoregionally advanced head and neck cancers, with comparable efficacy and patterns of failure to alternative regimens.

▶ The high toxicity of concurrent chemoradiotherapy for advanced head and neck cancer has prompted modification of currently used platinum-based regimens by reducing the dose, increasing the frequency, and/or adding other chemotherapeutic agents. This selected single-institution study offers interesting data on the tolerability and therapeutic value of low-dose weekly cisplatin and paclitaxel chemotherapy administered concomitantly with radiotherapy for advanced head and neck cancer. This study has shown that not only was the tolerability of chemotherapy improved as compared with full-dose cisplatin regimens but the disease control, patterns of failure, and survival of patients with advanced head and neck cancer was not different from those achieved with full-dose cisplatin protocols. These are very encouraging data, which may expand the indications for concurrent chemoradiotherapy also to patients with lower performance status who otherwise might have not qualified to undergo such therapy and patients with borderline renal function who would be at increased risk for renal failure on standard cisplatin protocols. Further research in this field will undoubtedly produce safer, less toxic, and better tolerated chemoradiotherapy.

M. Gapany, MD

General

A prospective study of the clinical impact of a multidisciplinary head and neck tumor board
Wheless SA, McKinney KA, Zanation AM (Univ of North Carolina Hosps, Chapel Hill)
Otolaryngol Head Neck Surg 143:650-654, 2010

Objective.—There have been no studies undertaken on the effect of the multidisciplinary head and neck tumor board on treatment planning. The objective of this study was to determine the efficacy of the multidisciplinary tumor board in altering diagnosis, stage, and treatment plan in patients with head and neck tumors.

Study Design.—Case series with planned data collection.

Setting.—Comprehensive cancer center and tertiary academic hospital.

Subjects and Methods.—A prospective study of the discussions concerning 120 consecutive patients presented at a multidisciplinary head and neck tumor board was performed. As each patient was presented, a record was made of the "pre-conference" diagnosis, stage, and treatment plan. After case discussion, the "post-conference" diagnosis, stage, and treatment plan were recorded. Results are compared between malignant and benign tumor cohorts.

Results.—The study population comprised 120 patients with new presentations of head and neck tumors: 84 malignancies and 36 benign tumors. Approximately 27 percent of patients had some change in tumor diagnosis, stage, or treatment plan. Change in treatment was significantly more common in cases of malignancy, occurring in 24 percent of patients versus six percent of benign tumors ($P = 0.0199$). Changes in treatment were also noted to be largely escalations in management ($P = 0.0084$), adding multi-modality care.

Conclusion.—A multidisciplinary tumor board affects diagnostic and treatment decisions in a significant number of patients with newly diagnosed head and neck tumors. The multidisciplinary approach to patient care may be particularly effective in managing malignant tumors, in which treatment plans are most frequently altered.

▶ It is hard to imagine delivery of contemporary high-quality care of patients with head and neck cancer within any other framework but the framework of the multidisciplinary head and neck oncology team. At the heart of such a team is the multidisciplinary tumor board. The complexities of multimodality therapy and the logistics of delivery require decision making on so many levels, that 1 single specialty is not able to handle it single-handedly. Furthermore, there can be more than 1 approach to managing a certain cancer, and the input of variety of specialists can help to choose the best method of therapy for a given patient. Factors such as patient's performance status, comorbidities, pretherapy speech and swallowing status, occupation, and personal preference, just to mention a few, can influence the choice of therapy. Such a multidisciplinary team will most often include a surgeon, radiation oncologist, medical oncologist, radiologist, pathologist, oral maxillofacial surgeon, patient care coordinator, prosthodontist, nutritionist, psychologist, physical therapist, and speech and swallowing specialist. This selected article for the first time demonstrates the benefits of the multidisciplinary head and neck tumor board in a formal study, adding factual evidence to what used to be until now only conventional wisdom.

M. Gapany, MD

Complications of esophagoscopy in an academic training program

Tsao GJ, Damrose EJ (Stanford Univ Med Ctr, CA)
Otolaryngol Head Neck Surg 142:500-504, 2010

Objective.—To assess the efficacy and safety of flexible versus rigid esophagoscopy in an academic training setting.

Study Design.—Case series with chart review.

Setting.—Tertiary academic training center.

Subjects and Methods.—A retrospective medical record review was performed on all adult patients undergoing esophagoscopy from 2002 to 2007.

Results.—A total of 546 procedures were performed with flexible (n = 276) or rigid (n = 270) endoscopes. Seven esophageal perforations (2.6%) occurred, all in association with rigid endoscopy and all in patients with a history of head and neck cancer. Esophageal perforation rates were associated with attending level of experience. There were no deaths. No synchronous esophageal cancers were found in any patient undergoing panendoscopy for the evaluation of a head and neck cancer.

Conclusion.—The 2.6 percent esophageal perforation rate observed in this study is higher than that typically reported for rigid esophagoscopy. When performed as part of routine panendoscopy, no synchronous esophageal tumors were found, questioning the value of esophagoscopy in this setting. All perforations occurred in patients with a history of head and neck cancer and were associated with the level of the surgeon's experience in performing rigid endoscopy.

▶ This is an important study to review, especially for faculty of otolaryngology training programs, but also for otolaryngologists in general otolaryngology practice. In their article, the authors bring up several important points pertaining to the skill and role of rigid esophagoscopy in otolaryngology practice. First, rigid esophagoscopy is not an easy slam-dunk surgical procedure, which in unskilled hands can result in an unacceptable rate of esophageal perforations. Second, in head and neck cancer, synchronous esophageal tumors are very rare; therefore, in the absence of localizing symptomatology, routine esophagoscopy is difficult to justify. Third, office endoscopy (including transnasal flexible esophagoscopy) is becoming standard of care for evaluation and staging of head and neck cancer, obviating the need for routine operative endoscopy. Lastly, when taught to residents in an academic setting, rigid esophagoscopy should be relegated to senior staff members. In general, flexible esophagoscopy (including transnasal office esophagoscopy) appears to be a safer and more economic diagnostic procedure, which in most cases (with the exception of foreign body removal) can replace rigid esophagoscopy.

M. Gapany, MD

Demographics and efficacy of head and neck cancer screening
Shuman AG, Entezami P, Chernin AS, et al (Univ of Michigan Med School, Ann
Arbor; Univ of Michigan, Ann Arbor)
Otolaryngol Head Neck Surg 143:353-360, 2010

Objective.—This study was designed to 1) describe the demographics
and 2) determine the efficacy of a head and neck cancer screening program
to optimize future programs.

Study Design.—Database analysis plus chart review.

Setting.—Tertiary care academic medical center.

Subjects and Methods.—After Institutional Review Board approval, we
reviewed our 14-year experience (1996-2009) conducting a free annual
head and neck cancer screening clinic. Available demographic and clinical
data, as well as clinical outcomes, were analyzed for all participants
(n = 761). The primary outcome was the presence of a finding suspicious
for head and neck cancer on screening evaluation.

Results.—Five percent of participants had findings suspicious for head
and neck cancer on screening evaluation, and malignant or premalignant
lesions were confirmed in one percent of participants. Lack of insurance
($P = 0.05$), tobacco use ($P < 0.001$), male gender ($P = 0.03$), separated
marital status ($P = 0.03$), and younger age ($P = 0.04$) were the significant
demographic predictors of a lesion suspicious for malignancy. Patients
complaining of a neck mass ($P < 0.001$) or oral pain ($P < 0.001$) were
significantly more likely to have findings suspicious of malignancy. A
high percentage (40%) was diagnosed with benign otolaryngologic pathol
ogies on screening evaluation.

Conclusion.—A minority of patients presenting to a head and neck
cancer screening clinic will have a suspicious lesion identified. Given
these findings, to achieve maximal potential benefit, future head and
neck cancer screening clinics should target patients with identifiable risk
factors and take full advantage of opportunities for education and
prevention.

▶ Head and neck cancer, when detected early, carries an excellent prognosis,
with cure rates as high as 90% for T1N0 tumors. A logical conclusion that
follows is that the main effort for improving outcomes of head and neck cancer
should focus on early detection of the disease. This, however, is easier said than
done. There are several reasons for this failure. First, head and neck cancer is
a relatively rare disease, and screening general population proves to not be
cost-effective. Second, head and neck cancer afflicts patients of lower socio-
economic level who seldom seek medical attention before becoming highly
symptomatic. Third, otolaryngologists–head and neck surgeons, who are best
equipped to detect early cancers of the head and neck, do not have the time
or the capacity to provide routine screening even for patients who fall into
the high-risk group (males older than 40 years, who smoke and consume
excessive amount of alcohol), to say nothing about general population. This
selected article represents a commendable effort at achieving the elusive goal

of early detection of head and neck cancer and exemplifies the difficulties associated with achieving this goal. It is definitely worth reviewing.

M. Gapany, MD

Diagnostic accuracy of fine-needle aspiration cytology in Warthin tumors
Veder LL, Kerrebijn JDF, Smedts FM, et al (Erasmus Univ Med Ctr, Rotterdam, The Netherlands)
Head Neck 32:1635-1640, 2010

Background.—Our aim was to evaluate the diagnostic accuracy of fine-needle aspiration cytology (FNAC) for Warthin tumors of the parotid gland.

Methods.—All cytologic diagnoses of Warthin tumor between 1990 and 2007 were correlated with available histology. In addition, our results were compared to current literature.

Results.—In 310 cases, Warthin tumor was diagnosed by FNAC. In 133 cases, (43%) both cytology and histology were available. In 127 of these 133 cases (95.5%), the diagnosis Warthin tumor was confirmed by histology. In 4 cases (3%), a benign lesion was diagnosed and 2 (1.5%) revealed a malignant lesion. On review, those cytologic diagnoses were not certain. In the literature, 11 missed malignancies (5.4%) in 202 cases were reported.

Conclusion.—The diagnostic accuracy of FNAC for the diagnosis of Warthin tumor is high and the percentage of missed malignant tumors is very low. Our results imply that a cytologic diagnosis of Warthin tumor may justify conservative treatment.

▶ Over the years, my approach to managing Warthin tumor has grown progressively conservative. In part because in the majority of cases, I find that the risks of the operation for removal of this tumor outweigh the benefits; most of my patients are asymptomatic elderly individuals, who had a stable mass in their parotid gland for a few years. Furthermore, the report of the cytopathologist on the fine-needle aspiration (FNA) of the mass in the vast majority of cases is resoundingly definitive, leaving little doubt about the correctness of the diagnosis. Most of my patients are relieved when I tell them that the operation is optional and that observation is a very reasonable alternative. I follow up my patients for a few years to ascertain that the mass does not progress in size and then discontinue the follow-up. Over the years, I have learned from my cytopathology colleagues that they, as a rule, are very confident (as confident as one can be with cytopathology) of the diagnosis of Warthin tumor. It was very reassuring to read this selected large retrospective study confirming the accuracy of FNA in diagnosing this particular salivary gland tumor.

M. Gapany, MD

Esophageal pathology in patients after treatment for head and neck cancer

Farwell DG, Rees CJ, Mouadeb DA, et al (Univ of California Davis School of Medicine, Sacramento; Wake Forest Univ School of Medicine, Winston-Salem, NC; et al)
Otolaryngol Head Neck Surg 143:375-378, 2010

Objective.—To determine the prevalence of esophageal pathology following treatment for primary head and neck cancer (HNCA).

Study Design.—Case series with planned data collection.

Setting.—Academic medical practice.

Subjects and Methods.—Subjects comprised HNCA survivors. Esophagoscopy was prospectively performed on 100 patients at least three months after treatment for HNCA. Patient demographics including cancer stage, cancer treatment, use of reflux medications, symptoms surveys, and esophageal findings were prospectively determined.

Results.—The mean age of the cohort was 64 (± 10) years; 75 percent were male. The mean time between the end of treatment and endoscopy was 40 (± 51) months. Eighty-one percent of HNCA was advanced stage (3 or 4). The distribution of site of the primary HNCA was as follows: oropharynx (38%), larynx (33%), oral cavity (17%), unknown primary (10%), hypopharynx (1%), and nasopharynx (1%). Treatment modalities included surgery alone (15%), surgery with radiation (34%), radiation alone (6%), chemoradiation alone (24%), and chemoradiation with surgery (20%). The findings on esophagoscopy included peptic esophagitis (63%), stricture (23%), candidiasis (9%), Barrett metaplasia (8%), gastritis (4%), and carcinoma (4%). Only 13 percent had a normal esophagoscopy.

Conclusion.—Esophageal pathology is extremely common in patients treated for HNCA. These findings support routine esophageal screening after HNCA treatment.

▶ This is an interesting study, supporting routine screening transnasal esophagoscopy (TNE) in patients treated for head and neck cancer. In the past, it was standard practice to perform routine preoperative rigid esophagoscopy as part of pretherapy operative endoscopy. More recently, however, routine rigid esophagoscopy in the absence of any localizing symptoms fell out of favor. The main reasons for that are 2-fold: first, in head and neck cancer patients, synchronous esophageal tumors are rare and second, rigid esophagoscopy is not an easy or completely innocuous operation associated with a relatively high risk for esophageal perforation. On the other hand, TNE is a safe office procedure, which in most cases can replace rigid esophagoscopy. While in this study the authors failed to routinely perform pretreatment TNE, they were able to show that esophageal pathology was very common in treated head and neck cancer patients. My conclusion from reading this study is that TNE should definitely be performed as part of initial evaluation of the head and neck cancer patients and probably subsequently, during follow-up, when indicated.

M. Gapany, MD

Evaluating the role of prophylactic gastrostomy tube placement prior to definitive chemoradiotherapy for head and neck cancer
Chen AM, Li B-Q, Lau DH, et al (Univ of California Davis Cancer Ctr, Sacramento)
Int J Radiat Oncol Biol Phys 78:1026-1032, 2010

Purpose.—To determine the effect of prophylactic gastrostomy tube (GT) placement on acute and long-term outcome for patients treated with definitive chemoradiotherapy for locally advanced head and neck cancer.

Methods and Materials.—One hundred twenty consecutive patients were treated with chemoradiotherapy for Stage III/IV head and neck cancer to a median dose of 70 Gy (range, 64–74 Gy). The most common primary site was the oropharynx (66 patients). Sixty-seven patients (56%) were treated using intensity-modulated radiotherapy (IMRT). Seventy patients (58%) received prophylactic GT placement at the discretion of the physician before initiation of chemoradiotherapy.

Results.—Prophylactic GT placement significantly reduced weight loss during radiation therapy from 43 pounds (range, 0 to 76 pounds) to 19 pounds (range, 0 to 51 pounds), which corresponded to a net change of -14% (range, 0% to -30%) and -8% (range, +1% to -22%) from baseline, respectively ($p < 0.001$). However, the proportion of patients who were GT-dependent at 6- and 12-months after treatment was 41% and 21%, respectively, compared with 8% and 0%, respectively, for those with and without prophylactic GT ($p < 0.001$). Additionally, prophylactic GT was associated with a significantly higher incidence of late esophageal stricture compared with those who did not have prophylactic GT (30% vs. 6%, $p < 0.001$).

Conclusions.—Although prophylactic GT placement was effective at preventing acute weight loss and the need for intravenous hydration, it was also associated with significantly higher rates of late esophageal toxicity. The benefits of this strategy must be balanced with the risks.

▶ This is a second article in this year's selection that challenges the concept of prophylactic percutaneous endoscopic gastrostomy (PEG) in patients undergoing radiochemotherapy for head and neck cancer. The concept of prophylactic PEG in these patients has developed to address the problem of excessive weight loss and malnutrition during radiochemotherapy. No doubt, prophylactic placement of PEG allows maintenance of proper nutrition and hydration through the course of therapy, prevents interruptions of treatment due to dysphagia and odynophagia, and helps with the management of acute toxicity of radiochemotherapy. On the other hand, several recent studies, including this article, have shown that prophylactic PEG is associated with significant higher incidence of high-grade dysphagia, long-term PEG dependence, and esophageal stricture formation. In this series, like in other published studies, only one-third of patients who did not have a prophylactic PEG placed before initiation of therapy required PEG during the course of radiochemotherapy. It is, therefore, reasonable to assume that with careful monitoring of weight and nutritional status, a PEG could be avoided in two-thirds of patients who undergo radiochemotherapy.

M. Gapany, MD

Extent of neck dissection required after concurrent chemoradiation for stage IV head and neck squamous cell carcinoma
Cannady SB, Lee WT, Scharpf J, et al (Oregon Health Sciences Univ, Portland; Duke Univ School of Medicine, Durham, NC; Cleveland Clinic Head and Neck Inst, OH; et al)
Head Neck 32:348-356, 2010

Background.—The management of initially bulky nodal disease after primary nonsurgical treatment for stage IV head and neck squamous cell carcinoma (HNSCC) continues to be a subject of debate.

Methods.—A retrospective chart review of neck management in patients after chemoradiation was performed.

Results.—Of the initially positive necks analyzed, 210/329 (65%) had a complete clinical response to treatment and 161 necks underwent neck surgery. Patients were pathologically positive 13.8% and 39.6% of the time after clinical complete or partial response, respectively. Regional recurrence was more frequent in necks with partial clinical ($p = .04$) or pathologic responses ($p < .01$) and with primary site recurrences ($p < .01$).

Conclusions.—It is still safest at our institution to perform selective neck dissection on patients with $\geq$N2 neck disease when initially observed to prevent unsalvageable regional recurrence until more accurate interval assessment tools are confirmed.

▶ This is an excellent and a very important retrospective study authored by a highly respected head and neck oncology team. This study addresses several controversial issues highly relevant to management of metastatic cervical lymphadenopathy in head and neck cancer following concomitant chemoradiotherapy. First, is the question of validity of posttherapy imaging in determining the need for neck dissection. While positron emission tomography (PET)-CT appears to be a highly sensitive method to detect residual neck disease, it is definitely very dependent on the expertise of the nuclear medicine specialist interpreting the results. It is therefore understandable that in some institutions the head and neck oncologic surgeon might feel uncomfortable observing patients with N2-N3 pretreatment cervical lymphadenopathy, despite complete clinical response and negative PET-CT. The data in this study support the approach of neck dissection for more advanced neck disease. Second, there is the question regarding the extent of the neck dissection (comprehensive cervical lymphadenectomy vs selective cervical lymphadenectomy). This study confirms the safety of selective neck dissection with respect to overall survival, disease-free survival, and regional control.

In my practice, I have adopted a CT-PET surveillance protocol, based on an excellent prospective study from the Netherlands, recently published in *The Journal of Nuclear Medicine* and reviewed last year.[1]

M. Gapany, MD

Reference

1. Krabbe CA, Pruim J, Dijkstra PU, et al. 18F-FDG PET as a routine posttreatment surveillance tool in oral and oropharyngeal squamous cell carcinoma: a prospective study. *J Nucl Med.* 2009;50:1940-1947.

Future of the TNM classification and staging system in head and neck cancer

Takes RP, Rinaldo A, Silver CE, et al (Radboud Univ Nijmegen Med Ctr, The Netherlands; Univ of Udine, Italy; Albert Einstein College of Medicine, Bronx, NY; et al)
Head Neck 32:1693-1711, 2010

Staging systems for cancer, including the most universally used TNM classification system, have been based almost exclusively on anatomic information. However, the question arises whether staging systems should be based on this information alone. Other parameters have been identified that should be considered for inclusion in classification systems like the TNM. This is all the more important, as a shift toward nonsurgical treatments for head and neck cancer has been made over the years. For these treatment modalities tumor/biologic characteristics next to anatomic information may be particularly important for treatment choice and outcome. The shortcomings of the current TNM classification system will be discussed, along with suggestions for improvement and expansion of the TNM system based on tumor, patient, and environment-related factors. Further improvement of the TNM classification is expected to result in better treatment choices, outcome and prognostication of patients with head and neck cancer.

▶ The currently used TNM staging of head and neck cancer is based only on anatomical considerations and fails to include any factors that could determine the biological behavior of the tumor. The most vivid example of such a glaring deficiency can be the recently discovered association between tumor human papillomavirus (HPV) status and prognosis of oropharyngeal and oral cavity cancers. Tumors that are staged identically using TNM classification might exhibit completely different biological behavior in nonsmokers and nondrinkers when they are HPV positive, as compared with tumors in smokers and/or drinkers with HPV-negative tumors. This selected article is an excellent review of this topic. It provides a thorough analysis of the shortcomings of the existing TNM classification, points out the relevant prognostic factors that are not, but probably should be, considered for inclusion, and discusses the future of head and neck tumor staging. This article is a very useful reading for general otolaryngologists as well as for otolaryngologists who treat head and neck cancer.

M. Gapany, MD

Primary care perceptions of otolaryngology
Domanski MC, Ashktorab S, Bielamowicz SA (The George Washington Univ, DC)
Otolaryngol Head Neck Surg 143:337-340, 2010

Objective.—To identify diseases of the head and neck for which primary care physicians may underappreciate the role of the otolaryngologist.
Study Design.—Cross-sectional analysis.
Setting.—With increasing subspecialization in the world of medicine, there is the potential for confusion about the scope of practice for different specialties by primary care physicians. These clinicians are often faced with patients who have disease processes in which otolaryngologists are trained but may end up referring patients to other specialists.
Subjects and Methods.—A brief, web-based survey was administered via e-mail to resident physicians of family medicine, pediatrics, and internal medicine programs in the United States. The survey asked responders which specialist they believed was an expert for particular clinical entities: allergies, oral cancer, restoring a youthful face, sleep apnea, thyroid surgery, and tracheostomy. Respondents could choose from a dermatologist, general surgeon, ophthalmologist, oral maxillofacial surgeon, orthopedic surgeon, otolaryngologist, and plastic surgeon. The responder was able to choose more than one specialist for each question.
Results.—A total of 1064 completed surveys were analyzed. The percentage of primary care residents who picked otolaryngologists as experts was 13.8 percent for allergies, 73.6 percent for oral cancer, 2.7 percent for restoring a youthful face, 32.4 percent for sleep apnea, 47.2 percent for thyroid surgery, and 72.5 percent for tracheostomy.
Conclusion.—This study demonstrates that many primary care residents are not aware of the scope of expertise that an otolaryngologist may offer. Increased exposure to otolaryngology during primary care residency training may increase understanding of the specialty among primary care physicians.

▶ This selected article raises a question, which is of critical importance to the future of our specialty and reflects the basic flaw in medical education in most medical schools in the United States. In most of them, the specialty of otolaryngology is relegated to elective category, and in the best-case scenario, only about one-fourth of graduates from medical schools in the United States will have any exposure to our specialty. This lack of education in otolaryngology then carries through into primary care residency and into primary care practice. The lack of understanding of basic principles in otolaryngology and often lack of knowledge of basic terminology impairs significantly the communication between the specialist and the consulting primary care physician, to say nothing about the timeliness and appropriateness of those consultations. To improve the consulting service to primary care physicians in the Minneapolis Veterans Affairs Medical Center, I personally triage all consults to otolaryngology, which are submitted through the electronic medical record system, allowing me to communicate directly and in real time with the consulting physician or non-MD practitioner. Through this process, I also attempt to educate primary care physicians as much as I can. However, unless some changes are introduced into the curricula in medical schools in the United States, I do not see how things could improve in the future.

M. Gapany, MD

Outcomes

Comparison of pharyngocutaneous fistula between patients followed by primary laryngopharyngectomy and salvage laryngopharyngectomy for advanced hypopharyngeal cancer

Tsou Y-A, Hua C-H, Lin M-H, et al (China Med Univ Hosp, Taichung City, Taiwan, Republic of China; et al)
Head Neck 32:1494-1500, 2010

Background.—We analyzed the incidence rate, possible etiology, and management of pharyngocutaneous fistula after laryngopharyngectomy between hypopharyngeal cancer patients who received surgery first and subsequently concurrent chemoradiation therapy (CCRT) and those who received CCRT first followed by surgical salvage.

Methods.—This is a case cohort, retrospective study collected in a tertiary medical center from January 1996 to July 2007.

Results.—From the total of 160 patients, 52 patients (32.5%) developed pharyngocutaneous fistula. There is a significant difference between the pharyngocutaneous fistula rate of those with initial CCRT and the initial surgery groups. By univariate analysis and multiple logistic regression, tests revealed that preoperative radiation and hypo-albuminemia are risk factors for pharyngocutaneous fistula. A prolonged hospital course was noted among patients in the fistula group, especially when they received surgical repair, had hypo-albuminemia (albumin, <2.5 g/dL), or received preoperative radiation therapy (pre-OPRT).

Conclusions.—Preoperative radiation therapy and hypo-albuminemia increase the fistula rate significantly. A prolonged hospital course was noted among all fistula patients.

▶ Salvage surgery for failed radiochemotherapy has become an integral part of head and neck oncologic surgery practice. With it, we have observed an increased incidence of pharyngocutaneous fistulae and other wound-healing problems. In our institution, where we perform most of our oncologic surgery, we are under constant pressure from the National Surgical Quality Improvement Program (NSQUIP) officers to reduce our wound complication rate, which, for the last several years, has been a high outlier compared with the national average. Unfortunately, by NSQUIP criteria, risk adjustment for radiotherapy only applies for surgery performed within 3 months following completion of radiotherapy; operations performed later than 3 months are not risk adjusted. Because our first positron emission tomography/CT evaluation for response to radiochemotherapy is performed at 3 months after completion of treatment, we almost exclusively operate later than the set risk adjustment criteria. So far, our request for review of the existing risk adjustment criteria for radiotherapy has fallen on deaf ears. It is our hope that studies like this one will change the minds of NSQUIP policy makers regarding the late effects of radiotherapy (and especially radiochemotherapy) on surgical wound healing.

M. Gapany, MD

Does Postoperative Thyrotropin Suppression Therapy Truly Decrease Recurrence in Papillary Thyroid Carcinoma? A Randomized Controlled Trial
Sugitani I, Fujimoto Y (Cancer Inst Hosp, Tokyo, Japan)
J Clin Endocrinol Metab 95:4576-4583, 2010

Context.—TSH suppression therapy has been used to decrease thyroid cancer recurrence. However, validation of effects through studies providing a high level of evidence has been lacking.

Objective.—This single-center, open-label, randomized controlled trial tested the hypothesis that disease-free survival (DFS) for papillary thyroid carcinoma (PTC) in patients without TSH suppression is not inferior to that in patients with TSH suppression.

Design.—Participants were randomly assigned to receive postoperative TSH suppression therapy (group A) or not (group B). Before assignment, patients were stratified into groups with low- and high-risk PTC according to the AMES (age, metastasis, extension, size) risk-group classification.

Interventions and Outcome Measures.—For patients assigned to group A, L-T$_4$ was administered to keep serum TSH levels below 0.01 μU/ml. TSH levels were adjusted to within normal ranges for patients assigned to group B. Recurrence was evaluated by neck ultrasonography and chest computed tomography.

Results.—Eligible participants were recruited from 1996–2005, with 218 patients assigned to group A and 215 patients to group B. Analysis was performed on an intention-to-treat basis. DFS did not differ significantly between groups. The 95% confidence interval of the hazard ratio for recurrence was 0.85–1.27 according to Cox proportional hazard modeling, within the margin of 2.12 required to declare 10% noninferiority.

Conclusions.—DFS for patients without TSH suppression was not inferior by more than 10% to DFS for patients with TSH suppression. Thyroid-conserving surgery without TSH suppression should be considered for patients with low-risk PTC to avoid potential adverse effects of TSH suppression.

▶ It is time for endocrinologists and surgeons in the United States, who manage well-differentiated thyroid cancer, to start paying more attention to how our colleagues in Japan are treating this disease. While in the United States even low-risk well-differentiated thyroid carcinomas are most commonly treated with total thyroidectomy, radioiodine ablation, and thyroid-stimulating hormone (TSH) suppression, in Japan a more conservative approach yields equally good outcomes. There, thyroid lobectomy for unilateral disease is the standard operation, in conjunction with ipsilateral central compartment lymph node sampling. Total thyroidectomy is performed only for multifocal disease involving both lobes or in cases of bilateral neck metastases. Radioactive iodine ablation is considered only in patients with high-risk well-differentiated thyroid cancer.

This selected article is a landmark study that challenges the concept of TSH suppression in well-differentiated thyroid cancer. It is the first open-label, randomized, controlled study to assess this therapeutic modality and render level 1 evidence-based data on this subject. Because the disease-free survival in the absence of TSH suppression was not inferior to that in the presence of TSH suppression in this study, the authors propose to manage low-risk well-differentiated thyroid cancer with conservative surgery, without radioiodine ablation and without TSH suppression. We should be taking note of their approach.

M. Gapany, MD

Human papillomavirus predicts outcome in oropharyngeal cancer in patients treated primarily with surgery or radiation therapy
Hong AM, Dobbins TA, Lee CS, et al (Royal Prince Alfred Hosp, Sydney, New South Wales, Australia; Univ of New South Wales, Sydney, Australia; Univ of Western Sydney, Sydney, New South Wales, Australia; et al)
Br J Cancer 103:1510-1517, 2010

Objective.—This study examines the prognostic significance of human papillomavirus (HPV) in patients with locally advanced oropharyngeal squamous cell carcinoma (SCC) treated primarily with surgery or definitive radiotherapy.

Methods.—One hundred and ninety-eight patients with Stage 3/4 SCC were followed up for recurrence in any form or death from any cause for between 1 and 235 months after diagnosis. HPV status was determined using HPV E6-targeted multiplex real-time PCR/p16 immunohistochemistry. Determinants of recurrence and mortality hazards were modelled using Cox's regression with censoring at follow-up dates.

Results.—Forty-two per cent of cancers were HPV-positive (87% type 16). HPV predicted loco-regional control, event-free survival and overall survival in multivariable analysis. Within the surgery with adjuvant radiotherapy ($n = 110$), definitive radiotherapy-alone ($n = 24$) and definitive radiotherapy with chemotherapy ($n = 47$) groups, patients with HPV-positive cancers were one-third or less as likely to have loco-regional recurrence, an event or to die of any cause as those with HPV-negative cancers after adjusting for age, gender, tumour grade, AJCC stage and primary site. The 14 patients treated with surgery alone were considered too few for multivariable analysis.

Conclusion.—HPV status predicts better outcome in oropharyngeal cancer treated with surgery plus adjuvant radiotherapy as well as with definitive radiation therapy ± chemotherapy.

▶ Recent studies have shown that 45% to 70% of oropharyngeal cancers will be positive for human papillomavirus (HPV) DNA. Furthermore, evidence has been mounting that HPV infection constitutes an independent etiologic factor for causing oropharyngeal cancer and that HPV-associated oropharyngeal cancer has different epidemiologic, biologic, and clinical characteristics from non-HPV cancer. Furthermore, they confirm a better response to chemoradiotherapy and better survival in patients with HPV-associated cancer. Most recent studies are now suggesting that the effect of HPV on the outcome of oropharyngeal cancer might not be influenced by the choice of therapy. This selected study has shown that HPV-positive oropharyngeal cancers treated with surgery and adjuvant radiotherapy had also better outcomes, which were at least as good as those treated with organ preservation modalities. At this point, however, data from routine screening for HPV infection can be used primarily for patient counseling and do not have any immediate therapeutic implications. Future studies might produce modifications in strategies for treating HPV-associated head and neck cancer.

M. Gapany, MD

Management of the N0 Neck in Recurrent Laryngeal Squamous Cell Carcinoma
Bohannon IA, Desmond RA, Clemons L, et al (Univ of Alabama at Birmingham)
Laryngoscope 120:58-61, 2010

Objectives/Hypothesis.—To evaluate the utility of neck dissections in patients undergoing salvage laryngectomy with a clinically negative neck.

Study Design.—Retrospective cohort study.

Methods.—This retrospective review identified 71 patients with N0 necks who underwent salvage laryngectomy from 2001 to 2007. The standard practice of surgeons within our institution was different, thus neck dissections were performed on approximately one half of the patients, creating two groups for comparison. The number of neck dissections with positive metastasis were examined. Postoperative complications, overall survival, and site of recurrence were compared between patients with neck dissection and no neck dissection.

Results.—Thirty-eight patients underwent 71 neck dissections concurrently with salvage laryngectomy. A total of 33 patients had salvage laryngectomy without neck dissection. Only three of 71 neck dissections (4%) had positive nodal metastasis. The rate of fistula, wound infection, hematoma/bleeding, chyle leak, wound dehiscence, and flap failure did not reveal any statistical differences. However, the overall complication rate in neck dissections patients was higher (42.2 %) than no neck dissections (21.3%; $P =.04$). Neck dissection patients had a higher proportion of fistulas (32%) than no dissections (18%; $P =.2$). Regional failure occurred in 7.9% of the patients with neck dissections and 15% of patients without neck dissection ($P =.5$). There was no survival advantage for patients who underwent neck dissection compared to no neck dissection ($P =.47$).

Conclusions.—There was no survival advantage gained by performing neck dissection in the clinically negative neck. However, a trend toward reduced regional failure with neck dissection must be balanced by the increased potential for complications and fistulae.

▶ Salvage laryngectomy is an integral part of organ-preservation approach, reserved for cases of recurrent or persistent cancers. On the other hand, the management of N0 neck in the setting of salvage laryngectomy is subject to controversy. The truth of the matter is that there are no solid data to support the thought that a more aggressive surgical approach, which includes either unilateral or bilateral neck dissections, will improve patient survival. On the contrary, all the studies published so far (including this selected one) show that prophylactic neck dissection for N0 neck in cases of local failures of laryngeal cancer treated with radiotherapy or radiochemotherapy will not improve patient survival but may improve regional control. We also know that neck dissections (unilateral or bilateral), performed concomitantly with the salvage laryngectomy, significantly increase the rate of complications. Thus, improved regional control without a significant survival advantage has to be balanced against an increased risk of surgical complications. For those of us who are under strict scrutiny of surgical quality improvement programs, such as Veterans Administration Surgical Quality Improvement Program, increased risk of surgical complications can be a serious deterrent against more aggressive operative approach, especially in patients whose general health status further increases operative risk.

M. Gapany, MD

Neck Dissection After Chemoradiotherapy: Timing and Complications

Goguen LA, Chapuy CI, Li Y, et al (Brigham and Women's Hosp, Boston, MA; Dana-Farber Cancer Inst, Boston, MA)
Arch Otolaryngol Head Neck Surg 136:1071-1077, 2010

Objectives.—To determine the incidence of postchemoradiotherapy (post-CRT) neck dissection (ND) complications; to ascertain whether timing (<12 vs ≥12 weeks) from CRT to ND or other factors are associated with increased complications; and to determine whether ND timing influences disease control or survival.
Design.—Ten-year retrospective analysis.
Setting.—Tertiary care center.
Patients.—One hundred five patients with head and neck cancer undergoing ND after CRT.
Main Outcome Measures.—Complications and survival variables compared between groups undergoing ND less than 12 weeks (less-than-12-weeks ND group) and 12 weeks or more (12-weeks-or-more ND group) after CRT.
Results.—Sixty-seven NDs were performed less than 12 weeks and 38 were performed 12 weeks or more after CRT. Patient characteristics, treatment, and ND pathology results were comparable between the 2 ND groups. The incidence of complications between the less-than-12-weeks and the 12-weeks-or-more ND groups included major wound complications in 8 of 67 (11.9%) vs 1 of 38 (2.6%; $P = .15$), minor wound complications in 11 of 67 (16.4%) vs 4 of 38 (10.5%; $P = .56$), airway complications in 7 of 67 (10.4%) vs 2 of 38 (5.3%; $P = .48$), and systemic complications in 9 of 67 (13.4%) vs 2 of 38 (5.3%; $P = .32$). The number of patients with at least 1 complication was significantly smaller in the 12-weeks-or-more ND group ($P = .04$). Multivariate analysis showed that radical ND was significantly associated with an increased number of complications, and higher radiation doses approached significance ($P = .05$). Induction chemotherapy was associated with fewer wound complications ($P = .01$). There were no significant differences in overall survival ($P = .82$), progression-free survival ($P = .77$), or regional relapse ($P = .54$) between groups. Positive ND findings were associated with diminished progression-free and overall survival.
Conclusion.—These findings indicate that ND can be safely performed 12 weeks or more after CRT without adversely affecting surgical complications or survival variables.

▶ This article deals with surgery for salvage after radiochemotherapy. While retrospective in its design, this article provides some valuable information regarding the expected impact of delaying the decision on salvage neck dissection on patients with initial metastatic neck disease for 3 months after completion of radiotherapy. The vast majority of data in the literature are now supporting CT/positron emission tomography coregistration at 3 months as the most accurate way to determine the need for salvage neck dissection. The

question whether this delay will unfavorably affect the postoperative complication rates or impact the neck recurrence rates or the disease-free and overall
survivals, however, remains subject to controversy. This article provides reassuring data. The authors found that delaying the neck dissection for 3 months after
completion of radiochemotherapy was not associated with increased rate of
surgical complications and had no untoward effect on disease control or survival
rates. Well-designed prospective studies are needed to confirm these findings.

M. Gapany, MD

**The Assessment of Pharyngocutaneous Fistula Rate in Patients Treated
Primarily With Definitive Radiotherapy Followed by Salvage Surgery of
the Larynx and Hypopharynx**
Dirven R, Swinson BD, Gao K, et al (Royal Prince Alfred Hosp and Univ of
Sydney, Australia)
Laryngoscope 119:1691-1695, 2009

Objectives/Hypothesis.—To determine whether definitive radiotherapy
prior to surgery increases the rate of pharyngocutaneous fistula (PCF)
following laryngectomy or hypopharyngectomy and to determine if differences in duration of time between definitive radiotherapy and surgery
alters PCF rate.

Study Design.—A retrospective review of 152 patients treated surgically
for primary laryngeal or hypopharyngeal squamous cell carcinoma.

Methods.—Following previous definitive radiotherapy treatment 38
patients underwent salvage surgery and 114 patients underwent primary
surgery with curative intent. The PCF rate was assessed in both groups.

Results.—The rate of PCF was found to be significantly higher in the
salvage surgery group than those undergoing primary surgery (34.2%
vs. 15.7%) ($P < .05$). Fistula rate was also higher in the subgroup that
received concurrent chemoradiation to radiotherapy alone ($P = .002$).
The patients who developed PCF in the salvage surgery group had significantly lower median time to surgery (5.8 months) than the nonfistula
group (9.8 months) ($P = .032$). PCF rate was 75% within 4 months of
radiotherapy to salvage surgery compared to 25% after 4 months
($P = .034$). Within 12 months of radiotherapy this percentage was 48%
compared to 0% after 12 months ($P = .014$). The median radiotherapy
dose was significantly higher in those whose surgery was complicated by
PCF (70 Gy) compared to patients who did not develop a fistula (64 Gy)
($P = .001$).

Conclusions.—Patients undergoing salvage surgery within 12 months,
and in particular within 4 months, who have received high dose radiotherapy (>64 Gy) or concurrent chemoradiation are at high risk of developing PCF.

▶ Salvage surgery for failed radiochemotherapy has become an integral part of
head and neck oncologic surgery practice. With it, we have observed an

increased incidence of pharyngocutaneous fistulae and other wound healing problems. In our institution, where we perform most of our oncologic surgery, we are under constant pressure from the National Surgical Quality Improvement Program (NSQUIP) officers to reduce our wound complication rate, which for the last several years, has been a high outlier compared with the national average. Unfortunately, according to the NSQUIP criteria, risk adjustment for radiotherapy only applies for surgery performed within 3 months following completion radiotherapy; operations performed later than 3 months are not risk adjusted. Because our first positron emission tomography/CT evaluation for response to radiochemotherapy is performed at 3 months after completion of treatment, we almost exclusively operate later than the set risk-adjustment criteria. So far, our request for review of the existing risk-adjustment criteria for radiotherapy has fallen on deaf ears. It is our hope that studies like these 2 articles (see pages 31 and 37) will change the minds of NSQUIP policy makers regarding the late effects of radiotherapy (and especially radiochemotherapy) on surgical wound healing.

M. Gapany, MD

Radiotherapy

Mature results of a randomized trial of accelerated hyperfractionated versus conventional radiotherapy in head-and-neck cancer
Saunders MI, for the Chart Trial Collaborators (Mount Vernon Hosp, Northwood, UK; et al)
Int J Radiat Oncol Biol Phys 77:3-8, 2010

Purpose.—To evaluate long-term late adverse events and treatment outcome of a randomized, multicenter Phase III trial of continuous, hyperfractionated, accelerated radiotherapy (CHART) compared with conventional radiotherapy (CRT) in 918 patients with advanced squamous cell carcinomas of the head and neck.

Methods and Materials.—Survival estimates were obtained for locoregional relapse-free survival, local relapse-free survival, overall survival, disease-specific survival, disease-free survival and for late adverse events.

Results.—The 10-year estimates (± 1 standard error) for locoregional relapse-free survival, overall survival, disease-free survival, and disease-specific survival were 43% $\pm$ 2% for CHART and 50% $\pm$ 3% with CRT (log-rank $p = 0.2$); 26% $\pm$ 2% and 29% $\pm$ 3% ($p = 0.4$), respectively; 41% $\pm$ 2% and 46% $\pm$ 3% ($p = 0.3$), respectively; and 56% $\pm$ 3% and 58% $\pm$ 3% ($p = 0.5$), respectively. There was a small but significant reduction in the incidence of slight or worse and moderate or worse epidermal adverse events with CHART ($p = 0.002$ to 0.05). Severe xerostomia, laryngeal edema, and mucosal necrosis were also significantly lower with CHART ($p = 0.02$ to 0.05).

Conclusions.—Despite the reduction in total dose from 66 Gy to 54 Gy, control of locoregional disease and survival with CHART were similar to those with CRT. These findings, together with the low incidence of long-term severe adverse events, suggest that CHART is a treatment option for patients with low-risk disease and for those unable to withstand the toxicity of concurrent chemoradiotherapy.

▶ This is an important article because it provides level I evidence confirming positive long-term results of accelerated hyperfractionated radiotherapy. In this publication, the authors of the initial randomized trial, comparing accelerated hyperfractionation with conventional radiotherapy for head and neck cancer (published in 1997), report their mature results of long-term follow-up. It is very encouraging to see that 10 years after completion of the randomized study, the initial results still hold true; that is, despite significant reduction of the total radiation dose and thus radiation therapy-associated side effects, the locoregional control, disease-free survival, disease-specific survival, and overall survival have not been compromised. While the search for ideal radiotherapy protocol for head and neck cancer continues, several strategies are emerging, which improve response and/or decrease side effects of the therapy. These include the use of chemotherapeutic or immunologic agents as radiosensitizers, the use of positron emission tomography imaging to improve preradiotherapy planning, and intensity-modulated radiotherapy, to mention just a few. Accelerated hyperfractionation appears to be a good alternative to standard radiotherapy, offering uncompromised therapeutic outcomes and reduced side effects.

M. Gapany, MD

Multi-institutional trial of accelerated hypofractionated intensity-modulated radiation therapy for early-stage oropharyngeal cancer (RTOG 00-22)

Eisbruch A, Harris J, Garden AS, et al (Univ of Michigan, Ann Arbor; American College of Radiology, Reston, VA; MD Anderson Cancer Ctr, Houston, TX; et al)

Int J Radiat Oncol Biol Phys 76:1333-1338, 2010

Purpose.—To assess the results of a multi-institutional study of intensity-modulated radiation therapy (IMRT) for early oropharyngeal cancer.

Patients and Methods.—Patients with oropharyngeal carcinoma Stage T1–2, N0–1, M0 requiring treatment of the bilateral neck were eligible. Chemotherapy was not permitted. Prescribed planning target volumes (PTVs) doses to primary tumor and involved nodes was 66 Gy at 2.2 Gy/fraction over 6 weeks. Subclinical PTVs received simultaneously 54–60 Gy at 1.8–2.0 Gy/fraction. Participating institutions were preapproved for IMRT, and quality assurance review was performed by the Image-Guided Therapy Center.

Results.—69 patients were accrued from 14 institutions. At median follow-up for surviving patients (2.8 years), the 2-year estimated local-regional failure (LRF) rate was 9%. 2/4 patients (50%) with major underdose deviations had LRF compared with 3/49 (6%) without such deviations ($p = 0.04$). All cases of LRF, metastasis, or second primary cancer occurred among patients who were current/former smokers, and none among patients who never smoked. Maximal late toxicities Grade ≥ 2 were skin 12%, mucosa 24%, salivary 67%, esophagus 19%, osteoradionecrosis 6%. Longer follow-up revealed reduced late toxicity in all categories. Xerostomia Grade ≥ 2 was observed in 55% of patients at 6 months but reduced to 25% and 16% at 12 and 24 months, respectively. In contrast, salivary output did not recover over time.

Conclusions.—Moderately accelerated hypofractionatd IMRT without chemotherapy for early oropharyngeal cancer is feasible, achieving high tumor control rates and reduced salivary toxicity compared with similar patients in previous Radiation Therapy Oncology Group studies. Major target underdose deviations were associated with higher LRF rate.

▶ The search for ideal radiotherapy protocol for head and neck cancer continues. In recent years, several strategies have emerged, which improve response and/or decrease side effects of the therapy. These include the use of chemotherapeutic or immunologic agents as radiosensitizers, the use of positron emission tomography imaging to improve preradiotherapy planning, accelerated hyperfractionation, and intensity-modulated radiotherapy (IMRT), to mention just a few. This multi-institutional prospective trial (Radiation Therapy Oncology Group 00-22) was designed to evaluate the efficacy of hyperfractionated IMRT for oropharyngeal cancer. Implications of this study were limited to early oropharyngeal cancers because concurrent chemoradiotherapy for advanced oropharyngeal cancer cannot be tolerated when delivered in the setting of IMRT protocol. The trial also used a centralized quality assurance process to assure the quality of participating IMRT plans. The importance of this study is that it sets clear target dose prescriptions and tissue dose constraints for IMRT for early oropharyngeal cancer, demonstrating that adherence to protocol guidelines is a significant factor associated with improved local-regional control and low rate of side effects.

M. Gapany, MD

Surgical Technique

Postoperative Complications After Extracapsular Dissection of Benign Parotid Lesions With Particular Reference to Facial Nerve Function
Klintworth N, Zenk J, Koch M, et al (Univ of Erlangen-Nuremberg, Germany)
Laryngoscope 120:484-490, 2010

Objectives/Hypothesis.—The desirable extent of surgical intervention for benign parotid tumors remains a matter of controversy. Superficial or total parotidectomy as a standard procedure is often said to be the gold standard; however, with it the risk of intraoperative damage to the facial nerve cannot be ignored. For some time now, extracapsular dissection without exposure of the main trunk of the facial nerve has been favored as an alternative for the treatment of discrete parotid tumors. Data on the incidence of facial nerve lesions and other acute postoperative complications of extracapsular dissection have been lacking until now.

Study Design.—Retrospective analysis.

Methods.—We performed a retrospective analysis of the data from patients in whom extracapsular dissection of a benign parotid tumor had been performed under facial nerve monitoring and as a primary intervention in our department between 2000 and 2008.

Results.—A total of 934 patients were operated on for a newly diagnosed benign tumor of the parotid gland. Three hundred seventy-seven patients (40%) underwent extracapsular dissection as a primary intervention. The most common postoperative complication was hypoesthesia of the cheek or the earlobe, as reported by 38 patients (10%). Eighteen patients (5%) developed a seroma and 13 patients (3%) a hematoma. A salivary fistula formed in eight patients (2%). Secondary bleeding occurred in three patients (0.8%). In 346 patients (92%) facial nerve function was normal (House-Brackmann grade I) in the immediate postoperative period, whereas 23 patients (6%) showed temporary facial nerve paresis (House-Brackmann grade II or III) and eight patients (2%) developed permanent facial nerve paresis (seven patients House-Brackmann grade II, one patient House-Brackmann grade III).

Conclusions.—Extracapsular dissection of benign parotid tumors is associated with a low rate of postoperative complications, a fact that is confirmed by the available literature. We therefore recommend that use of this technique always be considered as a means of treating benign parotid tumors as conservatively, that is, as uninvasively, as possible.

▶ A number of recent publications from around the world have challenged the operation of superficial parotidectomy as the only correct approach to resecting benign tumors of the parotid gland. Concepts such as limited parotidectomy, partial parotidectomy, and, finally, extracapsular tumor dissection were all advocated as safe when it comes to long-term recurrence rates and preservation of facial nerve function. These studies have shown that staying close to the capsule of benign parotid gland tumors does not increase the rate of tumor recurrence, as long as the capsule is kept intact and no spillage of the tumor occurs. The operation of extracapsular tumor dissection as a rule is performed without identification of the facial nerve, albeit with intraoperative facial nerve monitoring. In my commentaries to those articles in the past, I was skeptical of the surgical soundness of such an approach (skipping the identification of the facial nerve), citing a time-tested surgical principle, namely, that the safest way to prevent injury to an anatomical structure is to identify that structure. This very large retrospective study (on 370 extracapsular dissections of benign parotid gland tumors) confirmed that facial nerve injury in extracapsular tumor dissection operation was less likely to occur than in a standard superficial parotidectomy and thus appeared to be safer when it comes to preservation of facial nerve function. I stand corrected.

M. Gapany, MD

3 Laryngology

Basic and Clinical Research

Ergonomic Analysis of Microlaryngoscopy

Statham MM, Sukits AL, Redfern MS, et al (Univ of Pittsburgh Voice Ctr, PA)
Laryngoscope 120:297-305, 2010

Objectives/Hypothesis.—To apply ergonomic principles in analysis of three different operative positions used in laryngeal microsurgery.

Study Design.—Prospective case-control study.

Methods.—Laryngologists were studied in three different microlaryngeal operative positions: a supported position in a chair with articulated arm supports, a supported position with arms resting on a Mayo stand, and a position with arms unsupported. Operative positions were uniformly photographed in three dimensions. Full body postural data was collected and analyzed using the validated Rapid Upper Limb Assessment (RULA) tool to calculate a risk score indicative of potential musculoskeletal misuse in each position. Joint forces were calculated for the neck and shoulder, and compression forces were calculated for the L5/S1 disc space.

Results.—Higher-risk postures were obtained with unfavorably adjusted eyepieces and lack of any arm support during microlaryngeal surgery. Support with a Mayo stand led to more neck flexion and strain. Using a chair with articulated arm supports leads to decreased neck strain, less shoulder torque, and decreased compressive forces on the L5/S1 disc space. Ideal postures during microlaryngoscopy place the surgeon with arms and feet supported, with shoulders in an unraised, neutral anatomic position, upper arms neutrally positioned 20° to 45° from torso, lower arms neutrally positioned 60° to 100° from torso, and wrists extended or flexed <15°.

Conclusions.—RULA and biomechanical analyses have identified lower-risk surgeon positioning to be utilized during microlaryngeal surgery. Avoiding the identified high-risk operative postures and repetitive stress injury may lead to reduced occupationally related musculoskeletal pain and may improve microsurgical motor control.

▶ This is a very important article, and the first in otolaryngology literature, to address the issue of ergonomics in the operating room. For a long time now, ergonomics in the workplace has been a subject of extensive research, resulting in adoption by the National Institute of Occupational Safety and Health of stringent recommendations for workstation design. Until now, literally nothing has been done to address the occupational hazards encountered by otolaryngologists in the operating room and, to a lesser degree, in the clinic. While our colleagues in dentistry are well aware of the work-related musculoskeletal disorders, otolaryngologists, as a rule, are oblivious to those problems. Yet, the problem of occupational injuries among otolaryngologists, particularly severe neck and back injuries, is very prevalent. In a mail survey of 700 members of American Academy of Otolaryngology-Head and Neck Surgery, which I conducted a few years ago, more than 50% reported incapacitating neck and/or back injuries at least once in their professional career. The importance of this selected publication cannot be overemphasized because it has the potential of raising the awareness of otolaryngologists to the hazards of their profession. Furthermore, the article makes some useful suggestions on how to avoid musculoskeletal strain in microlaryngeal surgery.

M. Gapany, MD

Anatomical landmarks for endosonography of the larynx
Kraft M, Mende S, Arnoux A, et al (Kantonsspital Aarau, Switzerland; et al)
Head Neck 32:326-332, 2010

Background.—A precise knowledge of anatomy is necessary to allow a correct interpretation of sonographic images when investigating a particular region of the body. The objective of the present study was to establish anatomical landmarks for endosonography of the larynx.

Methods.—In an experimental study, a total of 32 normal human larynges were examined endosonographically, and the classical landmarks

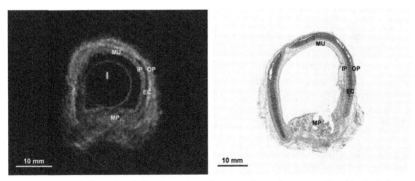

FIGURE 1.—Trachea. Correlation between endosonography and corresponding histological cross section (hematoxylin-eosin stain, original magnification ×1). IP, inner perichondrium of trachea; OP, outer perichondrium of trachea; EC, elastic cartilage; MP, membranous portion of trachea; MU, tracheal mucosa. (Reprinted from Kraft M, Mende S, Arnoux A, et al. Anatomical landmarks for endosonography of the larynx. *Head Neck.* 2010;32:326-332 copyright 2010. Reprinted with permission of John Wiley & Sons, Inc.)

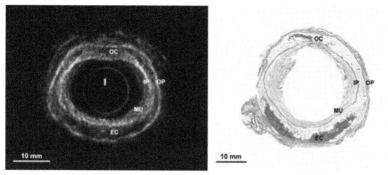

FIGURE 2.—Cricoid. Correlation between endosonography and corresponding histological cross section (hematoxylin-eosin stain, original magnification ×1). IP, inner perichondrium of cricoid; OP, outer perichondrium of cricoid; EC, elastic cartilage; OC, ossified cartilage; MU, cricoidal mucosa. (Reprinted from Kraft M, Mende S, Arnoux A, et al. Anatomical landmarks for endosonography of the larynx. *Head Neck.* 2010;32:326-332 copyright 2010. Reprinted with permission of John Wiley & Sons, Inc.)

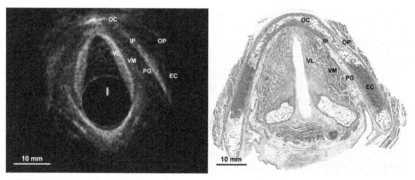

FIGURE 3.—Vocal fold. Correlation between endosonography and corresponding histological cross section (hematoxylin-eosin stain, original magnification ×1). IP, inner perichondrium of thyroid; OP, outer perichondrium of thyroid; EC, elastic cartilage; OC, ossified cartilage; PG, paraglottic space; VM, vocal muscle; VL, vocal ligament. (Reprinted from Kraft M, Mende S, Arnoux A, et al. Anatomical landmarks for endosonography of the larynx. *Head Neck.* 2010;32:326-332 copyright 2010. Reprinted with permission of John Wiley & Sons, Inc.)

were correlated to horizontal whole-organ sections of the scanned specimens.

Results.—All laryngeal specimens showed a similar and reproducible sonoanatomy, which could be verified consistently on corresponding histological cross sections. Anatomical structures readily identified included the laryngeal framework, the vocal ligament, the vocal muscle, the ventricular fold, the preepiglottic and paraglottic space, and the epiglottis.

Conclusions.—Due to a reproducible sonoanatomy of the larynx, endosonography might be an interesting complementary tool in the diagnostic investigation of laryngeal lesions such as medium-sized tumors, cysts, laryngoceles, and stenoses (Figs 1-3).

▶ Ultrasonography has made inroads into the field of otolaryngology through its use as a way to locate neck masses for fine-needle aspiration and discover and track the size of thyroid nodules. There are clear advantages to using ultra-sound (not using ionizing radiation) to visualize the deep laryngeal anatomy, but the effort had been hampered by the depth of penetration, limited resolution, and lack of expertise in reading the images. The authors were able to correlate the ultrasonography findings with histologic evaluation to identify the laryngeal framework, muscles, vocal ligament, and pre-epiglottic and paraglottic spaces. The resolution was sufficiently fine to resolve the inner and outer perichondrium of the epiglottis, cricoid, and thyroid cartilages. Since the system can be used only in the operating room at the time of microlaryngoscopy (since the lumen needs to be filled with fluid), the probe was sufficiently large (12 mm) to make it difficult in 22% and impossible to pass in 41% of cadaveric specimens. Using a 10- or 15-MHz transducer allows for images with resolution greater than CT. Miniaturization of the probe could make ultrasonography a viable intraoperative tool for mapping the extent of an endolaryngeal tumor (up to the thyroid cartilage).

R. A. Franco, Jr, MD

Auto-crosslinked hyaluronan gel injections in phonosurgery
Molteni G, Bergamini G, Ricci-Maccarini A, et al (Univ of Modena and Reggio Emilia, Italy; Ospedale Bufalini di Cesena, Italy)
Otolaryngol Head Neck Surg 142:547-553, 2010

Objectives.—To evaluate the clinical performance of an auto-cross-linked gel obtained from hyaluronic acid (ACP-based gel) as an anti-adhesive agent and/or augmentative agent in vocal cord surgery for the treatment of vocal fold (VF) atrophy, sulcus vocalis, and postsurgery scarring as well as its tolerability at short- and long-term follow-up.

Study Design.—This was a prospective multicenter trial conducted between 2007 and 2009.

Setting.—Academic center.

Subjects and Methods.—Inclusion criteria were patients with glottic gap due to previous endoscopic phonosurgery, VF scars, vocal cord atrophy, and sulcus vocalis. Forty patients who underwent endoscopic injection of hyaluronic acid under general anesthesia were enrolled. Two different injections sites were used: the thyroarytenoid muscle in cases of glottic gap for augmentative purposes, and the lamina propria for treatment of scars and sulcus vocalis. A voice-evaluation protocol was performed before surgery, at the first follow-up visit (3 mo), and at the final follow-up (12 mo).

Results.—Follow-up data at three months were available for 38 patients, while data at 12 months follow-up were available for 27 patients. No side effects, hematoma, or infection and allergic reactions were reported in either the perioperative or postoperative period. Patients had statistically significant improvement in voice parameters compared with the baseline data at the first follow-up visit and at the 12-month follow-up.

Conclusion.—ACP-based gel seems to be a new tool in the challenging treatment of VF scarring, functioning as both an anti-adhesive product and an augmentation agent. Improvements in all glottal parameters and in both objective and subjective evaluation of voice performance were observed.

▶ There is a plethora of available materials for injection in the vocal folds. In many ways, these materials, as diverse as they are, end up providing very similar effects by acting as bulking agents that are inserted deep to the vocal ligament. Hyaluronic acid (HA) is a native constituent of the vocal fold superficial lamina propria and has the most ideal viscoelastic properties of the various augmentation materials now available. The major drawback to using HA is that it is easily and quickly degraded. To combat this, HA can be cross-linked to make it more resistant to breakdown. This cross-linking also makes it stiffer and less ideal as a superficial lamina propria substitute. The authors found statistically significant improvements in the voice parameters (as would be expected with most augmentation materials) with the added potential benefits of the HA minimizing postoperative superficial lamina propria scarring. Rheological and histological studies will need to be performed to establish that the mucosa is truly more pliable and less scarred with the use of HA at the time of surgery.

R. A. Franco, Jr, MD

Brainstem Pathology in Spasmodic Dysphonia
Simonyan K, Ludlow CL, Vortmeyer AO (Natl Insts of Health, Bethesda, MD)
Laryngoscope 120:121-124, 2010

Spasmodic dysphonia (SD) is a primary focal dystonia of unknown pathophysiology, characterized by involuntary spasms in the laryngeal muscles during speech production. We examined two rare cases of post-mortem brainstem tissue from SD patients compared to four controls. In the SD patients, small clusters of inflammation were found in the reticular formation surrounding solitary tract, spinal trigeminal, and ambigual nuclei, inferior olive, and pyramids. Mild neuronal degeneration and depigmentation were observed in the substantia nigra and locus coeruleus. No abnormal protein accumulations and no demyelination or axonal degeneration were found. These neuropathological findings may provide insights into the pathophysiology of SD (Fig 1).

▶ Spasmodic dysphonia (SD) is still a mysterious disorder. The exact location of injury in patients with SD is not yet established, and the exact genes responsible have yet to be identified. The authors found histological evidence of differences between the brainstem of patients with SD (2) and that of controls (4) that are very interesting. They found microglia and macrophage activation clustered around the lower brainstem nuclei and degeneration and depigmentation in the substantia nigra and locus coeruleus. More studies are required to

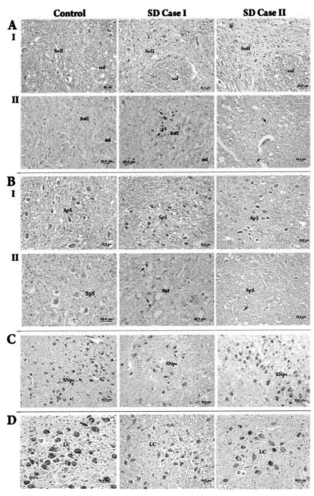

FIGURE 1.—Microphotographs of the brainstem regions in the controls and both spasmodic dysphonia cases show normal cell morphology in the interstitial part of the solitary tract nucleus (SolI) (A-I), and the spinal trigeminal nucleus (Sp5) (B-I) (hematoxylin and eosin [H&E] stain); clusters of microglial/macrophage activation (arrows) in the reticular formation surrounding the SolI (A-II) and Sp5 (B-II) (CD68/KP1 immunostain); and mild neuronal degeneration and depigmentation in the substantial nigra, pars compacta (C), and the locus coeruleus (D) (H&E stain), respectively. (Reprinted from Simonyan K, Ludlow CL, Vortmeyer AO. Brainstem pathology in spasmodic dysphonia. *Laryngoscope*. 2010;120:121-124, with permission from The American Laryngological, Rhinological and Otological Society, Inc.)

establish that this is a reliable finding and elucidate the mechanism underlying these findings.

R. A. Franco, Jr, MD

Calcium Hydroxylapatite Injection Laryngoplasty for the Treatment of Presbylaryngis: Long-Term Results

Kwon T-K, An S-Y, Ahn J-C, et al (Seoul Natl Univ College of Medicine, South Korea)

Laryngoscope 120:326-329, 2010

Objectives/Hypothesis.—Presbylaryngis is a normal part of the aging process, but many people visit hospitals with communication difficulties. The authors evaluated the efficacy of calcium hydroxylapatite (CaHA) injection laryngoplasty in patients with presbylaryngis.

Study Design.—Retrospective review.

Methods.—Thirty-three patients with diagnosed presbylaryngis were administered a CaHA injection, and 17 of these patients without other vocal pathologies were included in the analysis. All 17 were male (mean age 65.9 years), mean follow-up duration was 335 days, and all injections were performed through the cricothyroid membrane under local anesthesia in a clinic.

Results.—Subjective ratings, perceptual ratings, maximum phonation time, and closed quotients significantly improved after injection, and these improvements persisted without significant change for over 12 months. No major complications were encountered except for transient hematoma, pain, and a foreign body sensation.

Conclusions.—The authors conclude that CaHA injection laryngoplasty offers an effective and safe means of treating presbylaryngis (Figs 1 and 2).

▶ As the baby boomer population of the United States continues to age, many are coming to the otolaryngologist for treatment of their weak, raspy, and

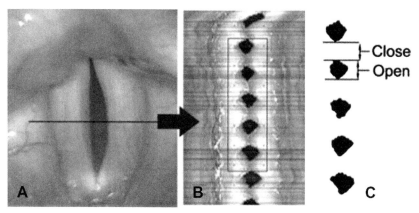

FIGURE 1.—Videostrobokymographic analysis. (A) A midvocal fold line was chosen for vocal fold vibration analysis. (B) Over five cycles of vocal fold vibration were selected. (C) Calculate closed quotient (CQ): CQ = closed phase/(open phase + closed phase) × 100. (Reprinted from Kwon T-K, An S-Y, Ahn J-C, et al. Calcium hydroxylapatite injection laryngoplasty for the treatment of presbylaryngis: long-term results. *Laryngoscope.* 2010;120:326-329, with permission from The American Laryngological, Rhinological and Otological Society, Inc.)

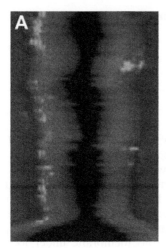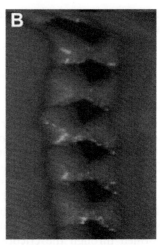

FIGURE 2.—Videostrobokymographic findings in preinjection and postinjection period of an 82-year-old male with presbylaryngis. (A) A preinjection videostrobokymography. Note that there is no vocal fold contact during phonation. (B) A 4-month postinjection videostrobokymography. A total of 0.3 cc of Radiesse was injected in the right vocal fold. Note that there are visible vocal fold contacts and decreased lateral excursion of the right vocal fold vibration. (Reprinted from Kwon T-K, An S-Y, Ahn J-C, et al. Calcium hydroxylapatite injection laryngoplasty for the treatment of presbylaryngis: long-term results. *Laryngoscope*. 2010;120:326-329, with permission from The American Laryngological, Rhinological and Otological Society, Inc.)

effortful voice stemming from an overall loss of superficial lamina propria (SLP) termed presbylaryngis. The natural history of the vocal folds is to lose bulk in the SLP layer. This is exemplified in the rapid changes seen in the immature larynx where the newborn true vocal fold is composed of the large SLP layer over muscle, whereas by age 13 the vocal fold takes on the adult trilaminar structure of SLP (much thinner than in the newborn), vocal ligament, and muscle. There appears to be a gradual loss in the volume of the SLP throughout life that eventually leads to an incompetent larynx (a persistent midmusculomembranous region gap) and the typical symptoms of presbylaryngis (effortful phonation and weak and raspy voice). Injection laryngoplasty can address the lack of bulk and the effortful and weak voice. The authors of this study used transcricothyroid injection of Radiesse Voice (calcium hydroxylapetite) under nasolaryngoscopic guidance to bulk the vocal folds in 33 patients diagnosed with presbylaryngis. They had a mean follow-up of nearly 1 year in 17 of these patients without major complications. There was videostrobokymographic evidence (Figs 1 and 2) for restoration of midmusculomembranous closure and improvements in the grade, roughness, breathiness, asthenia, strain scale and patient's subjective voice rating. It is encouraging that the results were intact at the 1-year mark.

R. A. Franco, Jr, MD

Chronic Vocal Fold Scar Restoration With Hepatocyte Growth Factor Hydrogel

Kishimoto Y, Hirano S, Kitani Y, et al (Kyoto Univ, Sakyo-ku, Japan; et al)
Laryngoscope 120:108-113, 2010

Objectives/Hypothesis.—Therapeutic challenges exist in the management of vocal fold scarring. We have previously demonstrated the therapeutic potential of hepatocyte growth factor (HGF) in the management

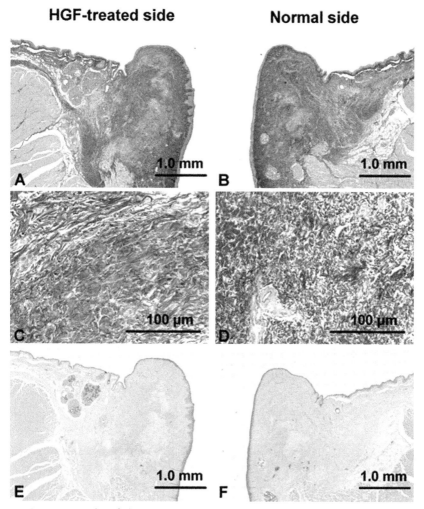

FIGURE 3.—Histologic findings in the hepatocyte growth factor (HGF)-treated group. (A–D) Elastica van Gieson stain. (E–F) Alcian blue stain. Tissue contraction and collagen deposition were found to be minimal (A, B), and elastin (C, D) and hyaluronic acid (E, F) were favorably restored. (Reprinted from Kishimoto Y, Hirano S, Kitani Y, et al. Chronic vocal fold scar restoration with hepatocyte growth factor hydrogel. *Laryngoscope.* 2010;120:108-113, with permission from The American Laryngological, Rhinological and Otological Society, Inc.)

of acute phase vocal fold scarring using a novel hydrogel-based HGF drug delivery system (DDS). However, the effect of HGF on matured vocal fold scarring remains unclear. The current study aims to investigate the effect of HGF-DDS on chronic vocal fold scarring using a canine model.
Study Design.—Animal model.
Methods.—Vocal folds from eight beagles were unilaterally scarred by stripping the entire layer of the lamina propria; contralateral vocal folds were kept intact as normal controls. Six months after the procedures,

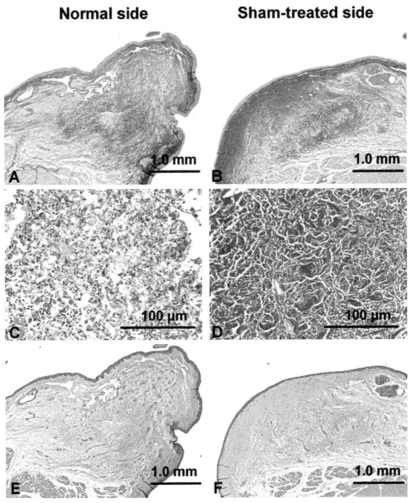

Normal side   **Sham-treated side**

FIGURE 4.—Histologic findings in the sham-treated group. (A–D) Elastica van Gieson stain. (E–F) Alcian blue stain. Severe tissue contraction and excessive collagen deposition were observed in sham-treated vocal folds (A, B). Elastin (C, D) and hyaluronic acid (E, F) were decreased in the superior portion of the treated vocal fold. (Reprinted from Kishimoto Y, Hirano S, Kitani Y, et al. Chronic vocal fold scar restoration with hepatocyte growth factor hydrogel. *Laryngoscope.* 2010;120:108-113, with permission from The American Laryngological, Rhinological and Otological Society, Inc.)

hydrogels (0.5 mL) containing 1 μg of HGF were injected into the scarred vocal folds of four dogs (HGF-treated group). Hydrogels containing saline solution were injected into the other four dogs (sham group). Histological and vibratory examinations on excised larynges were completed for each group 9 months after the initial surgery.

Results.—Experiments conducted on excised larynges demonstrated significantly better vibrations in the HGF-treated group in terms of mucosal wave amplitude. Although phonation threshold pressure was significantly lower in the HGF-treated group compared with the sham group, no significant differences were observed in the normalized glottal gap between HGF-treated and sham groups. Histological examinations of the HGF-treated vocal folds showed reduced collagen deposition and less tissue contraction with favorable restoration of hyaluronic acid.

Conclusions.—Results suggest that administration of HGF may have therapeutic potential in the treatment of chronic vocal fold scarring (Figs 3 and 4).

▶ Clinically, the treatment for vocal fold scarring is extremely challenging. Previous studies have demonstrated that hepatocyte growth factor (HGF) can decrease acute scarring, increase hyaluronic acid production, and decrease fibroblast collagen formation after vocal fold injury. This group examined the potential for HGF to modulate established scar through a canine model where vocal stripping caused scarring of an entire vocal fold. Six months later, the scar was injected with a hydrogel infused with HGF. They found significantly improved mucosal wave as evidenced by the amplitude of the wave in those dogs treated with the HGF as compared with the saline-injected scarred controls. The exciting aspect is the ability to modify established scar through the use of HGF. It is imperative that we attempt to bring these treatments to the clinic where the scarred vocal fold can potentially be treated with an awake injection of an HGF.

R. A. Franco, Jr, MD

Effect of a Novel Anatomically Shaped Endotracheal Tube on Intubation-Related Injury

Gordin A, Chadha NK, Campisi P, et al (The Hosp for Sick Children, Toronto, Ontario, Canada)
Arch Otolaryngol Head Neck Surg 136:54-59, 2010

Objectives.—To develop an anatomically shaped endotracheal tube (ETT) and to compare the degree of induced laryngeal injury of this ETT with that of a standard ETT using an animal model.

Design.—Randomized controlled animal study.

Subjects.—Eight *Sus scrofa* piglets (15-20 kg) randomly intubated with either a standard or a modified uncuffed ETT.

Interventions.—The modified ETT was handcrafted by gluing and then trimming dry polyvinyl acetate foam circumferentially to the distal end of a standard uncuffed ETT. After intubation, the foam quickly self-expanded as it absorbed the secretions of the laryngopharynx and adopted the shape of the intraluminal airway. This conforming shape also sealed the larynx to allow for positive pressure ventilation. Both groups were intubated for 4 hours under constant hypoxic conditions (mean oxygen saturation <70%) to enhance and accelerate intubation damage. They were then humanely killed, and the larynx and trachea were harvested for histologic examination.

Main Outcome Measures.—The severity of laryngeal injury graded on a scale from 0 to 4 (0 indicates normal; 1, epithelial compression; 2, epithelial loss; 3, subepithelial and glandular necrosis; and 4, perichondrium involvement).

Results.—All of the specimens histologically demonstrated areas of inflammation and epithelial loss. The standard ETT caused substantial deep damage, with a mean (SD) severity score of 2.79 (0.74). The modified ETT caused mainly superficial damage, with a mean (SD) severity score of 1.65 (0.56) ($P < .001$).

Conclusion.—The modified ETT objectively caused less laryngotracheal damage compared with the standard ETT and may be of potential clinical benefit.

▶ The most common cause for laryngotracheal stenosis is injury from prolonged intubation. The airway lining is disrupted or devitalized secondary to the inhibition of perfusion from an overly inflated endotracheal tube. This leads to a focal stenosis that can become critical enough to require surgical correction. Obviously, the creation of an endotracheal tube that could decrease the incidence of injury during intubation would go a long way toward eradicating the very worrisome consequences of this iatrogenic injury. A modified endotracheal tube wrapped in a 5-cm long segment of dry polyvinyl acetate (PVA) (Merocel) was compared with standard endotracheal tubes in the larynges of piglets. Histologic evaluation after 4 hours of intubation revealed significantly less injury of the mucosa from the level of the trachea to the supraglottis ($P = .001$) in those piglets in which the modified tube was used. The PVA effectively sealed the airway to pressures of 40 cm H_2O through self-expansion by absorbing the laryngotracheal secretions without causing focal deep injuries to the lining of the larynx or trachea.

R. A. Franco, Jr, MD

Electromyographic Laryngeal Synkinesis Alters Prognosis in Vocal Fold Paralysis
Statham MM, Rosen CA, Smith LJ, et al (Univ of Pittsburgh, PA)
Laryngoscope 120:285-290, 2010

Objectives/Hypothesis.—Synkinesis, or misdirected reinnervation, is likely a confounder when predicting return of function of an immobile vocal fold. Currently, no information exists on the incidence of synkinesis in unilateral vocal fold immobility (UVFI) or the effect synkinesis has on prognosis and treatment. Our objective was to examine a vocal fold adductor synkinesis screening protocol using diagnostic laryngeal electromyography (LEMG). We aim to determine the effect of synkinesis on prognosis of recovery of purposeful vocal fold motion.

Study Design.—Retrospective review of LEMG data and patient charts from laryngology practice.

Methods.—A standardized LEMG analysis method to diagnose vocal fold adductory synkinesis was performed in 124 consecutive laryngeal electromyographic exams.

Results.—Synkinesis testing was positive in 12/124 patients (9.7%). Post hoc quantitative analysis of electromyographic recordings to compare motor unit potential amplitude in the thyroarytenoid/lateral cricoarytenoid complex during sustained phonation to those in the same muscle during a "sniff " revealed a significant difference in motor unit potential amplitude ratio for control subjects (0.32), those who recovered purposeful vocal fold motion (0.40), and those with vocal fold paralysis (0.96) ($P = .001$). The presence of synkinesis in patients with UVFI improved the negative predictive value of LEMG from 53% to 100% and the sensitivity from 56% to 100%.

Conclusions.—Presence of laryngeal synkinesis using motor amplitude ratio criteria, in the setting of good voluntary motor unit recruitment and UVFI, downgrades a patient's prognosis to one that is poor for recovery. We propose this screening protocol as an adjunct to diagnostic LEMG (Fig 2).

▶ The use of electromyography (EMG) in the larynx has proven difficult. Laryngeal EMG findings in patients with vocal fold immobility appear to mean most in a negative predictive capacity. It is felt that synkinetic reinnervation confuses the

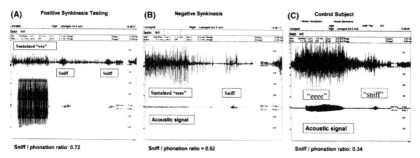

Sniff / phonation ratio: 0.72   Sniff / phonation ratio = 0.52   Sniff / phonation ratio: 0.34

FIGURE 2.—(A) Demonstrates LEMG tracing in patient with VF paralysis and large ratios of motor unit potential amplitude sniff/phonation during synkinesis testing. We delineate this as an example of a positive exam. (B) LEMG tracing in patient with VF immobility and ratio of MUP amplitude sniff/phonation during synkinesis testing similar to than noted for controls. We provide this as an example of negative synkinesis exam. (C) LEMG tracing in a control subject with a mobile VF. LEMG = laryngeal electromyography, VF = vocal fold. (Reprinted from Statham MM, Rosen CA, Smith LJ, et al. Electromyographic laryngeal synkinesis alters prognosis in vocal fold paralysis. *Laryngoscope*. 2010;120:285-290, with permission from The American Laryngological, Rhinological and Otological Society, Inc.)

EMG into predicting return of function (improved voice and motion) because of the presence of motor unit action potentials during vocalization tasks. This group found that when the ratio of the amplitude from the thyroarytenoid muscle/ lateral cricoarytenoid muscle complex during phonation and during a sniff was higher than 0.65, then this represented synkinesis. Recognizing the synkinesis improved the negative predictive value of the laryngeal EMG from 53% to 100% and the sensitivity from 56% to 100%.

R. A. Franco, Jr, MD

Gore-Tex medialization laryngoplasty for treatment of dysphagia
Hendricker RM, deSilva BW, Forrest LA (The Ohio State Univ, Columbus)
Otolaryngol Head Neck Surg 142:536-539, 2010

Objective.—Gore-Tex medialization laryngoplasty is a well described procedure for the management of glottal incompetence with associated phonatory disturbance. Limited literature exists describing the use of this procedure in the management of dysphagia. We describe our experience with Gore-Tex medialization laryngoplasty and the treatment of dysphagia.

Study Design.—Case series with chart review.

Setting.—Tertiary referral center.

Subjects and Methods.—Between April 2000 and September 2008, 189 Gore-Tex medialization laryngoplasties were performed on 180 patients by the senior author. Complete records and analysis were available for and performed on 121 procedures for 113 patients. The main outcome measures were discontinuation of gastrostomy tube (g-tube) use or avoidance of g-tube, as well as clinical subjective improvement in swallowing function.

Results.—Fifty-seven of 113 (50%) patients had complaints of dysphagia at presentation, with 47 of 57 (82%) having an objective swallowing evaluation. Thirty-two of 47 (68%) had documented penetration and/or aspiration. Twenty of 57 (35%) patients with dysphagia required g-tubes for alimentation. Eleven of 20 (55%) patients were able to discontinue g-tube use after Gore-Tex medialization laryngoplasty, and an additional five patients with aspiration were able to avoid need for g-tubes with Gore-Tex medialization laryngoplasty and swallowing therapy.

Conclusions.—Gore-Tex medialization laryngoplasty is a well tolerated and well described treatment for the management of glottal incompetence. The procedure is an appropriate adjunct in dysphagia management for the appropriate patient population.

▶ Swallowing is a physiologically complicated dynamic process that relies on precise timing and coordination to successfully and safely transfer an oral bolus into the esophagus without spilling any of it into the airway. Unilateral vocal fold mobility impairment can lead to dysphagia in certain cases. Surgical correction can lead to improvement in swallowing function in some patients. It must be stated that medialization laryngoplasty is considered to be a voice restorative procedure and not primarily a swallowing restorative procedure. Previous studies looking into the effects of type I medialization on aspiration as documented by videofluoroscopy revealed that as many as 25% to 40% of postprocedure medialization patients have evidence of aspiration. In this study, 32 of the 47 (68%) patients with preoperative dysphagia had evidence for penetration or aspiration. Twenty of the 57 patients with complaints of dysphagia (the 47 with testing and 10 more without testing but with symptoms) required g-tube feeding pre-op, with only 9 requiring g-tube feeding after surgery. We are not told how the milder dysphagia patients did post surgery. Although this improvement in the most severe swallowing-disordered patient group is very encouraging (from 20 down to 9 requiring g-tube feeding), the study did have some problems that do not allow us to make widespread claims about the efficacy of type I thyroplasty for the treatment of dysphagia. The study did not compare direct preoperative with postoperative videofluoroscopic examinations in the 57 patients with dysphagia, something important if we are to claim the surgery had anything to do with the improvement in symptoms. How do we know they are not still aspirating but just a small amount? The authors also do not reveal the clinical subjective improvement in swallowing function as data, so we do not know how many of the original 57 with preoperative dysphagia improved. Despite these deficiencies, the improvement in the g-tube–dependent subset should be seen as encouraging but not definitive.

R. A. Franco, Jr, MD

Histologic Study of Acute Vocal Fold Wound Healing After Corticosteroid Injection in a Rabbit Model
Campagnolo AM, Tsuji DH, Sennes LU, et al (Univ of São Paulo School of Medicine, Brazil)
Ann Otol Rhinol Laryngol 119:133-139, 2010

Objectives.—Injectable corticosteroids have been used in phonosurgery to prevent scarring of the vocal fold because of their effects on wound healing, and to ensure better voice quality. We histologically evaluated the effects of dexamethasone sodium phosphate infiltration on acute vocal fold wound healing in rabbits 3 and 7 days after surgically induced injury by quantification of the inflammatory reaction and collagen deposition.

Methods.—A standardized surgical incision was made in the vocal folds of 12 rabbits, and 0.1 mL dexamethasone sodium phosphate (4 mg/mL) was injected into the left vocal fold. The right vocal fold was not injected and served as the control. The larynges were collected 3 and 7 days after surgery. For histologic analysis, the vocal folds were stained with hematoxylin-eosin for quantification of the inflammatory response and with picrosirius red for quantification of collagen deposition.

Results.—There was no quantitative difference in the inflammatory response between vocal folds injected with the corticosteroid and control

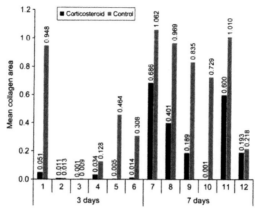

FIGURE 6.—Mean collagen area (square micrometers times 100) in control and corticosteroid-treatcd groups 3 and 7 days after injury. (Reprinted from Campagnolo AM, Tsuji DH, Sennes LU, et al. Histologic study of acute vocal fold wound healing after corticosteroid injection in a rabbit model. *Ann Otol Rhinol Laryngol.* 2010;119:133-139, with permission from Annals Publishing Company.)

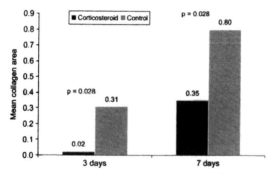

FIGURE 7.—Comparison between corticosteroid-treated and control groups in mean collagen area (square micrometers times 100) 3 and 7 days after injury. (Standard deviations were 0.02 for corticosteroid-treated group at 3 days 0.36 for control group at 3 days, 0.26 for corticosteroid-treated group at 7 days, and 0.31 for control group at 7 days.) (Reprinted from Campagnolo AM, Tsuji DH, Sennes LU, et al. Histologic study of acute vocal fold wound healing after corticosteroid injection in a rabbit model. *Ann Otol Rhinol Laryngol.* 2010;119:133-139, with permission from Annals Publishing Company.)

vocal folds. However, the rate of collagen deposition was significantly lower in the corticosteroid-treated group at 3 and 7 days after injury (p = 0.002).

Conclusions.—The present results suggest that dexamethasone reduces collagen deposition during acute vocal fold wound healing (Figs 6-8).

▶ Postsurgical scar formation along the medial surfaces of the vocal folds can cause disruption of mucosal wave propagation that leads to permanent hoarseness. Scar formation is a process that begins with an inflammatory response to injury and continues with collagen deposition and remodeling of the scar over

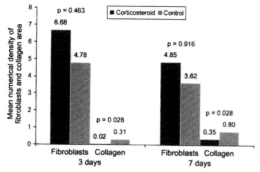

FIGURE 8.—Comparison between corticosteroid-treated and control vocal folds in number of fibroblasts and collagen area (square micrometers times 100) 3 and 7 days after injury. (Standard deviations for corticosteroid-treated group at 3 days were 5.2 for fibroblasts and 0.02 for collagen. Those for control group at 3 days were 3.34 for fibroblasts and 0.36 for collagen. Those for corticosteroid-treated group at 7 days were 3.97 for fibroblasts and 0.26 for collagen. Those for control group at 7 days were 2.49 for fibroblasts and 0.31 for collagen.) (Reprinted from Campagnolo AM, Tsuji DH, Sennes LU, et al. Histologic study of acute vocal fold wound healing after corticosteroid injection in a rabbit model. *Ann Otol Rhinol Laryngol.* 2010;119:133-139, with permission from Annals Publishing Company.)

the course of months. Given how difficult it is treating established vocal fold scar, the optimal time to intervene in the scarring process is at the start of the process. The authors found that local steroid injection into the vocal folds at the time of the phonomicrosurgical procedure led to a substantial decrease in the amount of collagen within the surgical site at day 3 and day 7 postprocedure (Figs 6-8). What is interesting is that despite the elevated number of fibroblasts in the wound at day 3 and day 7, there was a modulation in the collagen they produced leading to a decrease in the overall collagen output. Local steroid use is cheap and very feasible and may lead to further improvements in the surgical outcomes.

R. A. Franco, Jr, MD

Paced Glottic Closure for Controlling Aspiration Pneumonia in Patients With Neurologic Deficits of Various Causes

Broniatowski M, Moore NZ, Grundfest-Broniatowski S, et al (Case Western Reserve Univ School of Medicine, OH; Case Western Reserve Univ, OH; Cleveland Clinic Lerner College of Medicine at Case Western Reserve Univ, OH; et al)
Ann Otol Rhinol Laryngol 119:141-149, 2010

Objectives.—We undertook to determine whether paced vocal fold adduction can check aspiration in patients with various neurologic conditions.
Methods.—Five patients with fluoroscopically documented aspiration and repeated pneumonias were enrolled. Two previously reported patients with hemispheric stroke were compared to 3 additional subjects with brain

stem–basal ganglia and cerebellar stroke, cerebral palsy, and multiple sclerosis. A modified Vocare stimulator was implanted subcutaneously and linked to the ipsilateral recurrent laryngeal nerve via perineural electrodes. Vocal fold adduction and glottic closure were effected with pulse trains (42 Hz; 1.2 mA; 188 to 560 μs) and recorded with Enhanced Image J. Fluoroscopy results with and without stimulation were assessed by 2 independent blinded reviewers. Pneumonia rates were compared before, during, and after the 6- to 12-month enrollment periods.

Results.—There was statistically significant vocal fold adduction (p < 0.05) for all patients, further verified with bolus arrest (p < 0.05 for thin liquids, thick liquids, and puree depending on the speech-language pathologist). Pneumonia was prevented in 4 of the 5 patients during enrollment. In the fifth patient, who had brain stem–basal ganglia and cerebellar stroke, we were unable to completely seal the glottis and open the cricopharyngeus enough to handle his secretions.

Conclusions.—Vocal fold pacing for aspiration pneumonia from a variety of neurologic insults appears to be appropriate as long as the glottis can be sealed. It is not sufficient when the cricopharyngeus must be independently opened (Figs 1 and 2).

▶ Aspiration pneumonia is a serious medical condition that can afflict those patients who have difficulties creating a glottic seal during deglutition. It is important to remember that the clinical result of aspiration pneumonia is complex and dependent on many factors such as immune status, level of overall hydration and nutrition, degree of laryngeal sensation difficulties, level of consciousness, and inability to close the vocal folds. Many people tolerate

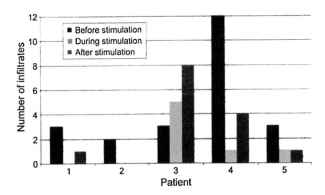

FIGURE 1.—Infiltrates and stimulation. Distribution of cumulated pulmonary infiltrates over time (see Table 3 for numbers). Average number of infiltrates was 4.6 before, 1.4 during, and 2.8 after stimulation for all patients. There was no infiltrate during stimulation in patients 1 and 2, and there was marked reduction in others except for patient 3. in whom infiltrates increased in number with time. Note high prestimulation number in patient 4. followed by sharp decline. Statistically significant differences were indicated by χ^2 test between prestimulation. stimulation, and poststimulation states (p = 0.001) when calculated for roughly equal observation times. (Reprinted from Broniatowski M, Moore NZ, Grundfest-Broniatowski S, et al. Paced glottic closure for controlling aspiration pneumonia in patients with neurologic deficits of various causes. *Ann Otol Rhinol Laryngol.* 2010;119:141-149, with permission from Annals Publishing Company.)

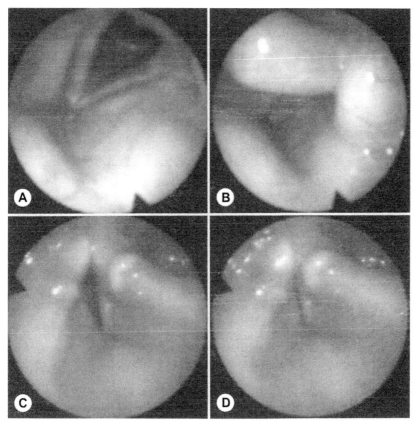

FIGURE 2.—A,B) Stimulation of right vocal fold resulted in tight glottic seal (B) in patient 5. C,D) In patient 3, stimulation of left vocal fold resulted in incomplete adduction (D) insufficient for tight glottic closure. Note poor abduction (C) in resting position in patient 3, who had cerebrovascular accident of brain stem, basal ganglia, and cerebellum. (Reprinted from Broniatowski M, Moore NZ, Grundfest-Broniatowski S, et al. Paced glottic closure for controlling aspiration pneumonia in patients with neurologic deficits of various causes. *Ann Otol Rhinol Laryngol.* 2010;119:141-149, with permission from Annals Publishing Company.)

a certain level of aspiration without manifesting pneumonia. Certainly, there does exist a line that is crossed in many people who have gross laryngeal incompetence leading to aspiration that overwhelms the ability to resist pneumonia. Although many physicians perform medialization laryngoplasty to reestablish gross laryngeal closure, this is a static procedure for a normally very dynamic organ. The procedure used in this study was the application of a paced electrical signal to the ipsilateral recurrent laryngeal nerve in 5 patients with severe dysphagia and recurrent aspiration pneumonias caused by multiple neurological insults (stroke, cerebral palsy, multiple sclerosis). All the patients were unable to ingest food prior to the study. The electrical stimulation caused forceful adduction, resulting in improved glottic closure in 4 of the 5 patients. There was a significant reduction in the number of pneumonias during and after the testing period in all but one subject who continued to have persistently incompetent glottic closure. This attempt to separate the airway from the alimentary tract during swallowing is a step in the direction of dynamic restoration of function that will hopefully have application for unilateral and bilateral vocal fold immobility for voice. As an overall plan to decrease aspiration pneumonia, it seems better to attack the motor system because it is much easier to effect a desired result (ie, movement of a vocal fold through electrical stimulation of the nerve) than the afferent sensory deficit many of these patients exhibit.

R. A. Franco, Jr, MD

Patients with Throat Symptoms on Acid Suppressive Therapy: Do They Have Reflux?
Khan A, Cho I, Traube M (New York Univ School of Medicine)
Dig Dis Sci 55:346-350, 2010

Purpose.—The aim of this study was to characterize the reflux events in patients with laryngeal symptoms unresponsive to proton pump inhibitor (PPI) therapy.

Background.—Gastroesophageal reflux disease (GERD) is commonly implicated as the cause of laryngeal symptoms.

Methods.—We retrospectively reviewed the pH/impedance records of 21 patients evaluated for persistent throat symptoms despite PPI therapy. They were compared to 30 others with typical reflux symptoms despite medication.

Results.—Five of 21 (24%) patients in the "throat group" had normal reflux values, 13 (62%) continued to have abnormal acid reflux, and three (14%) had abnormal nonacid reflux but normal acid reflux while on medication. These results did not differ from those with typical symptoms unresponsive to medication.

Conclusion.—In patients with chronic laryngeal symptoms despite PPI therapy, a substantial minority have no reflux at all, but the majority have abnormal amounts of acid reflux despite their taking PPI medication (Tables 1 and 2).

▶ Proton pump inhibitor (PPI) therapy is the accepted treatment for patients with the typical symptoms attributed to laryngopharyngeal reflux (LPR).

TABLE 1.—Mean Number of Reflux Events

	Throat ($n = 21$)	Typical ($n = 30$)	P-value
5 cm acid (normal <12)	15.2	15.8	0.93
5 cm nonacid (normal <44)	34.2	45.5	0.15
5 cm total (normal <48)	49.4	61.3	0.29
15 cm acid (normal <5)	9.5	11.2	0.78
15 cm nonacid (normal <18)	20.5	25.6	0.31
15 cm total (normal <19)	30.0	36.8	0.42

	5 CM Acid	5 CM Nonacid	5 CM Total	15 CM Acid	15 CM Nonacid	15 CM Total
	TABLE 2.—Number of Patients with Abnormal Reflux					
Throat ($n = 21$)	11 (52%)	6 (29%)	9 (43%)	13 (62%)	10 (48%)	13 (62%)
Typical ($n = 30$)	12 (40%)	15 (50%)	19 (63%)	16 (53%)	18 (60%)	20 (67%)

Despite the dissent regarding which examination signs, symptoms, and test findings define the presence of LPR, physicians make the diagnosis each day and struggle with those patients who return with persistent throat clearing, hoarseness, or globus despite PPI therapy. It is assumed that PPI treatment will reduce the acid production and alleviate the severity of the symptoms, but most patients with presumed LPR are not pH or impedance tested before PPI treatment and many are not even after failing a course of PPIs. This makes understanding what caused the failure impossible. In this study, patients who had persistent symptoms despite PPI treatment with throat symptoms were compared with those who had gastroesophageal reflux disease symptoms with the use of combined impedance and pH testing. One striking finding was that 24% of the throat group did not have evidence for reflux by gastroenterological standards despite symptoms most would attribute to LPR. It makes sense that these patients would not get better on PPI therapy. What makes less sense is that despite PPI treatment, many patients with persistent symptoms continue to have acid reflux. They also found that nonacid reflux is likely not a major contributor to symptoms in most subjects. What was most striking is that the pattern of reflux appears to be similar for the throat and typical groups, meaning that as of yet, discovered factors may be responsible for the differences between these groups. The authors mention the heightened sensation of reflux in those who are anxious compared with controls with the same objective amount of reflux. It is compelling evidence that we still have a lot of work to do before we understand LPR.

R. A. Franco, Jr, MD

Prevalence of penetration and aspiration on videofluoroscopy in normal individuals without dysphagia

Allen JE, White CJ, Leonard RJ, et al (Univ of California, Davis, Sacramento)
Otolaryngol Head Neck Surg 142:208-213, 2010

Objective.—To determine the prevalence of penetration and aspiration on videofluoroscopic swallow studies (VFSS) in normal individuals without dysphagia.

Study Design.—Case series with planned data collection.

Setting.—A tertiary urban university hospital.

Subjects and Methods.—Normal adult volunteers without dysphagia, neurological disease, or previous surgery underwent VFSS. Studies were recorded and then reviewed for evidence of penetration or aspiration.

The degree of penetration was assessed with the penetration-aspiration scale (PAS). The effect of age, bolus size, and consistency was evaluated.

Results.—A total of 149 VFSS (596 swallows) were reviewed. The mean age of the cohort was 57 years (± 19 years); 56 percent were female. Only one (0.6%) individual aspirated on VFSS. Seventeen (11.4%) individuals demonstrated penetration. The mean PAS for the entire cohort was 1.17 (± 0.66). Prevalence of penetration by swallow was 2.85 percent (17/596). Prevalence of penetration was 9.3 percent in elderly individuals aged >65 years and 14.3 percent in adults aged <65 years ($P = 0.49$). Prevalence of penetration on a liquid bolus was 3.4 percent (15/447) and on paste was 1.3 percent (2/149) ($P > 0.05$). Prevalence of penetration for a bolus <30 cc was 2.34 percent (7/298) and for a bolus >30 cc was 5.4 percent (8/149) ($P > 0.05$).

Conclusion.—Aspiration on VFSS is not a normal finding. Penetration is present in 11.4 percent of normal adults and is more common with a liquid bolus (Figs 1 and 2).

▶ Airway protection is the most important function of the larynx. It allows us to take an oral bolus of food and shuttle it safely into the esophagus, completely bypassing the airway on its way down. The presence of penetration, and certainly aspiration, would increase the risk of developing aspiration pneumonia, a potentially devastating pulmonary complication of altered laryngeal protection. But the lack of a history of pneumonia does not necessarily imply there is normal

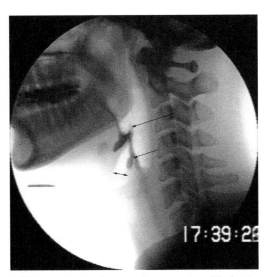

FIGURE 1.—Lateral fluoroscopic view demonstrating penetration while the airway is open (*doubled-ended arrow*), with arytenoid (*short arrow*) and epiglottis (*long arrow*) outlined by barium, which also fills the vallecula, and with bolus entering the airway. This finding would be graded at least 2 on the penetration-aspiration scale depending on patient response. (Reprinted from Allen JE, White CJ, Leonard RJ, et al. Prevalence of penetration and aspiration on videofluoroscopy in normal individuals without dysphagia. *Otolaryngol Head Neck Surg.* 2010;142:208-213, with permission from American Academy of Otolaryngology–Head and Neck Surgery Foundation.)

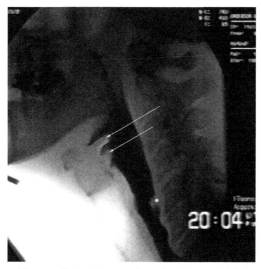

FIGURE 2.—Lateral fluoroscopic view demonstrating a closed airway with barium outlining the tip of the epiglottis (*long arrow*) and arytenoids (*short arrow*) but not entering the airway. Incidental non-obstructing cricopharyngeal bar is seen (*starburst*). (Reprinted from Allen JE, White CJ, Leonard RJ, et al. Prevalence of penetration and aspiration on videofluoroscopy in normal individuals without dysphagia. *Otolaryngol Head Neck Surg.* 2010;142:208-213, with permission from American Academy of Otolaryngology–Head and Neck Surgery Foundation.)

swallowing and no evidence of penetration or aspiration. The authors investigated the prevalence of penetration and aspiration in a normal population of individuals without a history of dysphagia. In this normal cohort, they found that 11% had evidence for penetration and less than 1% aspirated. Penetration itself is somewhat loosely defined and in many cases likely is an artifact of the impression of the epiglottis retroflexed onto the laryngeal vestibule with barium contrast on either side of the tip but not making its way into the laryngeal vestibule. It is likely we are overcalling the presence of penetration on these examinations. This study also makes it clear that the overwhelming majority of subjects do not have penetration or aspiration and that swallowing function can appear normal clinically even if there is evidence of aspiration/penetration.

R. A. Franco, Jr, MD

Scaffold-Free Tissue-Engineered Cartilage Implants for Laryngotracheal Reconstruction

Gilpin DA, Weidenbecher MS, Dennis JE (Case Western Reserve Univ, Cleveland, OH)

Laryngoscope 120:612-617, 2010

Objectives/Hypothesis.—Donor site morbidity, including pneumothorax, can be a considerable problem when harvesting cartilage grafts for laryngotracheal reconstruction (LTR). Tissue engineered cartilage may offer a solution to this problem. This study investigated the feasibility of using autologous chondrocytes to tissue-engineer scaffold-free cartilage grafts for LTR in rabbits to avoid degradation that often arises from an inflammatory reaction to scaffold carrier matrix.

Study Design.—Animal study.

Methods.—Auricular cartilage was harvested from seven New Zealand white rabbits, the chondrocytes expanded and loaded onto a custom-made bioreactor for 7 to 8 weeks to fabricate autologous scaffold-free cartilage sheets. The sheets were cut to size and used for LTR, and the rabbits were sacrificed 4, 8, and 12 weeks after the LTR and prepared for histology.

Results.—None of the seven rabbits showed signs of respiratory distress. A smooth, noninflammatory scar was visible intraluminally; the remainder of the tracheal lumen was unremarkable. Histologically, the grafts showed no signs of degradation or inflammatory reaction, were covered with mucosal epithelium, but did show signs of mechanical failure at the implantation site.

Conclusions.—These results show that autologous chondrocytes can be used to fabricate an implantable sheet of cartilage that retains a cartilage phenotype, becomes integrated, and does not produce a significant inflammatory reaction. These findings suggest that with the design of stronger implants, these implants can be successfully used as a graft for LTR (Fig 5).

▶ Laryngotracheal reconstruction with cartilage augmentation is a standard procedure performed to treat mild airway stenosis in the area of the subglottis and upper trachea. It involves incising the cricoid and upper trachea and inserting a cartilaginous graft that is wedged between the cut edges to focally expand the airway at the site of stenosis. Because the graft needs to be sturdy enough

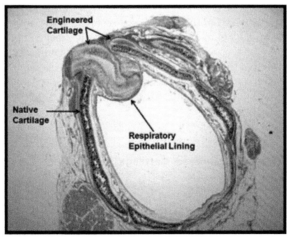

FIGURE 5.—Histologic section of laryngotracheal reconstruction (LTR) with implanted graft at level of the trachea (safranin-O/Fast Green stain). Viable engineered cartilage noted within the LTR defect with a layer of respiratory epithelium. (Reprinted from Gilpin DA, Weidenbecher MS, Dennis JE. Scaffold-free tissue-engineered cartilage implants for laryngotracheal reconstruction. *Laryngoscope.* 2010;120:612-617, with permission from The American Laryngological, Rhinological and Otological Society, Inc.)

to withstand the forces springing the cut edges back together, it is typically harvested from the ribcage and fashioned into the final graft after placing it into the wound and sculpting it to fit. Through the use of tissue engineering, it should be possible to harvest the patient's own chondrocytes and grow cartilage that can be grafted back in to treat the stenosis. This would obviate the need to harvest a piece of rib and avoids the possible complications of thoracic infection and pneumothorax. The authors created a scaffold-free cartilage implant that was used to successfully expand the airway in rabbits, without the need for immunosuppressive drugs. Because these grafts were relatively thin, there was some buckling and even some migration of the grafts, but all the procedures were successful in augmenting the airway in an average of 17%. It is envisioned that in the near future, custom tissue engineering of cartilage will make it possible to use 100% biocompatible tissue and avoid the need to harvest grafts.

R. A. Franco, Jr, MD

The Prevalence of Laryngeal Pathology in a Treatment-Seeking Population With Dysphonia
Van Houtte E, Van Lierde K, D'Haeseleer E, et al (Univ Hosp Ghent, Belgium)
Laryngoscope 120:306-312, 2010

Objectives/Hypothesis.—This article describes the prevalence of laryngeal pathology in a treatment-seeking population with dysphonia in the Flemish part of Belgium.

Study Design.—Retrospective investigation.

Methods.—During a period of 5 years (2004–2008), data were collected from 882 patients who consulted with dysphonia at the ear, nose, and throat department of the University Hospital in Ghent (Belgium). Laryngeal pathology was diagnosed using videostroboscopy. Ages ranged from 4 years to 90 years.

Results.—Functional voice disorders were most frequently diagnosed (30%), followed by vocal fold nodule (15%), and pharyngolaryngeal reflux (9%). The role of age, gender, and occupation was investigated. Pathologies were significantly more common in females than in males, representing 63.8% and 36.2% of the population, respectively. Professional voice users accounted for 41% of the workforce population, with teachers as main subgroup. In professional voice users, functional dysphonia occurred in 41%, vocal fold nodules in 15%, and pharyngolaryngeal reflux in 11%. Our data were compared with data from other countries.

Conclusions.—Functional voice disorders were overall the most common cause of voice disorders (except in childhood), followed by vocal fold nodules and pharyngolaryngeal reflux. Professional voice users accounted for almost one half of the active population, with functional voice disorders as the main cause of dysphonia.

▶ The voice has taken on a supreme role in our modern communications-based society. Professional voice users, such as physicians, lawyers, teachers, business executives, etc, require the use of their voices to effectively execute their professional duties. These professionals are also disproportionately impacted by disorders of the voice. It is important for the medical professionals who treat these disorders to understand the prevalence of the different laryngeal pathologies they may encounter to properly diagnose and counsel their patients. In this study, 882 patients were evaluated over 4 years. They were found to have functional disorders 30% of the time with vocal nodules accounting for 15% of diagnoses and 9% of laryngopharyngeal reflux. It is interesting to look at the distinct subpopulations within the 882 subjects. In children, vocal nodules were overwhelmingly responsible for the dysphonia (63%). Professional voice users comprised 41% of the subjects. In these patients, functional disorders accounted for 41% of the diagnoses, followed by nodules in 15% and reflux in 11%. It is interesting that the functional diagnosis jumped from 30% to 41% in the professional voice users, with nodules and reflux remaining stable. The study found that more women seek treatment than men, a fact that has been verified by many other studies and one that likely represents the differences in men and women more than in the rates of laryngeal pathology.

R. A. Franco, Jr, MD

Vocal cord dysfunction: Beyond severe asthma
Parsons JP, Benninger C, Hawley MP, et al (The Ohio State Univ Med Ctr, Columbus; et al)
Respir Med 104:504-509, 2010

Background.—Vocal cord dysfunction (VCD) is the abnormal adduction of the vocal cords during inspiration causing extrathoracic airway obstruction. VCD has been described as a confounder of severe asthma. The influence of VCD among less severe asthmatics has not been previously defined.

Methods.—We retrospectively reviewed the medical records of 59 patients with pulmonologist-diagnosed asthma who were referred for videolaryngostroboscopy (VLS) testing from 2006 to 2007.

Results.—A total of 44 patients had both asthma and VCD. 15 patients had asthma without concomitant VCD. Females were predominant in both groups. Overall, the majority of patients referred for VLS testing had mild-to-moderate asthma (78%) and 72% of these patients had VCD. Few patients from either group had "classic" VCD symptoms of stridor or hoarseness. Gastroesophageal reflux disease (GERD) and rhinitis were common in both groups.

Conclusions.—Vocal cord dysfunction occurs across the spectrum of asthma severity. There was a lack of previously described "classic" VCD symptoms among asthmatics. Symptoms were diverse and not easily distinguished from common symptoms of asthma, highlighting the need for a high index of suspicion for VCD in patients with asthma. Failure to consider and diagnose VCD may result in misleading assumptions about asthma control, and result in unnecessary adjustments of asthma

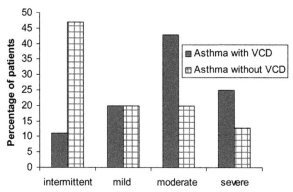

FIGURE 1.—Distribution of patients in each group stratified by asthma severity. (Reprinted from Parsons JP, Benninger C, Hawley MP, et al. Vocal cord dysfunction: beyond severe asthma. *Respir Med.* 2010;104,504-509, with permission from Elsevier Ltd.)

medications. The high prevalence of GERD raises the question of the role of acid reflux in the pathogenesis of VCD in asthmatics (Fig 1).

▶ Vocal cord dysfunction, or VCD, is a paradoxical motion of the vocal folds (adduction on inspiration) that can lead to symptoms of difficulty in breathing with mild stridor and hoarseness. In patients with a preexisting diagnosis of asthma, the changes in the respiratory symptoms may be improperly ascribed to poor asthma control instead of VCD (Fig 1). VCD does not improve with the addition of more asthma medications, further confusing the practitioner who is not aware of this clinical entity. The authors found that a large percentage of the patients with VCD had clinically evident signs of untreated laryngopharyngeal reflux (LPR). There has been the suggestion that it is the irritation from the LPR that leads to the abnormal adduction during inspiration, and many practitioners call for the aggressive treatment of LPR with proton pump inhibitors when there is the suggestion of VCD and there are exam findings of reflux. It is not unusual to perform a videoendoscopic examination and not see evidence of paradoxical vocal fold motion because the abnormal motion is transient and paroxysmal. Examinations may need to be coupled to riding a stationary bicycle, running on a treadmill, or exposure to noxious smells in order to elicit VCD.

R. A. Franco, Jr, MD

General

Laryngeal sensory testing in the assessment of patients with laryngopharyngeal reflux
Dale OT, Alhamarneh O, Young K, et al (Derbyshire Royal Infirmary, Derby, UK)
J Laryngol Otol 124:330-332, 2010

Laryngopharyngeal reflux is commonly encountered in the ENT outpatient setting. It leads to impaired sensory capacity of the laryngeal mucosa. The sensory integrity of the laryngopharynx can be evaluated through endoscopic administration of pulsed air, which stimulates the laryngeal adductor reflex. The pressure of air needed to elicit this reflex indicates the degree of sensory impairment. Such laryngeal sensory testing gives a quantifiable means of assessment in patients with laryngopharyngeal reflux, and can be used to measure the response to treatment. Laryngeal sensory testing is safe and well tolerated by patients.

▶ There are few subjects in the ear, nose, and throat setting more contentious than laryngopharyngeal reflux (LPR). The controversy is fueled by the lack of an objective test that has sufficient sensitivity and reliability to diagnose LPR and the lack of consensus of how best to treat those patients who are symptomatic. Inclusion of patients who are symptomatic but do not have LPR in double-blinded randomized treatment protocols has confounded the data, leading to inconclusive results. Some have advocated using laryngeal sensory testing as a tool to diagnose LPR. In this study, the authors used small calibrated puffs of air to find the threshold for the laryngeal adductor reflex. From previous studies, we understand that LPR seems to alter the laryngeal sensation, making the subjects more insensate. The authors were able to stratify patients into 3 groups based on their responses to the laryngeal sensation testing. These authors did not correlate the reflux finding score, dual pH probe findings, or the reflux symptom index scores with the sensory testing findings to see if they correlated. The next logical step would be to find out how many of those who were considered positive for LPR improved with treatment. It may be that there is, in fact, not one single best test to diagnose LPR, but it requires a combination of results that are interrelated to come to the proper diagnosis of LPR.

R. A. Franco, Jr, MD

Rational Diagnostic and Therapeutic Management of Deep Neck Infections: Analysis of 233 Consecutive Cases
Marioni G, Staffieri A, Parisi S, et al (Univ of Padova, Italy; et al)
Ann Otol Rhinol Laryngol 119:181-187, 2010

Objectives.—Although deep neck infections are less common nowadays because of the widespread use of antibiotics, they continue to carry significant morbidity and mortality rates.

Methods.—Between 2000 and 2008, deep neck infections were treated in 233 patients at the University of Padova. Cases of peritonsillar abscess, superficial infections, infections due to external neck injuries, and infections in head and neck tumors were excluded. Clinical, radiologic, laboratory, and microbiological assessments were analyzed.

Results.—The site of origin was identified in 189 of the 233 cases (81.1%), and the most common cause of deep neck infection was dental infection (39.5%). Intravenous antibiotic therapy was given to 78 patients, and 155 required both medical and surgical procedures. The bacteria most often isolated were gram-positive anaerobic cocci. None of our patients died of the deep neck infection or its complications.

Conclusions.—It is worth emphasizing that airway support is the priority in patients with deep neck infections. Empirical antibiotic treatments must cover gram-positive and gram-negative aerobic and anaerobic pathogens. Surgical exploration and drainage may be mandatory in selected cases at presentation or in cases that fail to respond to parenteral antibiotics within the first 24 to 48 hours. It is important to perform cultures during operation to establish the pathogen(s) involved and to obtain an antibiogram to tailor the antibiotic treatment.

▶ Deep neck infections require efficient diagnosis and treatment to prevent serious sequelae such as airway obstruction, mediastinitis, pericarditis, or major vessel erosion that may lead to massive hemorrhage. The mainstay of diagnosis is the direct examination with contrast-enhanced CT scanning to visualize the extent of the problem. In 40% of cases, the origin was odontogenic, followed by the tonsillar region (16%) and the salivary glands (14%). Medical treatment with intravenous antibiotics was sufficient to treat 33% of patients, while the remaining two-thirds required surgical exploration and drainage. The bacterial cultures revealed gram-positive cocci, followed by *Streptococcus viridans* and *Staphylococcus epidermidis* and various others in lesser numbers. They were able to safely treat all 233 patients without any deaths from the deep neck infections, although there were sequelae such as skin fistulization and mediastinitis that resolved. Patients need to continue antibiotic therapy after discharge to completely eradicate the risk of recurrence. It is important to note that clinical suspicion trumps the radiological findings in that nearly 20% of patients had no identifiable source for their deep neck infection. Clinical examination also underestimates the extent of disease in many cases.

R. A. Franco, Jr, MD

Supraglottic Swelling May Not Correlate With Tongue Swelling in Angiotensin Converting Enzyme Inhibitor-Induced Angioedema
Saxena S, Gierl B, Eibling DE (Univ of Pittsburgh School of Medicine and VA Pittsburgh Health Care System, PA)
Laryngoscope 120:62-64, 2010

Angioneurotic edema of upper airway tissues due to angiotensin converting enzyme inhibitor (ACEI) usage is a known perioperative complication of this class of medications. Swelling can begin rapidly, and typically involves the tongue and oral cavity. We have recently encountered four cases in which supraglottic edema developed after onset of tongue swelling and progressed despite resolving tongue edema. We present a representative case. This observation suggests that all patients with ACEI-induced angioedema should undergo laryngeal fiberoptic examination and appropriate airway management (Fig 1).

▶ Angioedema of the airway can be a life-threatening condition if not properly recognized and treated. Airway angioedema has been described after intubation

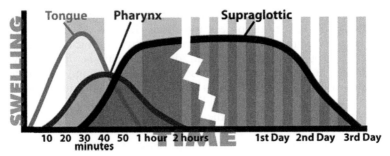

FIGURE 1.—Diagrammatic depiction of time course of asynchronous swelling of tongue, pharyngeal walls, and supraglottis in a representative patient with angiotensin converting enzyme inhibitor (ACEI)-induced angioedema. In this patient, tongue and pharyngeal swelling improved over 1 to 2 hours; however, the supraglottic swelling started worsening at around the same time and only resolved by the 3rd postoperative day. (Reprinted from Saxena S, Gierl B, Eibling DE. Supraglottic swelling may not correlate with tongue swelling in angiotensin converting enzyme inhibitor-induced angioedema. *Laryngoscope*. 2010;120:62-64, with permission from The American Laryngological, Rhinological and Otological Society, Inc.)

in patients who take angiotensin-converting enzyme (ACE) inhibitors for treatment of hypertension, likely secondary to higher levels of bradykinin, a protein that is usually inactivated by ACE. When there is evidence for tongue edema, the patient should have an endoscopic evaluation of the airway to look for supraglottic edema. The laryngeal edema can continue to worsen despite a substantial decrease in the tongue edema to the steroids and antihistamines (Fig 1). Early, elective fiberoptic-assisted orotracheal intubation may be necessary to avoid the potential for a surgical airway. The patient is extubated when the clinical parameters are met with a sufficient air leak and a favorable fiberoptic examination of the supraglottis.

R. A. Franco, Jr, MD

Surgical Technique

'Steam-boat' supraglottic laryngoplasty for treatment of chronic refractory aspiration: a modification of Biller's technique
Ku PKM, Abdullah VJ, Vlantis AC, et al (Chinese Univ of Hong Kong, Shatin, New Territories)
J Laryngol Otol 123:1360-1363, 2009

Objective.—The surgical treatment of intractable aspiration usually requires sacrifice of the patient's natural voice to prevent food entering the airway. Biller described a tubed supraglottic laryngoplasty to control aspiration while allowing patients to phonate with their larynx. Our preliminary experience with this technique in Chinese patients has been disappointing, as tension in the mucosa on wound closure led to wound dehiscence. Our objective was to modify Biller's technique in order to achieve a better outcome.

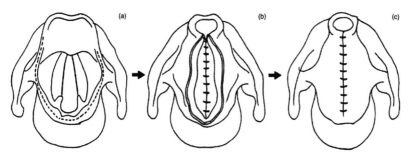

FIGURE 1.—The original technique of supraglottic laryngoplasty described by Biller. (a) The mucosa of the epiglottis, aryepiglottic folds and arytenoids is undermined after making the mucosal incision. (b & c) The supraglottis is rolled and tubed and secured by a two-layer closure using absorbable sutures, leaving an opening at its tip. (Reprinted from Ku PKM, Abdullah VJ, Vlantis AC, et al. 'Steam-boat' supraglottic laryngoplasty for treatment of chronic refractory aspiration: a modification of Biller's technique. *J Laryngol Otol.* 2009;123:1360-1363, with permission of Cambridge University Press.)

Method.—We modified Biller's technique by trimming the epiglottic cartilage and by inserting a tibial periosteal graft to reinforce closure of the mucosa, creating an arrangement resembling a Chinese steam boat.

Results.—Three Chinese patients underwent the modified Biller's technique. No wound dehiscence occurred, the surgery controlled aspiration, and the patients were able to phonate with their own larynx. All patients resumed oral feeding, and previously placed gastrostomy tubes were removed.

Conclusion.—The 'steam-boat' supraglottic laryngoplasty is a viable surgical alternative to total laryngectomy or tracheal diversion for controlling intractable aspiration, and preserves a phonating larynx (Fig 1).

▶ Intractable aspiration is a deadly condition leading to recurrent aspiration pneumonias, progressive scarring of the lungs, and eventual death. Treatments devised to treat this condition have surgically separated the airway from the alimentary tract, effectively sacrificing the ability to phonate for the safety of an airway that will not allow the passage of food/drink. Hugh Biller and Bill Lawson devised a procedure that would tubularize the supraglottic structures (Fig 1) to afford more airway protection while leaving an opening for the patient to breathe and phonate. When others attempted to replicate Biller and Lawson's results, they found a high degree of dehiscence of the supraglottic flaps. The authors of this article reinforced the reconstruction with a tibial periosteal flap and removed a strip of the lateral epiglottis to decrease the tension on the reconstruction with good initial results in the 3 subjects. The advantages to the patient are obvious when one considers the alternatives that are readily available today consist of total laryngectomy or a laryngeal diversion procedure that separates the airway from the alimentary tract, both of which make natural phonation impossible and require the patient to live with a stoma.

R. A. Franco, Jr, MD

A New Thread Guide Instrument for Endoscopic Arytenoid Lateropexy

Rovó L, Madani S, Sztanó B, et al (Univ of Szeged, Hungary)
Laryngoscope 120:2002-2007, 2010

Objectives/Hypothesis.—The varied etiology of bilateral vocal cord immobility (BVCI) requires a wide range of surgical approaches. A new endolaryngeal thread guide instrument (ETGI) is presented here for a minimally invasive endoscopic lateropexy of the arytenoid cartilage, which might serve as a basis for a simple solution for the main types of BVCI.

Study Design.—Prospective study of BVCI patients who underwent surgery, including 22 bilateral vocal cord paralyses (BVCP), 12 mechanical fixations (MF), 10 posterior glottic stenoses, and two rheumatoid ankyloses.

Methods.—The ETGI is based on a built-in movable curved blade with a hole at its tip to guide a thread in and out again between the skin and the laryngeal cavity. The loops formed around the arytenoid cartilage cause abduction. In cases of fixations, the cricoarytenoid joints were properly mobilized as a first step with a combination of cold technique and CO_2 laser.

Results.—As spirometric tests proved, 32 patients achieved improved breathing ability. One temporary tracheostomy was necessary and one patient with ongoing radiotherapy could not be decannulated. Subjectively, twelve patients' voices improved or approximated normal quality due to complete vocal cord recoveries on at least one side after lateropexy was ceased. Incomplete recovery with more or less impaired voice was observed in 16 cases. Three MF patients and two BVCP patients with poor overall health condition had severe dysphonia.

Conclusions.—Combined with simple and readily available methods, endoscopic arytenoid lateropexy is an effective solution for BVCIs with various etiologies. The ETGI facilitates this procedure with rapid and safe creation of fixating loops at the proper position.

▶ Bilateral vocal cord immobility, in many cases, causes dyspnea and stridor that require surgical treatment to correct. Although tracheotomy does establish an excellent airway, the cosmetic deformity and the added care it comes with deter many patients from choosing this as a viable long-term option. Endoscopic treatments are preferable, and those that are nondestructive are even better. These authors describe a new instrument that endoscopically passes a needle through the arytenoid and thyroid cartilage where a suture is threaded through the hole at the tip of the needle. This is withdrawn back into the lumen of the airway, and the needle is passed back through the arytenoid to be tied on the outside of the thyroid cartilage. This effectively lateralizes the arytenoid, increasing the cross-sectional area at the glottis (Figs 1-4 in the original article). The patients treated with this technique saw improved peak inspiratory flows of 62% in the first day and close to double the preoperative values a year later, placing objective data to what the patients subjectively claimed was improved easier breathing. The fact that this is a nondestructive procedure (not a CO_2 laser partial arytenoidectomy) that can be performed quickly and it passes 2 sutures at once to provide better security makes it extremely appealing and useful.

R. A. Franco, Jr, MD

Airway Injury During Emergency Transcutaneous Airway Access: A Comparison at Cricothyroid and Tracheal Sites

Salah N, El Saigh I, Hayes N, et al (Rotunda Hosp, Dublin, Ireland)
Anesth Analg 109:1901-1907, 2009

Background.—Oxygenation via the cricothyroid membrane (CTM) may be required in emergencies, but inadvertent tracheal cannulation may occur. In this study, we compared airway injury between the tracheal and CTM sites using different techniques for airway access.

Methods.—Anesthesiologists performed 4 airway access techniques on excised porcine tracheas. The techniques were 1) wire-guided (WGT), 2) trocar (TT), 3) needle cannula (NCT), and 4) surgical—scalpel with endotracheal tube (ST). Participants performed each technique at both the CTM and tracheal sites. Specimens were assessed for injury.

Results.—Injury was observed in 8 of 40 and 27 of 40 specimens at the CTM and tracheal sites, respectively ($P < 0.001$). Injury was more frequent at the tracheal site compared with the CTM in both the TT and ST groups ($P = 0.02$) but not for the NCT and WGT. The rank order for any injury at the tracheal site was ST (9 of 10) = TT (9 of 10) > WGT (6 of 10) > NCT (3 of 10) ($P = 0.02$, highest versus lowest), whereas there was no difference in injury at the CTM. The rank order for posterior injury at the tracheal site was TT (9 of 10) = ST (9 of 10) > WGT (5 of 10) > NCT (2 of 10) ($P = 0.005$, highest versus lowest). The rank order for penetrating injury at the tracheal site was ST (6 of 10) = TT (6 of 10) > WGT (2 of 10) > NCT (1 of 10) ($P = 0.057$, highest versus lowest). There was no difference in the incidence of lateral, superficial, or perforating injuries among sites and techniques. Fractures were more common at the tracheal site (15 of 40 vs 0 of 40, $P < 0.001$) and differed by technique. The rank order of fracture incidence at the tracheal site was ST (6 of 10) > WGT (5 of 10) > TT (4 of 10) > NCT (0 of 10) ($P = 0.011$, highest to lowest). Compression of >50% was seen in 10 of 40 vs 28 of 40 ($P < 0.001$) specimens at the CTM and tracheal sites, respectively. The rank order of compression of >50% of airway lumen for both sites was TT > ST > WGT > NCT ($P = 0.03$, $P < 0.001$, CTM and tracheal sites, respectively, highest versus lowest).

Conclusion.—Airway injury and luminal compression were more common at the tracheal site than at the CTM. The ST and TT were associated with the highest incidence of injury. This has implications for emergency airway access in cases in which it may be difficult to accurately identify the CTM.

▶ In the emergency protocol (ABC), obtaining and maintaining the airway stands as the first order of business. In the emergency setting, establishing an airway via the cricothyroid membrane is seen as a more reliable and quicker method than a surgical tracheotomy. The subjects in this study were anesthesia trainees (with previous cricothyroidotomy training using a simulation mannequin) who were asked to establish an emergency airway on excised porcine larynges and tracheas. The techniques used were wire guided, trocar, needle cannula, and a traditional surgical method with a scalpel. They found posterior tracheal injuries with all techniques but more with the scalpel and trocar than with the needle or wire-guided methods. They also found more injuries associated with attempts at tracheal insertion than cricothyroid membrane insertion. According to this study, there is a much higher risk of collateral damage when performing tracheal cannulation.

A key point that should not be overlooked is that cricothyroidotomy, regardless of technique, is meant to be an emergency procedure that is temporary. It is not a substitute for tracheotomy. An artificial airway should never be left in the cricothyroid space for days because of the very devastating and lingering effects of the resultant subglottic stenosis that can leave the patient tracheostomy tube dependent. When a cricothyroidotomy is performed, either it must be converted to a tracheotomy or the patient should be intubated, as soon as possible, to avoid the long-term sequelae from cricothyroidotomy.

R. A. Franco, Jr, MD

Awake Upper Airway Surgery
Macchiarini P, Rovira I, Ferrarello S (Univ of Barcelona, Spain; Azienda Ospedaliera Careggi, Firenze, Italy)
Ann Thorac Surg 89:387-391, 2010

Background.—The need to compromise between surgical and anesthetic access in airway surgery is an important clinical problem. We wanted to determine the feasibility of performing upper airway surgery under awake anesthesia and spontaneous respiration.

Methods.—This was a prospective, clinical feasibility study. Patients with upper tracheal stenosis were managed through cervical epidural anesthesia and conscious sedation, and atomized local anesthetic. No intraoperative intubation or jet ventilation was required. Outcome measures were ease of surgery, observer-rated functional result, early (less than 30 days) complications, and patient-reported satisfaction.

Results.—Twenty consecutive patients with idiopathic (n = 4) or postintubation (n = 16) complete (n = 3) or severe (>80%, n = 17) subglottic (n = 12) or upper trachea (n = 8) stenosis were enrolled. Operations included 12 subglottic and 8 segmental resections with primary anastomosis. Permissive hypercapnia was well tolerated. Median length of resection was 4.5 cm (range, 2 to 6 cm), and 12 releases (8 thyrohyoid, 4 suprahyoid) were required. One patient required a nasotracheal tube for 36 hours. All but 1 were able to cough and talk immediately, and to swallow fluids and solids, and were fully mobilized at 6 hours. There were no early complications. Median hospitalization was 3.1 days (range, 2 to 15). Patients had excellent (n = 16) or good (n = 4) functional (n = 20) outcomes, with no early relapse of stenosis. Median self-reported satisfaction at median 12 months was 9.5 ± 1.0 (scale, 0 to 10). All patients indicated that they would be happy to repeat the procedure.

Conclusions.—Awake and tubeless upper airway surgery is feasible and safe, and has a high level of patient satisfaction. If supported by random-ized controlled trial, this method will change the way airway stenosis surgery is approached by both surgeons and anesthesiologist.

▶ There has been a growing trend toward moving procedures from the oper-ating room into the awake outpatient setting. There has also been a realization that not all surgical procedures require the use of general anesthetics. There are many otolaryngological procedures that are performed with the use of local anesthesia such as local awake tracheotomy, tonsillectomy, laryngeal frame-work surgery, mastoidectomy, and thyroidectomy. Historically, airway recon-struction has not been performed under local.

In this case series, 20 patients underwent subglottic (12) and segmental (8) resection with primary anastomosis while awake through the administration of ropivacaine via a cervical epidural block. There were no major complications, and follow-up evaluations revealed that all 20 patients would choose to undergo surgery in the awake fashion rather than with the administration of general anesthesia.

R. A. Franco, Jr, MD

Effects of type II thyroplasty on adductor spasmodic dysphonia
Sanuki T, Yumoto E, Minoda R, et al (Kumamoto Univ, Japan)
Otolaryngol Head Neck Surg 142:540-546, 2010

Objectives.—Type II thyroplasty, or laryngeal framework surgery, is based on the hypothesis that the effect of adductor spasmodic dysphonia (AdSD) on the voice is due to excessively tight closure of the glottis, hampering phonation. Most of the previous, partially effective treatments have aimed to relieve this tight closure, including recurrent laryngeal nerve section or avulsion, extirpation of the adductor muscle, and botulinum toxin injection, which is currently the most popular. The aim of this study was to assess the effects of type II thyroplasty on aerodynamic and acoustic findings in patients with AdSD.

Study Design.—Case series.

Setting.—University hospital.

Subjects and Methods.—Ten patients with AdSD underwent type II thyroplasty between August 2006 and December 2008. Aerodynamic and acoustic analyses were performed prior to and six months after surgery. Mean flow rates (MFRs) and voice efficiency were evaluated with a phonation analyzer. Jitter, shimmer, the harmonics-to-noise ratio (HNR), standard deviation of the fundamental frequency (SDF0), and degree of voice breaks (DVB) were measured from each subject's longest sustained phonation sample of the vowel /a/.

Results.—Voice efficiency improved significantly after surgery. No significant difference was found in the MFRs between before and after surgery. Jitter, shimmer, HNR, SDF0, and DVB improved significantly after surgery.

Conclusions.—Treatment of AdSD with type II thyroplasty significantly improved aerodynamic and acoustic findings. The results of this study suggest that type II thyroplasty provides relief from voice strangulation in patients with AdSD.

▶ Adductor spasmodic dysphonia (SD) is a rare neurological disorder that results in the transmission of excessive neural signals to the laryngeal adductors that can be heard as a strangled or strained voice. The current standard treatment is repeated botulinum toxin injection into the thyroarytenoid muscle every 3 to 4 months. Although it can restore normal function, Botox treatment usually leaves the patient hypophonic for several days to weeks until the full strength returns to the voice (without spasms) anywhere from 6 to 12 weeks. There are patients who are not accepting the roller-coaster function offered by Botox and wish for a surgical solution that may offer them a long-term solution. Type II thyroplasty is a procedure where the larynx is opened vertically in the midline (midline thyrotomy) and the 2 halves of the thyroid cartilage are distracted laterally. This is performed with the patient awake to gauge the amount of distraction that is necessary to eliminate the spasms and still produce a relatively strong voice. The authors present data that show that in the short term, type II thyroplasty is effective. Long-term studies are necessary because of the reports that the SD symptoms return in some patients. The feeling is that Botox works effectively because its roller-coaster effects are always changing the dynamics of the afferent-efferent system, constantly making the brain guess what is happening, and giving patients with SD periods of normal voice. When the larynx is at a steady state, even after sacrifice of a recurrent laryngeal nerve, the spasms can return. Although type II thyroplasty does not alter the laryngeal innervation, it may suffer a similar fate to the other static procedures with delayed return of spasms.

R. A. Franco, Jr, MD

Endoscopic Airway Management of Laryngeal Sarcoidosis
Butler CR, Nouraei SAR, Mace AD, et al (Charing Cross Hosp, London, England)
Arch Otolaryngol Head Neck Surg 136:251-255, 2010

Objective.—To report the results of treating laryngeal sarcoidosis with intralesional steroids and minimally invasive laser surgery. Sarcoidosis is a rare multisystem inflammatory disorder of unknown cause. Laryngeal involvement is extremely rare, and its optimal management remains controversial.

Design.—Retrospective medical chart review.

Settings.—Tertiary care center/national referral airway reconstruction center.

Patients.—Ten consecutive patients treated for laryngeal sarcoidosis between 2004 and 2008.

Main Outcome Measures.—Demographic and clinical information including extralaryngeal manifestations obtained from patient records, laryngeal anatomic subsite manifestation of disease, intraoperative findings, and scores from the Medical Research Council (MRC) dyspnea outcome assessment instrument (which was administered preoperatively, at the first postoperative outpatient visit 4-6 weeks later, and at last follow-up).

Results.—The patients included 9 women and 1 man, a total of 2.8% of the unit's adult surgical airway case mix (10 of 353). Mean (SD) age at presentation was 37 (17) years. All patients presented with dyspnea and dysphonia; 2 required emergency tracheostomy prior to treatment. Six patients presented with isolated laryngeal sarcoid. Supraglottis and arytenoids were affected in all patients. The median number of endoscopic treatments was 2 (range, 1-4). Significant improvement in MRC dyspnea grading was found postoperatively ($P < .05$), and patients with tracheostomy were successfully decannulated. The mean (SD) follow-up time was 24 (18) months. There were no adverse effects of surgery. Nine patients had a substantial dose reduction or discontinuation of their systemic corticosteroid therapy following endoscopic treatment.

Conclusions.—Minimally invasive endoscopic surgery with intralesional corticosteroid injection and laser reduction is an effective method of controlling laryngeal sarcoid. It improves symptoms immediately with minimal morbidity and, most importantly, reduces the need for systemic steroid administration in most patients. This study supports early recognition and endoscopic intervention in the management of laryngeal sarcoidosis.

▶ Sarcoidosis is a rare entity encountered by otolaryngologists, typically in young African American females. It is mainly a pulmonary disorder with occasional laryngeal manifestations that are difficult to manage because of progressive laryngeal (supraglottic) stenosis. Although systemic steroids are the accepted treatment for this idiopathic inflammatory disorder when large organ systems are involved, the chronic use of steroids is not without the real dangers of adrenal suppression. Although there are systemic alternatives to steroids, these in turn have side-effect profiles that are also not ideal. The managing otolaryngologist must find a suitable alternative that can include suspension laryngoscopy and the local infiltration of steroids with carbon dioxide laser cytoreduction/ablation. The authors in this study were successfully able to manage the dyspnea in these patients with this combination leading to a reduction in the Medical Research Council dyspnea score. It is important to think in terms of managing this disorder with these relatively conservative measures than curing this, as of yet, idiopathic disorder.

R. A. Franco, Jr, MD

Granulation Formation Following Tracheal Stenosis Stenting: Influence of Stent Position
Ko P-J, Liu C-Y, Wu Y-C, et al (Chang Gung Univ, Tao-Yuan, Taiwan)
Laryngoscope 119:2331-2336, 2009

Objectives/Hypothesis.—To determine whether stent-to-vocal fold distance influences morbidity following stent placement for tracheal stenosis.

Methods.—Fifty-five stent procedures (46 Montgomery T-tube [Boston Medical Products, Westborough, MA] and 9 Dumon stents [Novatech, Grasse, France]) were performed in 40 patients enrolled in this study.

Results.—The most common complication of stenting for tracheal stenosis was granulation (23 procedures, 41.82%). Of 43 procedures where the stent upper edge was located at or below the vocal folds, granulation occurred in 21 procedures (48.84%). Of 12 procedures where the stent edge was located above the vocal fold, granulation occurred in two procedures, or 16.67% (odds ratio $= 4.773$, $P = .0458$, χ^2 test). Among patients in whom the stent edge was located at or below the vocal folds, the granulation complication rate was higher in those with a stent-to-vocal fold distance of <10 mm. Multivariate analysis revealed that the stent-to-vocal fold distance independently predicted granulation formation; an inverse correlation was identified between stent-to-vocal fold distance and granulation severity (n $= 43$, $r = -.501$, $P = .0006$; Spearman ranking test). Receiver operating characteristic curve analysis further demonstrated that a stent-to-vocal fold distance cutoff value between 9.5 and 11 mm had the best accuracy in predicting granulation formation.

Conclusions.—A stent-to-vocal fold distance of 10 mm was found to be a critical distance for discriminating granulation formation. Optimal stent-to-vocal fold distance should routinely be evaluated before stent placement.

▶ One versatile weapon we have in the battle against laryngotracheal stenosis is the T-tube. This device can be used in conjunction with an open reconstructive procedure as a temporary stent or as a permanent fix for the airway stenosis.

Because T-tubes are left in situ for weeks to months, and even years, the surgeon must anticipate the possible consequences of tube placement, specifically the proximal (closest to the vocal folds) tip. The authors found that granulation tissue formation was greatest when the proximal tip to vocal fold distance was less than 10 mm (granulation tissue in 10 of 16 when the tube was less than 10 mm and 4 of 18 when greater than 10 mm). They also found very little (2 of 12) granulation tissue when the tube went above the level of the true vocal folds. Although these patients were spared granulation tissue formation, when the proximal T-tube tip was 10 mm above the level of the true vocal folds, they had much higher rates of aspiration (9 of 12). Care must be taken when placing the T-tube in the subglottis because of the potential for mechanical trauma in this sensitive area that can lead to obstructive granulation tissue. It is important to have a healthy level of respect for granulation tissue and offer treatment even when it is nonobstructive because untreated granulation tissue can lead to a new focus of stenosis. A very effective method is videoendoscopic surveillance with the injection of steroids into the base of the granulation tissue.

R. A. Franco, Jr, MD

Intralesional Corticosteroid Injection and Dilatation Provides Effective Management of Subglottic Stenosis in Wegener's Granulomatosis
Wolter NE, Ooi EH, Witterick IJ (Univ of Toronto, Ontario, Canada)
Laryngoscope 120:2452-2455, 2010

Objectives/Hypothesis.—To describe our experience with the use of intralesional corticosteroid injection and dilatation (ILCD) in the management of subglottic stenosis (SGS).

Study Design.—Retrospective chart review.

Methods.—A retrospective chart review was performed of all patients with SGS requiring ILCD, from 2003 to 2008, at the Department of Otolaryngology–Head and Neck Surgery, Mount Sinai Hospital, Toronto, Canada.

Results.—Twelve patients with SGS underwent 36 ILCD operations with a mean of three procedures per patient. We identified eight patients with Wegener's granulomatosis (WG) and four patients without WG. The eight WG patients received an average of 3.37 procedures, whereas non-WG patients required an average of 2.25 procedures. This maintained airway patency and symptom control for an average of 11.9 and 8.1 months, respectively. Only one complication was identified, and no long-term sequelae were found. No patients required new tracheotomies and one patient with a previous tracheotomy was successfully decannulated.

Conclusions.—Our data supports the use of ILCD as a safe and effective treatment of SGS in both WG and non-WG patients (Fig 1).

▶ Wegener granulomatosis is a vasculitis affecting small- and medium-sized vessels that can manifest clinically as subglottic stenosis. In new cases of

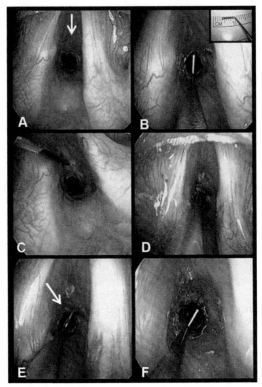

FIGURE 1.—Intraoperative photographs of intralesional corticosteroid injection and lysis. (A) Subglottic stenosis with a predominant anterior component (arrow). (B) A right-angle hook of known length is used as a measuring device (inset). Anteroposterior and transverse measurements are made with the measuring device. (C) Injection of the corticosteroid into the stenosis. (D and E) Incision of the stenotic segment using endoscopic laryngeal scissors. Previous incision indicated by arrow. (F) Following dilatation with bougie dilators, the final airway dimensions are remeasured. [Color figure can be viewed in the online issue, which is available at wileyonlinelibrary.com.] (Reprinted from Wolter NE, Ooi EH, Witterick IJ. Intralesional corticosteroid injection and dilatation provides effective management of subglottic stenosis in Wegener's granulomatosis. *Laryngoscope*. 2010;120:2452-2455, with permission from The American Laryngological, Rhinological and Otological Society, Inc.)

subglottic stenosis without a defined mechanism, Wegener granulomatosis should be ruled out. Subglottic stenosis affects about 1 in 5 patients with Wegener granulomatosis, but if left untreated it can be fatal. The subglottic stenosis does not always respond to systemic treatments, requiring surgical manipulation in many patients. Although large open airway reconstructions can be performed (cricotracheal resection), the most conservative approach possible is typically used because of fears of causing uncontrolled scarring leading to a tighter stenosis from disrupting the already inflamed subglottic mucosa. These authors describe their technique (Fig 1) for increasing the size of the subglottic airway in patients with Wegener and non-Wegener subglottic stenosis. While under general anesthesia, intralesional steroid injection is followed by the creation of radial cuts in the stenosis and dilation using Maloney dilators to the largest possible size. They found that Wegener granulomatosis patients typically go nearly a year between procedures, longer than the similarly treated non-Wegener granulomatosis patients. Because of the small sample size of 12 patients, comparisons cannot be made between the 2 groups (9 patients with Wegener granulomatosis and 3 patients with non-Wegener granulomatosis).

R. A. Franco, Jr, MD

Modified supracricoid laryngectomy
Garozzo A, Allegra E, La Boria A, et al (Univ of Catanzaro, Italy)
Otolaryngol Head Neck Surg 142:137-139, 2010

Supracricoid laryngectomy in its most common modalities, cricohyoidopexy (CHP) and cricohyoidoepiglottopexy (CHEP), is a conservative surgical technique whose principal objective is the natural restoration of the respiratory function. However, both swallowing and phonation undergo important modifications. The objective of this study was to maintain the surgical strategy of supracricoid laryngectomy while focusing on reconstruction of the glottic plane. An essential part of the study was to recreate the anatomical conditions that allow phonation using the sternohyoid muscles for neoglottis reconstruction (Fig 1).

▶ The supracricoid laryngectomy is an open procedure that involves the removal of the thyroid cartilage with the paraglottic space, sometimes the

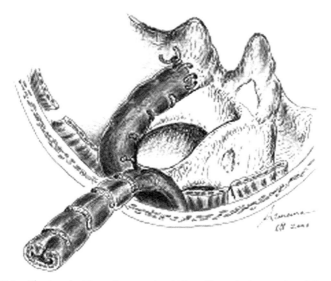

FIGURE 1.—The sternohyoid muscles were placed bilaterally on the free margins of the cricoid and anchored to the vocal apophysis of the arytenoids. (Reprinted from Garozzo A, Allegra E, La Boria A, et al. Modified supracricoid laryngectomy. *Otolaryngol Head Neck Surg.* 2010;142:137-139. Copyright 2010, American Medical Association. All Rights Reserved.)

epiglottis and the pre-epiglottic space for T1b, T2, and select T3 and T4 tumors. The true vocal folds are removed up to the anterior face of the arytenoids leaving the arytenoids on the cricoid. Reconstruction typically involves bringing the cricoid up to the hyoid bone and allowing the base of tongue to contact the edematous supraglottic arytenoid region to create airway closure for airway protection during swallowing and to create voice. Obviously, the loss of the true vocal folds has major implications for voice quality after the supracricoid laryngectomy, limiting its appeal to both physicians and patients. These authors describe a technique that preserves the sternohyoid muscles, tubularizes them, and attaches them to the anterior face of the arytenoids to re-establish tissue at the glottic level. Although there is no comparison to nonmodified supracricoid voices, the authors feel there is an improvement in the vocal function in these patients. Certainly there appears to be a theoretical advantage to this reconstruction, as there is a neocord that can later be injected as required to improve closure. It is encouraging that the patients did not have any difficulties breathing, despite the reconstruction. The technique is simple and makes use of structures that would ordinarily be sacrificed and discarded with the thyroid cartilage specimen.

R. A. Franco, Jr, MD

Superior Thyroid Cornu Syndrome: An Unusual Cause of Cervical Dysphagia
Mortensen M, Ivey CM, Iida M, et al (Univ of Virginia Health System, Charlottesville; Mount Sinai School of Medicine, NY; Jikei Univ, Tokyo, Japan)
Ann Otol Rhinol Laryngol 118:833-838, 2009

Objectives.—Ossification of a superior thyroid cornu in men may cause pharyngeal airway impingement and result in cervical dysphagia. We report on a clinical case series of this rare condition, called superior thyroid cornu syndrome. This is the first report of a case series of this entity as a possible cause of cervical dysphagia that was successfully treated with an endoscopic procedure.

Methods.—A clinical case series of 12 patients were identified as having superior thyroid cornu syndrome (years 2001 to 2006). Eleven patients were male and 1 was female; their mean age was 54.6 years. They complained of unresolved throat pain, difficulty swallowing, and/or pain on swallowing. On flexible laryngoscopy, there was an asymmetric indentation of the pharynx due to a prominent superior thyroid cornu. Laryngeal manipulation produced the pain and exposed the prominent cornu in the airway. Computed tomographic evidence of calcification of the superior thyroid horn without other abnormality was noted.

Results.—After maximal medical treatment with proton pump inhibitors, anti-inflammatory agents, nasal steroids, antihistamines, and/or other allergy treatments, 8 of the patients who had persistent symptoms were treated by transoral pharyngotomy and resection of an approximately 2.0 × 0.5-cm segment of a thyroid cornu. Vast improvement in symptoms

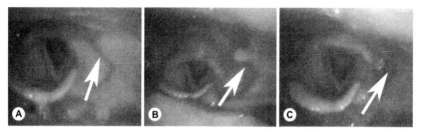

FIGURE 2.—Flexible fiberoptic laryngoscopy depicts prominence of left superior thyroid cornu. A) Area of left thyroid cornu at rest (arrow). B) Significant prominence of left cornu during Valsalva maneuver (arrow). C) Postoperative view of left pharynx during Valsalva maneuver demonstrates resolution of impaction (arrow). (Reprinted from Mortensen M, Ivey CM, Iida M, et al. Superior thyroid cornu syndrome: an unusual cause of cervical dysphagia. *Ann Otol Rhinol Laryngol.* 2009;118:833-838, with permission from Annals Publishing Company.)

occurred in 6 patients, and complete symptom resolution occurred in 3 of those 6. Two of 8 patients reported improvement in swallowing, but persistent pain. The follow-up duration was between 2 and 15 months from the time of surgery.

Conclusions.—Superior thyroid cornu syndrome may be a rare cause of cervical dysphagia. It may be diagnosed by careful laryngoscopy with laryngeal palpation followed by a computed tomography scan. Surgical resection of the affected superior thyroid cornu by transoral pharyngotomy appears to be effective in relief of symptoms (Fig 2).

▶ Cervical dysphagia is typically a complaint in which finding the causative factor can be very difficult. Ill-defined sensations in the pharynx can be associated with laryngopharyngeal reflux (LPR), mucosal lacerations from ingested foreign bodies, and laryngeal framework fractures. The authors present the elongated superior thyroid cartilage (Fig 2) as a potential cause for persistent and reproducible pain in the area of the upper thyroid cartilage. It is important to palpate to reproduce the sensation and correlate this to what is seen on the endoscopic examination. The authors used an endoscopic operative approach to remove the superior cornu with satisfactory results. Six of the 12 patients reported resolution of their symptoms, while 2 of the 12 patients did not have significant changes. It is important to consider that surgical treatment was instituted only after exhausting treatment for LPR, allergies, and cough. Given the 50% response rate, it may make sense to first infiltrate local anesthesia into this area to see if this reduces the symptoms before committing to resecting the superior cornu.

R. A. Franco, Jr, MD

Vocal fold paralysis: role of bilateral transverse cordotomy

Bajaj Y, Sethi N, Shayah A, et al (York Hosp, UK)
J Laryngol Otol 122:1348-1351, 2009

Objective.—Although modern endoscopic laser techniques aim to avoid a permanent tracheostomy by augmenting the glottic aperture in cases of bilateral vocal fold palsy, loss of tissue from the posterior glottis risks compromising voice quality and swallowing function. The objective of this study was to describe our experience with bilateral transverse posterior cordotomy.

Methods.—This was a retrospective analysis of functional outcomes in a series of consecutive patients undergoing a simple modification of the classical laser cordectomy procedure, which avoids tissue loss. The procedure was confined to the complete release of the vocal ligament from the arytenoid cartilage on both sides, while avoiding any significant loss of mucosa or cartilage.

Results.—Post-operative voice quality and quality of life were rated as good by most patients, which makes bilateral transverse cordotomy an attractive treatment option for bilateral vocal fold paralysis.

Conclusion.—Bilateral transverse cordotomy is a reliable treatment option for patients with bilateral vocal fold paralysis, and aims to avoid the morbidity associated with a permanent tracheostomy (Figs 1 and 3).

▶ As with many serious clinical problems, there is more than one surgical solution available with pros and cons that are valid. Since bilateral vocal fold immobility can lead to a narrow glottic aperture with dyspnea and air hunger, a procedure that can reliably establish a safe and adequate airway is desirable.

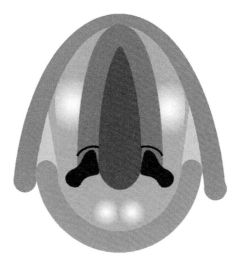

FIGURE 1.—Diagram showing bilateral transverse cordotomy. (Reprinted from Bajaj Y, Sethi N, Shayah A, et al. Vocal fold paralysis: role of bilateral transverse cordotomy. *J Laryngol Otol.* 2009;122:1348-1351, with permission of Cambridge University Press.)

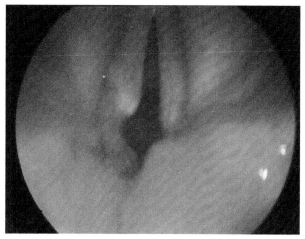

FIGURE 3.—Post-operative stroboscopic view, eight weeks after cordotomy. (Reprinted from Bajaj Y, Sethi N, Shayah A, et al. Vocal fold paralysis: role of bilateral transverse cordotomy. *J Laryngol Otol.* 2009;122:1348-1351, with permission of Cambridge University Press.)

Although tracheotomy can eliminate the dyspnea and air hunger, many patients are not willing to take on the added burden of stomal care and the detrimental cosmetic changes of having a plastic tube sticking out of their necks. Because of this, endoscopic procedures that can reasonably spare voice while improving airway size have gained favor. The authors propose that bilateral transverse cordotomy reliably improves airway while also maintaining adequate voice. The technique involves using a carbon dioxide laser to cut through the entire substance of the vocal fold (through the vocal ligament) anterior to the vocal process of the arytenoids (Figs 1 and 3). All patients with indwelling tracheostomy tubes were decannulated within 1 month of the procedure, and no one required a tracheotomy. One patient was readmitted for steroids and airway observation 48 hours after the procedure and was discharged home several days later. The procedure improves the airway size, and the patients seemed satisfied with their quality of life after the procedure, making this a viable option for bilateral vocal fold immobility leading to airway compromise.

R. A. Franco, Jr, MD

4 Otology

General

A Placebo-Controlled Trial of Antimicrobial Treatment for Acute Otitis Media

Tähtinen PA, Laine MK, Huovinen P, et al (Turku Univ Hosp, Finland; Univ of Turku, Finland)

N Engl J Med 364:116-126, 2011

Background.—The efficacy of antimicrobial treatment in children with acute otitis media remains controversial.

Methods.—In this randomized, double-blind trial, children 6 to 35 months of age with acute otitis media, diagnosed with the use of strict criteria, received amoxicillin–clavulanate (161 children) or placebo (158 children) for 7 days. The primary outcome was the time to treatment failure from the first dose until the end-of-treatment visit on day 8. The definition of treatment failure was based on the overall condition of the child (including adverse events) and otoscopic signs of acute otitis media.

Results.—Treatment failure occurred in 18.6% of the children who received amoxicillin–clavulanate, as compared with 44.9% of the children who received placebo (P<0.001). The difference between the groups was already apparent at the first scheduled visit (day 3), at which time 13.7% of the children who received amoxicillin–clavulanate, as compared with 25.3% of those who received placebo, had treatment failure. Overall, amoxicillin–clavulanate reduced the progression to treatment failure by 62% (hazard ratio, 0.38; 95% confidence interval [CI], 0.25 to 0.59; P<0.001) and the need for rescue treatment by 81% (6.8% vs. 33.5%; hazard ratio, 0.19; 95% CI, 0.10 to 0.36; P<0.001). Analgesic or antipyretic agents were given to 84.2% and 85.9% of the children in the amoxicillin–clavulanate and placebo groups, respectively. Adverse events were significantly more common in the amoxicillin–clavulanate group than in the placebo group. A total of 47.8% of the children in the amoxicillin–clavulanate group had diarrhea, as compared with 26.6% in the placebo group (P<0.001); 8.7% and 3.2% of the children in the respective groups had eczema (P = 0.04).

Conclusions.—Children with acute otitis media benefit from antimicrobial treatment as compared with placebo, although they have more side effects. Future studies should identify patients who may derive the greatest benefit, in order to minimize unnecessary antimicrobial treatment and the development of bacterial resistance. (Funded by the Foundation for Paediatric Research and others; ClinicalTrials.gov number, NCT00299455.)

▶ Although rarely a referral to the otolaryngologist, uncomplicated acute otitis media remains among the most common disorders of children. It has been considered largely a disorder of viral origin, and multiple prior studies and meta-analyses have shown limited to no benefit from antibiotics. Thus, many treatment guidelines have recommended observation before treatment. The results of this study change that paradigm. It also demonstrates the ability of well-designed and well-controlled studies to provide solid answers to focused clinical questions. Here, a relatively small sample size of slightly more than 300 subjects was used. The authors review the limitations of prior study designs and how they addressed these in their study. They also provide a straightforward and accurate power calculation to support their findings using this study size. Interestingly, they used a standard dose of amoxicillin of 40 mg/kg rather than the double dose that is often recommended. These results are best visualized in Fig 4 in the original article. In addition to their primary outcome measure, they also analyzed important secondary outcomes regarding patient comfort, such as resolution of fever, and quality of life, as well as their caregivers. In this regard, for those children in day care, their caregivers missed some 5.7% fewer workdays in the treatment group than in the placebo group. Complications such as tympanic membrane perforation were reduced in exchange for a higher rate of side effects. In summary, 2 main points are important from this study. First, when using strict diagnostic criteria, antibiotics can be of benefit in acute otitis media and should be prescribed early. Second, clinical answers can be obtained from well-designed tightly controlled studies much more readily than from retrospective reviews or poorly designed efforts. Thus, not only the results but also the approach makes this article worthy of review.

B. J. Balough, CAPT, MC, USN

Audiological Deficits After Closed Head Injury
Munjal SK, Panda NK, Pathak A (Post Graduate Inst of Med Education and Res, Chandigarh, India)
J Trauma 68:13-18, 2010

Background.—Damage to the peripheral auditory structures has long been recognized as a common component of head injury. It is estimated that a majority of patients with skull trauma have resultant hearing impairment. Damage to the peripheral and/or central auditory pathways can occur as a primary or secondary injury. Considering the high incidence of hearing loss, it was considered worthwhile to conduct an in-depth investigation by administering a comprehensive audiological test battery on head-injured patients.

Method.—The sample population consisted of 290 subjects with closed head injury (study group) and 50 subjects with otologically normal subjects (control group). The subjects in the study group were further divided into mild (n = 150), moderate (n = 100), and severe (n = 40) category on the basis of Glasgow Coma Scale score. The audiological assessment consisted of pure tone audiometry, speech audiometry, tympanometry, acoustic reflex testing, auditory brain stem response audiometry, and middle latency response audiometry.

Results and Conclusions.—It is concluded that there is higher prevalence of hearing impairment in the study group compared with control group. Majority of the patients who incur hearing loss after closed head injury have mild degree of hearing impairment. A significant difference between the study and control group observed on majority of the auditory brain stem response and middle latency response parameters studied (Table 1).

▶ Traumatic brain injury (TBI) after closed head injury has garnered a significant amount of public, media, and government attention over the past decade. Much of this is because of the injury patterns being seen from the military operations in southwest Asia. Attention too has come from the growing recognition of the impact from mild TBI due to recreational and sporting injuries and from motor vehicle accidents. There is growing recognition that even mild TBI can have lasting aftereffects on cognitive and sensory function and that repeated trauma can increase both the likelihood and severity of the sequella. For the otolaryngologist, 2 of the most common somatic symptoms after TBI are hearing and balance impairment. Given the increased public awareness, it is likely that these patients may present seeking evaluation and diagnosis for their complaints. Thus, this large, well-controlled, prospective study is a valuable resource and reference on the topic. Table 1 provides useful insight into the results. First, the hearing loss can be flat across all frequencies and not just limited to the high frequencies. Second, the degree of hearing loss is significant when compared with controls and is independent of the severity of TBI.

TABLE 1.—PTA—Right Ear: Comparison Between Control and Three Study Groups

Frequency (Hz)	Control Group (n = 50) Mean (dB)	SD	Mild CHI (n = 146) Mean (dB)	SD	Dunnet p	Moderate CHI (n = 73) Mean (dB)	SD	Dunnet p	Severe CHI (n = 18) Mean (dB)	SD	Dunnet p
250	11.00	5.05	23.97	13.65	0.0001	19.66	10.08	0.0001	23.75	12.49	0.001
500	11.50	4.87	23.86	12.73	0.0001	21.16	10.66	0.0001	23.13	10.88	0.001
1000	11.50	4.43	21.17	11.47	0.0001	20.82	10.80	0.0001	24.38	13.48	0.0001
2000	9.10	6.44	18.14	11.90	0.0001	20.34	11.19	0.0001	23.44	10.87	0.0001
4000	9.20	5.47	21.41	14.56	0.0001	25.27	14.33	0.0001	28.13	14.41	0.0001
8000	9.70	7.38	20.41	15.05	0.0001	27.26	15.09	0.0001	25.94	20.79	0.0001
12000	8.88	8.54	26.47	20.13	0.0001	31.98	18.38	0.0001	29.69	21.57	0.0001
PTA1	10.70	4.04	21.12	11.15	0.0001	20.78	10.20	0.0001	23.05	10.95	0.0001
PTA2	9.23	6.20	23.40	14.43	0.0001	28.17	14.70	0.0001	29.90	16.97	0.0001

This flat loss is consistent with reports from prior studies. Auditory brainstem response (ABR) testing also not surprisingly reveals increased latencies in waves I, III, and V. Combinations of ABR and somatosensory evoked potentials have previously been shown to provide prognostic information for recovery in patients with severe TBI. The middle latency response is discussed in this article and demonstrated a marked reduction in wave amplitude corresponding to decreased activity above the brainstem. This did show an increasing decline as severity increased. One limitation of this study is that no late cortical responses were performed. These too show decreases in other studies. A good commentary from the journal editor is provided at the end of the article.[1-3] In that, a comment is made that these results are from closed head injuries that were not exposed to blast type effects. In those patients, the hearing loss rates may be even higher. A variety of military studies are examining this at present. Given the > 300 000 military veterans with suspected TBI (many of whom were reservists or have left active duty), these may present to otolaryngologists outside the military or Veterans Affairs health care systems. Last, the patient with TBI often has cognitive impairment, other injuries, or other sensory deficits, thus making screening, identification, and treatment of their hearing loss of increased importance.

B. J. Balough, CAPT, MC, USN

References

1. Lew HL, Garvert DW, Pogoda TK, et al. Auditory and visual impairments in patients with blast-related traumatic brain injury: effect of dual sensory impairment on Functional Independence Measure. *J Rehabil Res Dev.* 2009;46:819-826.
2. Lew HL, Jerger JF, Guillory SB, Henry JA. Auditory dysfunction in traumatic brain injury. *J Rehabil Res Dev.* 2007;44:921-928.
3. Lew HL, Poole JH, Castaneda A, Salerno RM, Gray M. Prognostic value of evoked and event-related potentials in moderate to severe brain injury. *J Head Trauma Rehabil.* 2006;21:350-360.

Evaluation of the Universal Newborn Hearing Screening and Intervention Program
Shulman S, Besculides M, Saltzman A, et al (Blue Cross Blue Shield of Massachusetts Foundation, Boston; Mathematica Policy Res, Inc, Cambridge, MA; et al)
Pediatrics 126:S19-S27, 2010

During the last 20 years, the number of infants evaluated for permanent hearing loss at birth has increased dramatically with universal newborn hearing screening and intervention (UNHSI) programs operating in all US states and many territories. One of the most urgent challenges of UNHSI programs involves loss to follow-up among families whose infants screen positive for hearing loss. We surveyed 55 state and territorial UNHSI programs and conducted site visits with 8 state programs to evaluate progress in reaching program goals and to identify barriers to successful follow-up. We conclude that programs have made great strides in screening infants for hearing loss, but barriers to linking families of infants who do not pass the screening to further follow-up remain. We identified 4 areas in which there were barriers to follow-up (lack of service-system capacity, lack of provider knowledge, challenges to families in obtaining services, and information gaps), as well as successful strategies used by some states to address barriers within each of these areas. We also identified 5 key areas for future program improvements: (1) improving data systems to support surveillance and follow-up activities; (2) ensuring that all infants have a medical home; (3) building capacity beyond identified providers; (4) developing family support services; and (5) promoting the importance of early detection.

▶ This article represents a large and comprehensive examination of newborn hearing screening programs across the country. As such, it will likely serve as the reference article on this topic for years to come and thus is included in this year's list. For otolaryngologists engaged in cochlear implant programs, the observations and conclusions in this report will be of particular value. The most important of these is that while screening programs are indeed universally in place with some 92% screened, a great deal of work remains to be done in capturing those infants who fail initial screening and to have them return for follow-on testing to confirm the hearing loss and to receive early intervention (these rates were as low as 50%-60%). Otolaryngologists along with pediatricians can serve as medical advocates to improve these rates within their communities. Interestingly, these rates were less than the numbers of children identified as having a medical home in which to receive and coordinate care. The report lists 4 gaps to infants receiving this follow-up care of which an information gap was one of those factors identified. Education of primary care providers on the importance of early identification and intervention including cochlear implants for those profoundly deaf can be a role of the otolaryngologist in partnership with audiology, and this article provides the background information and data for those interested in that role.

B. J. Balough, CAPT, MC, USN

Hyperbaric oxygen therapy as salvage treatment for sudden sensorineural hearing loss: review of rationale and preliminary report
Muzzi E, Zennaro B, Visentin R, et al (Santa Maria della Misericordia Univ Hosp, Udine, Italy; OTI Services Hyperbaric Medicine Service, Venice, Italy; et al)
J Laryngol Otol 124:1-9, 2010

Background.—The management of sudden sensorineural hearing loss has not yet been standardised. Hyperbaric oxygen therapy influences recovery from sudden sensorineural hearing loss, but the underlying mechanism is unknown and the appropriate indications and protocols undetermined.

Materials and Methods.—Nineteen patients affected by sudden sensorineural hearing loss were treated after unsuccessful medical therapy, either in an acute or chronic setting. Pure oxygen inhalation at 2.5 atmospheres absolute pressure was administered for 90 minutes, for 30 sessions. Frequency-specific and average pure tone hearing thresholds were determined before and after hyperbaric oxygen therapy. The number of hyperbaric oxygen therapy sessions, the patient's age and any therapeutic delay were considered as quantitative variables possibly influencing outcome. Stepwise multivariate analysis was performed.

Results.—Salvage hyperbaric oxygen therapy appeared to improve patients' pure tone hearing thresholds, particularly at low frequencies. Positive results were more likely with increased patient age and reduced delay in receiving hyperbaric oxygen therapy.

Conclusion.—Hyperbaric oxygen therapy has a strong scientific rationale, and improves pure tone hearing thresholds in cases of sudden sensorineural hearing loss unresponsive to medical therapy. Further research may be able to identify those patients with sudden sensorineural hearing loss for whom hyperbaric oxygen therapy would be most cost-effective.

▶ Each year, several articles are published regarding the treatment of idiopathic sudden sensorineural hearing loss. Most of those are limited case series evaluating one treatment or another. This study, however, is worthy of review as it provides analysis of salvage therapy for those having failed standard medical treatment. Multiple references are provided to support the use of hyperbaric oxygen for this purpose. Further in the discussion, the authors carefully and thoroughly review the evidence to support the use of hyperbaric oxygen in treatment of sudden hearing loss at the organ, tissue, and cellular levels. A less detailed but still valuable review of the science behind the use of corticosteroids is also provided. This detailed discussion alone makes this an article worth reading. Given the rare nature of this disorder, this study suffers from many of the same problems that others on the topic do: small numbers, retrospective nature, and no control group. The authors do acknowledge these flaws and urge caution in interpretation of their results. One other limitation not mentioned is that the results provide only pure tone information without corresponding changes in word recognition scores. Some studies on transtympanic steroids have shown modest gains in pure tone levels but large improvements of word recognition to serviceable levels. This is a large flaw in an otherwise solid article. Two final points are worthy of note. The first was the analysis on effect of delay of treatment on outcome. Treatment within 30 days seems to be equally effective, whereas treatment after that time offers only modest benefit. This information is important in the design of future trials for this or other treatments. The second is that even after an initial failure, salvage treatment can provide benefit. This benefit appears to be independent of overall hearing level and appears as likely in those with minimal losses as those with severe loss. Doubtless there will be further work in this area.

B. J. Balough, CAPT, MC, USN

Prevalence and Characteristics of Tinnitus among US Adults

Shargorodsky J, Curhan GC, Farwell WR (Massachusetts Eye and Ear Infirmary, Boston; Brigham and Women's Hosp, Boston, MA; VA Boston Healthcare System, MA)
Am J Med 123:711-718, 2010

Background.—Tinnitus is common; however, few risk factors for tinnitus are known.

Methods.—We examined cross-sectional relations between several potential risk factors and self-reported tinnitus in 14,178 participants in the 1999-2004 National Health and Nutrition Examination Surveys, a nationally representative database. We calculated the prevalence of any and frequent (at least daily) tinnitus in the overall US population and among subgroups. Logistic regression was used to calculate odds ratios (OR) and 95% confidence intervals (CI) after adjusting for multiple potential confounders.

Results.—Approximately 50 million US adults reported having any tinnitus, and 16 million US adults reported having frequent tinnitus in the past year. The prevalence of frequent tinnitus increased with increasing age, peaking at 14.3% between 60 and 69 years of age. Non-Hispanic whites had higher odds of frequent tinnitus compared with other racial/ethnic groups. Hypertension and former smoking were associated with an increase in odds of frequent tinnitus. Loud leisure-time, firearm, and occupational noise exposure also were associated with increased odds of frequent tinnitus. Among participants who had an audiogram, frequent tinnitus was associated with low-mid frequency (OR 2.37; 95% CI, 1.76-3.21) and high frequency (OR 3.00; 95% CI, 1.78-5.04) hearing impairment. Among participants who were tested for mental health conditions, frequent tinnitus was associated with generalized anxiety disorder (OR 6.07; 95% CI, 2.33-15.78) but not major depressive disorder (OR 1.58; 95% CI, 0.54-4.62).

Conclusions.—The prevalence of frequent tinnitus is highest among older adults, non-Hispanic whites, former smokers, and adults with hypertension, hearing impairment, loud noise exposure, or generalized anxiety disorder. Prospective studies of risk factors for tinnitus are needed.

▶ This article represents a large analysis of adult tinnitus in the United States taken from survey data and then normalized to the characteristics of the general population. It provides important insight into the prevalence and relative risk factors for tinnitus but, because of the methodology, does not allow for determinations of causality. Despite this limitation, several valuable findings are present. First, although several smaller studies have reported associations between mental health disorders, this is the first large nationwide study to do so, with a 6 times relative risk for tinnitus in those with major depression or generalized anxiety. Second, vascular disease as a risk factor for tinnitus was shown to include both smoking and hypertension. In particular, the data on past and present smoking risk for tinnitus has not been previously shown. Third, race and ethnicity are independent risk factors for tinnitus suggestive of a genetic predisposition. Fourth, and perhaps most important, is that tinnitus is present in significant numbers even in the younger adult population. Furthermore, these risk factors are independent of age. Thus, as the authors conclude, prevention or early treatment of these disorders may be an effective means of reducing tinnitus in the population. The findings in this study will more than likely be used as a basis for further tinnitus research in the future, and as such, this is an important reference article for inclusion in this year's list.

B. J. Balough, CAPT, MC, USN

Three cases of inner ear damage after electrical burns
Choi DJ, Kim BG, Park I-S, et al (Hallym Univ, Seoul, Republic of Korea)
Burns 36:e83-e86, 2010

Background.—Electrical burns produce various kinds of tissue injuries, ranging from obvious thermal tissue destruction to the slow onset of neurologic defects even when no thermal injury is apparent. Multiple organ systems can be damaged and there may be neurologic and cardiovascular sequelae. Damage to the ear and related structures occurs when they are in the path of the electrical current, which preferentially travels along neurovascular bundles. Both early and delayed deep ischemic necrosis results from the vascular thrombosis induced by the electrical current's passage. Three patients who developed hearing disturbance, tinnitus, and dizziness after electrical burns were described.

Case Reports.—Case 1: Man, 42, was struck by a high-voltage wire carrying an estimated 22,900 V. He was unconscious for a brief period and suffered second-degree burns to both hands and the left lower leg. His chief complaint was of severe bilateral tinnitus and hearing loss, but no dizziness. Otologic examination showed normal ear canals and tympanic membranes, but the pure-tone audiogram revealed moderate downward-sloping sensorineural hearing loss in both ears. He was followed conservatively for 9 months and had moderate high-pitched tinnitus on tinnitogram and persistent bilateral sensorineural hearing loss.

Case 2: Man, 31, was burned by a 22,900 V overhead cable that fell over him. He had severe dizziness and tinnitus but no hearing loss. The external auditory canal was edematous, but audiogram detected normal hearing in both ears. The vestibular function test in electronystagmography revealed abnormal findings. Left canal paresis of 93% was found on the caloric test. The patient diligently performed Cawthorne-Cooksey exercises to help retrain his brain to recover from the vestibular disorders. The tinnitus completely resolved and dizziness was much improved subjectively after 6 months.

Case 3: Man, 52, had various electrical burns on his body and hearing loss. The injuries were sustained while he was working at high-voltage current. Physical examination revealed a second-degree burn on the left hand and both feet. The left ear had a hyperemic and mildly edematous auricle. Pure-tone audiometry showed an 80-dB sensorineural-type hearing loss. After 6 months the auricle had healed completely but the sensorineural hearing loss remained.

Conclusions.—Electrical injuries result when electrical energy is converted into heat energy, with the heat generated directly proportional to the resistance of the tissues that are traversed. The electrical energy alters cell membrane permeability, and the heat causes tissue proteins to become denatured. When there is contact with a high electrical energy arc, the patient often suffers a blunt mechanical injury with a strong thermoblastic effect. Treatment of ear injury caused by electrical burn differs depending on the type and severity of the injury. Early otologic examination is performed once any blood and debris has been cleaned from the external auditory canal. After aural hygiene the patient is given otic drops (unless he or she has cerebrospinal otorrhea) and systemic antibiotics. Surgery is delayed for 6 months because spontaneous healing may occur within this time frame. Sensorineural hearing loss seldom recovers spontaneously.

▶ Fortunately electrical burns are rare injuries. However, because of this rare nature, this article was selected for review to familiarize otolaryngologists should they encounter such an injury in their practice. As the authors state, the literature is very sparse in regard to discussing otologic sequela from electric injury. The first point they make is key, namely, that these injuries can represent a spectrum of disorders from obvious thermal injuries to gradual onset of neurological defects even in the absence of apparent injury. They explain this further in the article when they discuss that the damage to individual tissues is independent of the heat generated by the current passage. Therefore, neural tissues that should have low resistance and thus low thermal generation can readily be injured by current passage. No patient in this series had cardiac or other neurologic injury except to the ear. Entrance and exit wounds were not in proximity to the ear or head and neck. Two of the 3 cases presented had hearing loss as their complaint, but the other had only unilateral acute vestibular loss without apparent hearing injury (other than tinnitus). Thus, the absence of hearing loss does not exclude electrical injury to the inner ear, though a routine audiogram is advised in all cases. Lastly, it is important to remember that in all cases presented, there were high-voltage injuries in excess of 22 000 V. For common household electrical current injuries, the findings presented here may not be the same.

B. J. Balough, CAPT, MC, USN

Tinnitus in children: an uncommon symptom?

Shetye A, Kennedy V (St Ann's Hosp, London, UK; Halliwell Health and Children's Centre, Bolton, UK)

Arch Dis Child 95:645-648, 2010

Tinnitus in children is regarded as an uncommon problem rarely noted by general paediatricians. Its reported prevalence varies from 12% to 36% in children with normal hearing thresholds and up to 66% in children with hearing loss and approximately 3–10% of children have been reported troubled by tinnitus.

Some children do not spontaneously complain of it, but may demonstrate behavioural problems at school and home. A careful history, in conjunction with clinical findings, should guide the appropriate management approach. Even very young children are able to provide insights into what troubles them allowing children's thoughts and fears regarding this symptom to be addressed.

We review the available literature on the nature and impact of tinnitus and as guidelines for this do not exist, suggest a pragmatic approach to the management of tinnitus in children. Children with troublesome tinnitus, however, should be referred on to a paediatric audiology department for further investigation and management (Tables 1, 3 and 4).

▶ Tinnitus in adults is a commonly covered topic in the medical literature. As such, there is a wealth of information regarding evaluation and treatment options. In children, however, this is an infrequently covered topic. Thus, this article is included as a useful review on the topic. Several important points are worth noting. First, tinnitus is not an uncommon problem even in normal hearing children. Table 1 lists studies on the topic, some of which are quite

TABLE 1.—Studies of Tinnitus in Children with Normal and Impaired Hearing

Authors	Number of Children in Study	Percentage of Children Reporting Tinnitus (%)	Study Setting
Normal hearing			
Mills et al[1]	93	29	Routine school and community medical examination and paediatric ENT clinic
Aksoy et al[2]	1039	15.1	Primary and junior high school medical examination
Holgers and Juul[10]	964	12	Routine school exam
Nodar and Lezak[23]	2000	15	Routine school exam
Hearing impaired			
Graham[4]	158	Overall 49 HI 66 D 29	Hearing impaired units School for the deaf
Aust[6]	1420	7	ENT clinic
Mills and Cherry[11]	109	38.5	Attending with ear disease

D, profound hearing loss; ENT, ear, nose and throat; HI, moderate to severe hearing loss.
Editor's Note: Please refer to original journal article for full references.

TABLE 3.—Questions Relating to History and Possible Associated and Co-Existing Factors in Children with Tinnitus

Questions Relating to Tinnitus	Possible Associated/Co-Existing Factors to Note
Do you ever hear noises in your ears? What do they sound like? What do you call the noises? What do you do when you have the noise? How does the noise affect you? When is it worse, eg, at school or home, time of the day? Where the noise – in one/both is ears or head? How long have you heard these noises?	Ear disease[1 2 4 5] including middle ear problems, ear operations Neuro-otological symptoms, eg, balance problems High dynamic flow rate conditions, eg, thyroid dysfunction, anaemia Potential sources of ototoxicity, eg, aminoglycosides cisplatin[31] and non-steroidal anti-inflammatory drugs[32] History of trauma, eg, head trauma,[33 34] noise exposure[5] History of headache and specific features relating to migraine[5]

Editor's Note: Please refer to original journal article for full references.

TABLE 4.—Logical Approach to Proceed for Children with Tinnitus

Listen, provide reassurance and support to enable the child to recognise that the tinnitus is a non-threatening condition
Identify: worries of child/parents
    Tinnitus-related difficulties—home/school
Consider amplification if there is hearing loss
Sound enrichment
Involve teachers of the deaf to monitor child's progress at school
Address other existing issues as the tinnitus symptoms decrease:
    Explore if associated problems provoking or caused by tinnitus
    Address underlying educational/psychological concerns
Counselling
    Provide clear simple information
    Build on coping skills, imagination of child
Formal therapy
    Relaxation
    Psychology, eg, narrative therapy
Education
    Identifying and learning to manage aggravating factors
    Prevention of environmental causes of noise-induced hearing loss
Consider sound generators

large. Even in routine school exams, 10% to 15% of children report tinnitus when asked. Second, while less than 1% of adults are reported to have severe tinnitus, this review reports a much higher rate of troubles caused by the tinnitus. Often this is manifested by emotional or behavioral problems. Thus, when present, tinnitus in children is a more significant problem. Third, the article addresses the issue of asking children about their tinnitus and dispels the myth that asking about it will enhance the symptom or that children will invent symptoms when asked about them. In fact, the converse is true; they are more likely to omit information that is not asked and in discussing their symptoms they are less likely to become distressed. Two references are provided from the article that addresses this in depth.[1,2] The article also gives a simple evaluation and management scheme that is useful and is found in Tables 3 and 4.

B. J. Balough, CAPT, MC, USN

References

1. Kentish RC, Crocker SR, McKenna L. Children's experience of tinnitus: a preliminary survey of children presenting to a psychology department. *Br J Audiol.* 2000; 34:335-340.
2. Fitzpatrick G, Reder P, Lucey C. The child's perspective. In: Reder P, Lucey C, eds. *Assessment in Parenting: Psychiatric and Psychological Contributions.* London, UK: Routledge; 1995.

Vestibular substitution: comparative study
Polat S, Uneri A (Acıbadem Oncology and Neurology Hosp, Istanbul, Turkey; Marmara Univ Inst of Neurological Science, Istanbul, Turkey)
J Laryngol Otol 124:852-858, 2010

Objective.—To determine the efficacy of vestibular rehabilitation with the electrotactile vestibular substitution system, as a new treatment modality in patients with bilateral vestibular disorders.

Study Design and Settings.—Nineteen patients with bilateral, chronic, idiopathic vestibulopathy were studied prospectively. Patients were divided to two groups. Patients in the first group were rehabilitated with the electrotactile vestibular substitution system, while patients in the second group were treated with standard vestibular rehabilitation therapy. The sensory organisation test and dizziness handicap inventory were used to compare the pre- and post-training results of both rehabilitative treatments.

Results.—All group one patients in the standardised testing subset demonstrated improved results for both the composite sensory organisation test and for the functional transfer aspect of the dizziness handicap inventory, after five days' training with the electrotactile vestibular substitution system. In contrast, group two patients showed no significant improvement in their composite sensory organisation test or dizziness handicap inventory scores after eight weeks of therapy, compared with pre-treatment levels.

Conclusion.—These preliminary results indicate the efficacy of the electrotactile vestibular substitution system in improving patients' symptoms of vestibulopathy, and constitute evidence of successful sensory substitution (Table 1).

▶ This article discusses a new technology for treating a difficult patient population, ie, those with chronic bilateral vestibulopathy. These patients are difficult to treat with standard vestibular rehabilitation, as the extent of their dysfunction

TABLE 1.—Group One Patients: Demographics and Test Results

Age (yrs)	Gender	Aetiology	SOT Pre	SOT Post	SOT Late	DHI Pre	DHI Post	DHI Late
30	F	Chr ves	47	80	55	88	12	66
62	M	Chr ves	27	50	35	60	12	52
51	F	Chr ves	72	87	65	62	10	76
58	F	Chr ves	33	55	43	84	18	68
66	F	Chr ves	48	70	45	84	16	72
54	F	Chr ves	64	77	60	66	4	78
75	F	Chr ves	51	72	55	98	18	80
49	F	Chr ves	45	69	51	76	8	76
64	M	Chr ves	46	80	46	92	16	88
85	M	Chr ves	36	64	41	92	8	78
28	F	Chr ves	48	78	50	94	12	94

Yrs = years; SOT = sensory organisation test; DHI = dizziness handicap inventory; pre = before training; post = first post-training day; late = seventh post-training day; F = female; M = male; chr ves = chronic, idiopathic vestibulopathy.

limits their ability to perform exercises and progress in therapy. Sensory substitution overcomes this limitation by providing sensory feedback via tactile sensation on the tongue to provide information on body position. Table 1 provides vestibular test and dizziness handicap results for the group of patients using this technology. Substantial early effects were seen in the posttreatment testing. However, these results declined over time when not continuing treatment, gradually returning to near-baseline levels by the seventh day. With training, motivated patients can perform home rehabilitation to maintain benefit. Thus, for these challenging patients who are often housebound, this is a promising advance. Currently the device is not approved for use within the United States, though it is commercially available in other countries. Our center has performed our own institutional review board–approved studies in subjects suffering balance disorders after closed head injuries with similar results. Further studies need to be performed to identify which patients will benefit the most and if this can accelerate the gains seen with standard vestibular rehabilitation to return patients back to normal activity. This article serves as a good introduction to the potential of this and similar technologies and is well referenced.[1,2]

B. J. Balough, CAPT, MC, USN

References

1. Kentish RC, Crocker SR, McKenna L. Children's experience of tinnitus: a preliminary survey of children presenting to a psychology department. *Br J Audiol.* 2000; 34:335-340.
2. Fitzpatrick G, Reder P, Lucey C. The child's perspective. In: Reder P, Lucey C, eds. *Assessment in Parenting: Psychiatric and Psychological Contributions.* London, UK: Routledge; 1995.

Surgical Technique

Device Fixation in Cochlear Implantation: Is Bone Anchoring Necessary?

Molony TB, Giles JE, Thompson TL, et al (Tulane Univ School of Medicine, New Orleans, LA)
Laryngoscope 120:1837-1839, 2010

Objectives/Hypothesis.—To compare complication rates between patients whose cochlear implants were secured by a bony tie-down technique versus those secured by a periosteal tie-down technique.

Study Design.—A retrospective review of 302 consecutive patients undergoing cochlear implantation (327 implants), including both adults and children, at a single institution by a single surgeon.

Methods.—Cochlear implantation was performed in the standard fashion with bony securement of the device in the first subset of patients. The surgical technique was then modified to exclude the bony tie-down step in favor of a periosteally placed suture tie-down in the next subset of patients. The patient's medical records were then reviewed to determine complications, which were then compared between groups using χ^2 testing.

Results.—The overall complication rate for the periosteally secured cochlear implant subset was 9.5%, with no significant difference noted when compared to the 12.2% overall complication rate seen with the bone-secured implants. Minor complication rates were 9.5% versus 8.1%, respectively, with major complications occurring in 0% versus 4.1% of periosteally secured versus bone-secured devices. There were no statistical differences between groups for major, minor, or any specific complications. There were no cases of device migration.

Conclusions.—Cochlear implant devices may be secured in place with periosteally anchored sutures in lieu of bone-anchored sutures without any significant increases in perioperative complications.

▶ As originally approved, cochlear implant manufacturers continue to recommend periosteal suture fixation of the device after the bone well is drilled. However, a variety of flap designs and fixation techniques have now been developed by surgeons. With the advent of minimal exposure techniques, periosteal suture fixation has become more commonly used by surgeons because of the limited access. This article is significant in that it provides data regarding complication rates between these 2 methods. One limitation in their findings, which the authors acknowledge, is the relatively short duration of follow-up in the periosteal suture fixation group. Given the typical healing times, however, the average duration of follow-up of 7 months should be adequate to account for most complications. Perhaps the most important issue is not addressed by this article: device migration. No radiographic analyses are performed, and the inclusion of that data would have made for a much stronger conclusion. Even still, the comparable rates of complications indicate that from that regard, periosteal fixation is safe, and thus, this article is worthy of review.

B. J. Balough, CAPT, MC, USN

Diagnostics

Sensory Dysmodulation in Vestibular Migraine: An Otoacoustic Emission Suppression Study

Murdin L, Premachandra P, Davies R (Natl Hosp for Neurology and Neurosurgery, Queen Square, London, UK)
Laryngoscope 120:1632-1636, 2010

Objectives/Hypothesis.—To seek evidence of sensory dysmodulation in auditory brainstem reflexes in patients with vestibular migraine by studying suppression of otoacoustic emissions (OAEs) by contralateral noise.

Study Design.—A prospective case-control study.

Methods.—The authors measured contralateral suppression of OAEs in a group of 33 interictal patients with definite vestibular migraine (migrainous vertigo) according to the strict diagnostic criteria of Neuhauser (2001), and compared them with 31 nonmigrainous controls with matching age and sex distributions. Suppression values were then compared with previously published departmental normative data. In three patients, recordings were compared in the ictal and interictal states.

Results.—OAE suppression was reduced in 11/33 patients, and 3/31 controls ($P = .022$ χ^2 test). Binary logistic regression analysis confirmed that the presence of vestibular migraine was significantly associated with abnormal suppression, but no such relationship was seen for symptoms of phonophobia or disease duration. The amplitude of variability between the ictal and interictal state was out of the normal range in 2 out of the 3 patients in whom such recordings were made.

Conclusions.—These results provide support for the notion of interictal auditory sensory dysmodulation in an as yet unidentified subset of migraineurs with vestibular migraine.

▶ Like most vestibular disorders, migraine-associated vertigo is a clinical diagnosis based on history. The vertigo is thought to arise from dysfunction induced by the migraine in the brainstem nuclei. The authors provide a good description of this proposed mechanism in the introduction. However, the actual pathophysiology is unclear. This article takes a novel approach to attempt to identify this brainstem nuclear dysfunction via clinical audiologic testing. In this case, otoacoustic reflexes are used, as the reflex arc involved occurs in the brainstem, and this study was undertaken to provide objective physiologic evidence of the proposed pathophysiology. The results suggest some evidence to support their theory in that contralateral noise suppression did reduce significantly more patients in the migraine group. Interestingly, this did not correlate to hearing-related symptoms. While not highly sensitive, this test when positive could help provide objective evidence for migraine as the source of vertigo; this would need to be worked out in larger series of patients before becoming clinically useful. In their discussion, the authors also mention that at the stimulation intensity of 83 dB, middle ear reflex responses could not be excluded as contributing to this effect. This raises the interesting possibility of evaluating acoustic reflex testing in a similarly controlled population as another method to identify brainstem nuclear dysfunction in the active migraine population as a testing modality.

B. J. Balough, CAPT, MC, USN

External Ear, Middle Ear and Mastoid

Can Radiologic Imaging Replace Second-Look Procedures for Cholesteatoma?

Lin JW, Oghalai JS (Baylor College of Medicine, Houston, TX; Stanford Univ School of Medicine, CA)
Laryngoscope 121:4-5, 2011

Background.—The goals of cholesteatoma surgery are to remove disease, provide a dry, safe ear, and restore hearing. Surgeons also try to minimize any recurrent or residual cholesteatoma. Recurrent cholesteatoma is a new lesion that develops from retraction of the tympanic membrane or ear canal skin, whereas residual cholesteatoma forms from microscopic or gross disease that was missed initially. Recurrent cholesteatoma is usually easy to diagnose in the office, but residual lesions are often hidden in the mastoid or middle ear cleft. The risk of both lesions can be reduced by using canal-wall-down procedures, but the patient then must return for regular checkups lifelong and is subject to lifestyle restrictions. Canal-wall-up procedures done in a planned process of two surgeries separated by 6 to 18 months avoid this problem and are especially useful for chronic ear situations. The staged approach permits mucosal healing to preserve the middle ear space, gives time for evaluation of residual cholesteatoma, and restores hearing using ossicular chain reconstruction (OCR). For severely diseased ears the planned second-stage surgery is clearly the best approach. However, for mildly diseased ears, the surgeon may choose to perform primary OCR with no further intervention. The evidence supporting this choice and guidelines for practice were assessed.

Treatment Selection.—Residual disease is difficult to detect in the office, so after a single-stage treatment an effective means to evaluate the site is important. Modern imaging techniques are minimally invasive and quite reliable in these cases. For simple cases of recurrent cholesteatoma pearls in an otherwise well-aerated space, computed tomography (CT) scans are useful, but somewhat limited in terms of resolution and difficulty differentiating between recurrent cholesteatoma, inflamed mucosa, and scar tissue. The sensitivity and specificity of CT have been about 50%. Newer magnetic resonance imaging (MRI) techniques using diffusion-weighted fast spin echo (DW-FSE) sequences can detect cholesteatoma as a hyperintense lesion, clearly contrasted to the hypointense air, bone, granulation tissue, and scar tissue. Three studies have shown a combined result for DW-FSE of 97% sensitivity, 97% specificity, 97% positive predictive value, and 97% negative predictive value.

Guidelines.—The sensitivity of MRI long term is as yet unavailable, which is a limiting factor for choosing this method of evaluation. Therefore single-stage surgery with follow-up monitoring by imaging is advised only for mildly diseased ears that are unlikely to have any residual cholesteatoma. It is not known whether imaging is either needed or sufficient after surgery that appears to be successful.

Conclusions.—For moderately to severely diseased ears, cholesteatoma should be addressed using the planned second-stage surgical approach. For mildly diseased ears in patients from whom cholesteatoma has probably been eradicated, surgeons can use a single-stage approach followed by DW-FSE MRI evaluation. Further refinement and expansion of these guidelines awaits high-quality prospective randomized study.

▶ This article was selected because it provides a quick review of the advances in imaging technology to detect recurrent cholesteatoma after surgical excision, a topic that has been of interest in recent reviews. Even despite careful dissection, recurrence rates in canal-wall-up series have been reported in excess of 30%. As the authors discuss, this has traditionally been addressed by second-look surgery often coupled with ossicular reconstruction at the same setting. However, as prostheses using more biocompatible materials such as hydroxyapatite and titanium became available, reconstruction of the ossicular chain became more frequently undertaken at the first surgery. This along with the expense and inconvenience of further surgery has driven the desire for an alternative surveillance strategy. Diffusion-weighted MRI as reviewed holds the potential to replace routine second-look surgery. Its major limitation is in resolution to reliably detect recurrence less than 5 mm in size. With this, it remains unclear what frequency scanning should be performed and for how long, as a single negative scan does not preclude the absence of recurrence. Doubtless, there will be those who advocate that second-look surgeries should be limited in favor of routine scanning. Thus, otolaryngologists should remain conversant with this emerging literature to advocate effectively.

B. J. Balough, CAPT, MC, USN

Cholesteatoma in three dimensions: a teaching tool and an aid to improved pre-operative consent
Morris DP, Van Wijhe RG (Dalhousie Univ, Nova Scotia, Canada)
J Laryngol Otol 124:126-131, 2010

Background.—Otological surgeons face two recurring challenges. Firstly, we must foster an appreciation of the complex, three-dimensional anatomy of the temporal bone in order to enable our trainees to operate safely and independently. Secondly, we must explain to our patients the necessity for surgery which carries the potential for serious complication.

Methods.—Amira® software was applied to pre-operative computed tomography images of temporal bones with cholesteatoma, to create three-dimensional computer images. Normal structures and cholesteatoma were displayed in a user-friendly, interactive format, allowing both trainee and patient to visualise disease and important structures within the temporal bone.

Results.—Three cases, and their three-dimensional computer models are presented. Zoom, rotation and transparency functions complemented the three-dimensional effect.

Conclusion.—These three-dimensional models provided a useful adjunct to cadaveric temporal bone dissection and surgical experience for our residents' teaching programme. Also, patients with cholesteatoma reported a better understanding of their pre-operative condition when the models were used during the consenting process (Figs 2 and 7).

▶ Despite the advances of the information age, very little of this has meaningfully translated into the physician's office to improve patient care. To be certain, administrative tools such as electronic medical records and online radiology and pharmacy services have become commonplace. In this article, the truly transformative nature of the digital age is illustrated in a new technique to visually educate patients about their pathology and treatment to move closer to truly informed consent. The benefit to surgical education of residents is also discussed. A basic representation of the technique is shown in Fig 2, though the

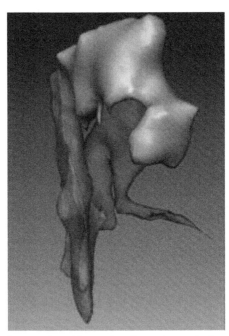

FIGURE 2.—Three-dimensional model rotated to show epitympanic disease wrapping around the head of the malleus and the body of the incus (case one). (Reprinted from Morris DP, Van Wijhe RG. Cholesteatoma in three dimensions: a teaching tool and an aid to improved pre-operative consent. *J Laryngol Otol.* 2010;124:126-131, with permission of Cambridge University Press.)

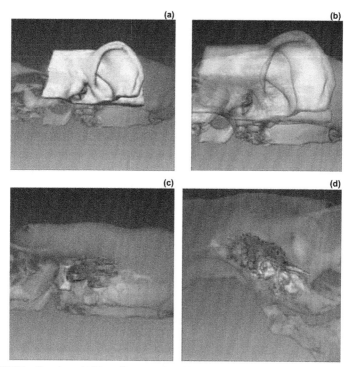

FIGURE 7.—Case three. (a) Three-dimensional model showing surface anatomy of the left pinna. Attic presentation of cholesteatoma can be seen through the ear canal. (b) Three-dimensional model with increased transparency of surface features. (c) Three-dimensional model with total transparency of surface soft tissues, revealing extensive mastoid involvement. (d) Three-dimensional model rotated to middle fossa view, showing invasion of the lateral semicircular canal. (Reprinted from Morris DP, Van Wijhe RG. Cholesteatoma in three dimensions: a teaching tool and an aid to improved pre-operative consent. *J Laryngol Otol.* 2010;124:126-131, with permission of Cambridge University Press.)

true power is best seen on ghosted 3-dimentional images of the whole temporal bone (Fig 7). The cost of the software is not described, though it is reported to import a standard digital imaging format. A main limitation for routine use is that even a basic study requires 1 hour to format by an operator. Given the complexity of the anatomy and surgical relevance, this would be physician time. Thus, the first uses of this in routine patient or resident education will likely be from libraries of standard pathologies that can then be used as interactive illustrations to complement current models. Further automation of the technology would be needed to make this useful on an individual patient basis.

B. J. Balough, CAPT, MC, USN

Combination Full- and Split-Thickness Skin Grafts for Superficial Auricular Wounds

Lear W, Odland P (Silver Falls Dermatology, Salem, OR; Skin Surgery Ctr, Seattle, WA)
Dermatol Surg 36:1453-1456, 2010

Background.—For aggressive, poorly defined, or recurrent basal cell carcinomas (BCCs) or squamous cell carcinomas (SCCs) involving the ear, Mohs micrographic surgery has achieved the highest cure rates. Although this approach preserves normal tissue, it creates a traumatic defect that must be repaired. Four categories of reconstructive options are possible for the helix and antihelix: healing by secondary intention, direct closure, flaps, and grafts. An antihelix with intact cartilage and a small or large defect can be allowed to heal by secondary intention. Direct closure and grafts are appropriate for smaller defects, and flaps are used for defects measuring 2.0 cm or larger. A novel approach combining a full-thickness skin graft (FTSG) and a single-thickness skin graft (STSG) has been developed to repair the helical rim and antihelix.

Method.—Patients are prepped and draped, then 1% lidocaine with epinephrine 1:200,000 is infiltrated around the defect and donor sites to achieve local anesthesia. The upper thigh is used for the STSG and the FTSG is taken from supraclavicular, preauricular, or postauricular skin, depending on patient preference and whether there has been previous surgery in these donor sites. The FTSG is harvested and trimmed of excess fat using sharp dissection. It is then immediately sutured into place using 6.0 fast-absorbing suture. The STSG is obtained manually using a Weck blade or electric dermatome. It is then trimmed and sutured into the remaining nonhelical part of the auricular defect. Interrupted 6.0 fast-absorbing gut suture is passed through the graft and cartilage and then looped back through the cartilage and graft to fix the STSG to the base of the defect so it follows the ear's contour. A bolster dressing is applied using cotton balls cut into small pieces, rolled in mupirocin ointment, and placed in the ear contours to immobilize and securely fix the grafts against the wound base. The graft and bolsters are to remain clean and dry. Patients are reevaluated 7 days after surgery, when the bolster is removed.

Results.—Four patients who had this technique had excellent results. Three had BCCs and one had an SCC. Defects ranged in size from 2.0 × 1.6 cm to 6.0 × 2.0 cm. The helical rim defect length was between 2.0 and 6.0 cm. On evaluation after 6 weeks, color match was excellent in all four patients, except for a small area of necrosis seen at the inferior edge of the FTSG in one patient.

Conclusions.—The single-stage option to reconstruct complex auricular defects combined FTSGs and STSGs quite effectively. This approach was

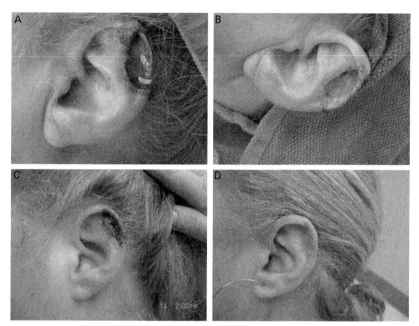

FIGURE 2.—Patient #4 (A) Mohs defect. (B) Immediate postoperative repair. (C) Day 7 postoperatively. (D) Week 6 postoperatively. (Reprinted from Lear W, Odland P. Combination full- and split-thickness skin grafts for superficial auricular wounds. *Dermatol Surg.* 2010;36:1453-1456, with acknowledgement of Blackwell Publishing.)

able to resurface and restore the ear's normal contour and normal anatomic appearance (Fig 2).

▶ The auricle is a complex structure of intricately folded skin over a cartilage framework with a distinctive cosmetic appearance. Given its exposed location, it is a frequent site for cutaneous malignancies accounting for nearly 10% of all skin cancers. As a result, there have been numerous descriptions for reconstruction of auricular defects depending on the size, shape, and location of the auricular remnant. The vast majority of these options involve advancement or rotational flaps largely because of the absence of the underlying cartilage framework. This article provides another option for repairing larger defects using full- and split-thickness skin grafts. While primarily for defects with remaining perichondrium, this technique can be used without intact perichondrium as well. It is particularly useful for the most common skin defects of the helix in which advancement of the remaining tissues would require resection of the intact cartilage framework. Fig 2 provides a good example of the type of defect in which this technique is used and very acceptable cosmetic result. Given the results obtained and that this type of defect is not infrequently encountered, this article is a useful addition to reconstructive options for the external ear.

B. J. Balough, CAPT, MC, USN

Do patients with sclerotic mastoids require aeration to improve success of tympanoplasty?

Toros SZ, Habesoglu TE, Habesoglu M, et al (Haydarpaşa Numune Education and Res Hosp, Istanbul; et al)
Acta Otolaryngol 130:909-912, 2010

Conclusion.—We could not find any significant difference in the results for graft success rate and functional hearing results between the myringoplasty and tympano-mastoidectomy groups. So mastoidectomy may not be necessary for successful tympanic membrane reconstruction and hearing improvement.

Objective.—To investigate the effect of aerating mastoidectomy on the surgical success rate of myringoplasty.

Methods.—This was a retrospective study. Data were analyzed from 92 patients who underwent surgical repair of tympanic membrane perforations due to chronic suppurative otitis media (CSOM) without cholesteatoma. Tympano-mastoidectomy was performed in 46 patients with a small sclerotic mastoid. The other 46 patients underwent myringoplasty without mastoidectomy. Patients were evaluated for success in tympanic membrane reconstruction and hearing levels after a minimum follow-up duration of 1 year.

Results.—Tympanic membrane perforation closure was successful in 76.1% ($n = 35$) of the 46 patients undergoing myringoplasty and in 78.3% ($n = 36$) of the 46 patients undergoing myringoplasty with mastoidectomy. The difference between the closure rates of the two groups was not statistically significant ($p > 0.05$). The difference between the two groups for hearing gain was also not statistically significant ($p > 0.05$).

▶ This article addresses another widely debated topic within otologic surgical treatment: whether to routinely perform mastoidectomy or not when repairing chronic tympanic membrane perforations. The bibliography provides several key articles that underpin the theory behind creating a larger pneumatized space to buffer the middle ear. More recent articles countering these theories are also presented. This concentrated discussion and list of relevant articles makes this a key article for reference on the subject. In this relatively large retrospective series of 92 patients, no benefit to mastoidectomy was observed. However, some other noteworthy things can be gleaned from their approach and results. Their overall success rate of tympanic membrane closure (76%) is low compared with most published series. Unfortunately, no stratification of middle ear risk such as the middle ear risk index or Bellucci scale is used in the series. Furthermore, it is not clear if there are revision cases in the series or—if there are—how many are in each group. This goes for pediatric cases as well. This lack of disease stratification presents a significant limitation in analysis and interpretation of the overall result and is not an uncommon failing in otologic literature. But all were performed via a postauricular approach to provide good visualization and in a uniform underlay technique. In my own practice, mastoidectomy accompanying tympanoplasty is reserved for revision cases. The theory here is not to improve aeration but rather to inspect the attic, antrum, and mastoid for residual inflammatory or cholesteatomatous disease that may have led to primary surgical failure. Thus, this article provides a good discussion and reference on the topic. It also tends to lend support against mastoidectomy in primary cases but is limited because of the methodological issues discussed.

B. J. Balough, CAPT, MC, USN

New treatment strategy and assessment questionnaire for external auditory canal pruritis: topical pimecrolimus therapy and Modified Itch Severity Scale
Acar B, Karabulut H, Sahin Y, et al (Kecioren Training and Res Hosp, Ankara, Turkey)
J Laryngol Otol 124:147-151, 2010

Objective.—We aimed to compare the efficacy of topical pimecrolimus versus hydrocortisone in treating external auditory canal pruritis, using the Modified Itch Severity Scale as an assessment tool.

Methods.—We included in the study 40 patients with isolated itching of the external auditory canal who had not received any benefit from previous topical and systemic treatments. Topical 1 per cent pimecrolimus or topical hydrocortisone was applied to each patient's external auditory canal for three months. A Modified Itch Severity Scale was developed and used to assess treatment response.

Results.—Compared with itching scores on initial assessment, the scores of patients receiving topical pimecrolimus had decreased by 52.3 per cent by the third week of treatment and by 77.6 per cent by the third month, whereas the scores of patients receiving topical hydrocortisone had decreased by 34.4 per cent by the third week and by 64.2 per cent by the third month.

Conclusions.—Topical pimecrolimus appears to be as effective as topical hydrocortisone in relieving external auditory canal pruritis. We used a novel scoring system, the Modified Itch Severity Scale, to evaluate external auditory canal pruritis; this is the first self-reporting questionnaire for the quantification of external auditory canal pruritis severity. Further studies are needed to validate this scoring system (Table 2).

▶ Otalgia and pruritis are frequent complaints for the otologist and otolaryngologist alike. Last year's review presented a study on the use of a new therapy for this condition. This represents a similar study but with some important differences, the first being the presentation of a quantifiable scale for the measurement of the symptom resolution. This Itch Severity Scale is found in Appendix 1 of the article and is a modification of a previously existing scale for use in evaluating symptoms in the external ear. This is valuable when directly comparing treatments. Despite the data demonstrating no statistically significant differences in treatment effects between the 2 agents studied, the authors claim in their

TABLE 2.—Modified Itch Severity Scale Scores Over Treatment Period

Score*	Baseline	3 Weeks	3 Months
Group 1	8.50 ± 7.66	4.05 ± 1.82	1.90 ± 1.29
Group 2	7.55 ± 1.63	4.95 ± 2.78	2.70 ± 2.67
p†	0.88	0.233	0.239

*Mean ± standard deviation.
†Wilcoxon test; group 1 vs group 2 at each time point.

conclusions that topical pimecrolimus was more effective. This is a significant flaw in an otherwise solid study. What is significant is that both treatments reduced itch severity by a significant amount within 3 weeks and this effect continued to improve until last studied at 3 months. These data are found in Table 2. Thus this study provides valuable information for evaluating effectiveness of treatment and time to symptom resolution for patients with this complaint. Furthermore, it validates pimecrolimus as an effective alternative to topical steroids and thus may find a role as a second-line therapy. Further study, however, is needed to determine if it can be used to similar benefit after steroids fail.

B. J. Balough, CAPT, MC, USN

Tympanoplasty in Chronic Otitis Media Patients With an Intact, but Severely Retracted Malleus: A Treatment Challenge
Hol MKS, Nguyen DQ, Schlegel-Wagner C, et al (Univ Med Centre, St Radboud, Nijmegen, The Netherlands; Cho Ray Hosp, Ho Chi Min City, Vietnam; Dept of Otorhinolaryngology, Lucerne, Switzerland)
Otol Neurotol 31:1412-1416, 2010

Objective.—To analyze the outcome of patients with chronic otitis media (COM) with an intact, but markedly medialized ossicular chain, treated by removing the malleus head and interposing an autologous incus and then an underlay myringoplasty.

Study Design.—Retrospective clinical study.

Setting.—Tertiary referral center.

Patients.—The search criteria within the prospective surgical database was COM with a central perforation (without cholesteatoma) with a markedly medialized malleus handle (the umbo adherent to the promontory) with an intact ossicular chain (study, n = 15) or an incus necrosis at the lenticular process (incus, n = 23). Only primary surgeries performed at our otorhinolaryngology department were included.

Intervention.—All patients underwent the same surgical procedure consisting of an autologous incus interposition and underlay myringoplasty with temporalis fascia.

Main Outcome Measure.—The patients' audiological and follow-up data were retrieved from the database. The postoperative audiogram (0.5–3 khz) with the longest follow-up was used.

Results.—The preoperative air-conduction thresholds were less impaired in the study group than in the incus group. After their surgery, all, except 3 patients, improved their hearing, and 97% had an intact tympanic membrane at a mean follow-up of 2 years. The air-bone gap was closed within 20 dB in 80% (study) and in 87% (incus), in one third of all patients even within 10 dB. Although the largest improvement was seen in the lower frequencies, closure of the air-bone gap at 4 khz was difficult to achieve.

Conclusion.—Patients presenting with COM, a (central) perforation, a medially rotated malleus and intact ossicular chain are a treatment challenge. Lateralizing the malleus handle may require disconnection of the ossicular chain and an autologous incus interposition to bring back the reconstructed tympanic membrane in its original position and improve the hearing.

▶ Long-term disease of the middle ear can result in a variety of problems. Among these are persistent perforations, conductive hearing loss, and retraction of the malleus to limit the depth of the middle ear space. This retraction of the malleus can confound typical reconstructive methods of tympanoplasty (underlay medial graft technique or lateral grafting), as in both cases the graft tissue is placed medial to the malleus and in the retracted position this may place the graft in very close proximity to the promontory. Thus, even with successful closure of the perforation, there may be a less than satisfactory hearing result because of adhesion and scarring of the graft and umbo to the promontory. The over-under graft technique can mitigate this to some degree, as in that case the graft is laterally placed to the malleus; however, even then in severely retracted cases hearing results may suffer from the limited movement of the ossicular chain. This article provides data to support a method to address this problem by disarticulating the ossicular chain to allow the malleus to be placed in a more natural position. It is important to note that the assembly reconstruction technique used here with an incus interposition supports the malleus and helps to maintain its position throughout the healing period. Columellar techniques using typical partial ossicular replacement prostheses will not achieve this same result. The data presented here support the disarticulation and reconstruction of the chain in these cases.

B. J. Balough, CAPT, MC, USN

Type 2 ossiculoplasty: prognostic determination of hearing results by middle ear risk index

Felek SA, Celik H, Islam A, et al (Ministry of Health Ankara Training and Res Hosp, Turkey; et al)
Am J Otolaryngol 31:325-331, 2010

Purpose.—The aims of this study were to investigate the prognostic impact of middle ear risk index on the postoperative hearing results in cases with type 2 ossiculoplasty; to compare the middle ear risk index results among primary, staged, and revision cases; and to compare the results of the prostheses used in ossicular reconstruction.

Material and Methods.—Records of 293 patients who had canal wall up tympanomasteidectomy and type 2 ossiculoplasty due to chronic otitis media between November 1995 and November 2007 were reviewed retrospectively.

Results.—The mean preoperative air-bone gap was 32.6 dB, and it decreased to 15.2 dB after a mean follow-up period of 26.8 months post-operatively. The mean change of air-bone gap was 17.4 dB. Postoperative air-bone gap was 20 dB or less in 79% of the cases. The patients with dry perforations were in the low-risk group, and 91% of them had an air-bone gap of 20 dB or less. This value was 86% in the ones with intact malleus. The patients who had primary surgery were found in moderate risk group, whereas staged and revision groups were in the high-risk group. The air-bone gap was 20 dB or less in 84%, 78%, and 59%, respectively, of those groups. The difference between the primary and the revision groups reached a statistical significance.

Conclusions.—We had the best ossicular reconstruction results with glass ionomer cement, whereas the worst results were obtained with allo-graft partial ossicular replacement prostheses. We determined that risk-reducing factors such as dry ear, minimal ossicular chain defect, and intact malleus were important to have successful results. The middle ear risk index is a valuable tool for the surgeon to judge the risks and the proba-bility success of the procedure as well as to make a good patient selection (Tables 1, 4 and 5).

▶ The otologic literature abounds with numerous case series of one particular reconstructive method or another. Unfortunately, nearly all do not stratify disease, so a particular method or prosthesis cannot be judged head-to-head with another. This is akin to evaluating cancer treatment methods regardless of staging or pathology. The same should be true for chronic ear disease to advance our understanding and techniques. In short, it is not the treatment from the surgeon that dictates the results but rather the status of the disease that the patient has. One such staging method for chronic ear disease used in this article is the middle ear risk index (MERI), which was originally described by Kartush in 1994 as shown in Table 1. This index combines several prior grading schemes into one weighted average. This was later revised in 2001 to include the risk from smoking on outcome.[1] This study provides a large series

TABLE 1.—Middle Ear Risk Index*

Risk Factor		Risk Value
Otorrhea	I, Dry	0
	II, Occasionally wet	1
	III, Persistently wet	2
	IV, Wet, cleft palate	3
Perforation	Absent	0
	Present	1
Cholesteatoma	O, M+ I+ S+	0
	A, M+ S+	1
	B, M+ S−	2
	C, M− S+	3
	D, M− S−	4
	E, Ossicle head fixation	2
	F, Stapes fixation	3
Middle ear (granulations or effusion)	No	0
	Yes	1
Previous surgery	None	0
	Staged	1
	Revision	2

The middle ear risk index is a term introduced by Kartush [7].
Editor's Note: Please refer to original journal article for full references.
*A value is assigned for each risk factor and then the values are added to determine the MERI. M: malleus; I: incus; S: stapes; +: present; −: absent.

TABLE 4.—Hearing Results According to MERI Categories

MERI Category	n	Mean Follow-Up X ± SD Median (Min-Max)	Preop ABG X ± SD Median (Min-Max)	Postop ABG X ± SD Median (Min-Max)	ABG Change X ± SD Median (Min-Max)	ABG ≤20 dB, n/%	ABG ≤10 dB, n/%
MERI (1–3), mild	96	27.3 ± 11.3 24 (6–84)	30.2 ± 8.9 30 (11–50)	12.3 ± 6.7 11 (0–37)	18 ± 8.4 19 (−14 to 34)	87/91	46/48
MERI (4–6), moderate	132	26.5 ± 11.1 24 (6–96)	32.8 ± 7.4 33 (12–54)	14.9 ± 7.5 14 (3–47)	18.5 (0 to 37)	112/85	36/27
MERI (7–12), severe	65	26.4 ± 13.1 24 (6–96)	36.1 ± 7.8 36 (17–55)	20.3 ± 9.8 20 (3–45)	15.9 ± 8.2 15 (−10 to 33)	33/51	14/22

n indicates number of patients; preop, preoperative; postop, postoperative.

using this indexing to predict postoperative outcomes. Table 4 demonstrates hearing results based on MERI stratification alone. While those with mild and moderate disease had similar good outcomes (air-bone gap < 20 dB), the excellent results (air-bone gap < 0 dB) are nearly twice as likely in the mild to moderate risk groups. This becomes even more apparent when staged versus primary surgical groups are compared in Table 5. Both have similar good results despite the difference in MERI of 3.9 to 6.7. Yet the excellent results are much higher in the primary group than the staged. In fact, those that were staged had an MERI similar to the revision cases, and their excellent results are similar. Thus, staging or primarily reconstruction likely has little to do with hearing outcome, but rather the MERI score does. Unfortunately, the impact of the

TABLE 5.—Middle Ear Risk Index and Hearing Results of the Surgical Procedures

Procedure	n	MERI (Min-Max)	Mean Follow-Up (mo) X ± SD Median (Min-Max)	Preop ABG X ± SD Median (Min-Max)	Postop ABG X ± SD Median (Min-Max)	ABG Change X ± SD Median (Min-Max)	ABG ≤20 dB, n/%	ABG ≤10 dB, n/%
Primary surgery	215	3.9 (1–10)	26.7 ± 11.7 24 (6–96)	31.8 ± 8.5 31 (11–55)	14.2 ± 8 13 (0–47)	17.7 ± 7.8 18 (−14 to 34)	180/84	79/37
Staged surgery	32	6.7 (4–11)	30 ± 12.6 24 (12–72)	36 ± 7.2 34 (23–52)	15.8 ± 6.5 16 (4–30)	20.2 ± 6.5 19.5 (5 to 32)	25/78	7/22
Revision surgery	46	6.8 (4–10)	25 ± 10.1 24 (6–60)	34.5 ± 7.3 36 (19–47)	19.4 ± 10 17 (3–36)	15.2 ± 7.6 13.5 (2 to 37)	27/59	10/22

n indicates number of patients; preop, preoperative; postop, postoperative.

analysis and use of the MERI is diluted by the various other analyses performed that do not account for MERI. One example is comparing autograft and allograft reconstructions. All yielded similar results in aggregate. The lack of stratification eliminates the ability to make distinctions between methods. Still, this article demonstrates the advantage of using a grading system to stratify extent of disease to more precisely judge the independent variables of surgical techniques and reconstructive methods.

B. J. Balough, CAPT, MC, USN

Reference

1. Becvarovski Z, Kartush JM. Smoking and tympanoplasty: implications for prognosis and the Middle Ear Risk Index (MERI). *Laryngoscope.* 2001;111:1806-1811.

Facial Nerve and Skull Base

Audiovestibular Factors Influencing Quality of Life in Patients With Conservatively Managed Sporadic Vestibular Schwannoma

Lloyd SKW, Kasbekar AV, Baguley DM, et al (Univ Dept of Otolaryngology–Head and Neck Surgery, Manchester, UK; Cambridge Univ Hosps NHS Foundation Trust, Cambridge, UK)
Otol Neurotol 31:968-976, 2010

Objectives.—To measure the health-related quality of life (QoL) of patients undergoing conservative management of a vestibular schwannoma and to identify audiovestibular factors that influence health-related QoL.
Study Design.—Cross-sectional case-control study.
Intervention.—Adult patients undergoing conservative management of a sporadic vestibular schwannoma were identified from a prospectively updated database. Each patient was asked to complete a series of questionnaires, including the Short Form 36 health-related QoL instrument, the Hearing Handicap Inventory, the Tinnitus Handicap Inventory, and the Dizziness Handicap Inventory. The QoL data obtained were compared

with UK normal data. Multiple linear regression was performed to identify audiovestibular factors influencing QoL.

Patients.—Of 241 patients still undergoing conservative management, 165 completed the questionnaires. The mean age was 66.6 years. Mean duration of follow-up was 5.7 years.

Results.—Physical component summary scores were significantly lower than those of the normal population. Mental component summary scores were significantly above the normal population. Regression analysis showed that dizziness handicap score and age were strong predictors of physical component summary (both $p < 0.0001$). Dizziness handicap score and tinnitus handicap score were significant predictors of mental component summary ($p = 0.0004$ and $p = 0.027$ respectively). However, the model only explained a small amount of the data, suggesting that there may be other factors influencing QoL.

Conclusion.—Dizziness is the most significant audiovestibular predictor of QoL in patients with vestibular schwannomas. Tinnitus also has an impact on mental QoL. Hearing loss does not seem to influence QoL. Other factors such as illness perception may have an important role to play in determining QoL.

▶ Management of vestibular schwannoma remains a widely debated topic with most of the attention based upon outcomes from surgery versus radiotherapy. Conservative management or watch and wait has also become a viable option. As with any treatment, the desired outcome is that the benefits exceed the risk. For watch and wait, this has primarily been no growth of tumor. This article is unique in that it seeks to evaluate the outcome from the patient's perspective in terms of quality of life (the effect of the disease and treatment from the patient's perspective) for conservative management alone as related to audiovestibular complaints. Numerous references are provided, and the introduction reviews the prior comparisons of outcomes between surgery, radiation, and conservative management very well. In their series, roughly 20% of the tumors grew, while the remainder remained the same or decreased in size. This is in keeping with other published series of conservative management. Although a large emphasis is placed by physicians on the hearing status of patients or its results after treatment, these data suggest that dizziness is of more importance to patients' overall sense of well being from a physical perspective and coupled with tinnitus a significant predictor of their mental functioning perspective. Thus, their results suggest that our emphasis on treatment should be focused in these areas as much, if not more so than in hearing. This is interesting in that complaints about hearing are frequently the cause for referral. The authors do mention that even large tumors were included in this data set, and this may limit the interpretation of their results for conservatively managed tumors that are typically small.

B. J. Balough, CAPT, MC, USN

Combinatorial Treatments Enhance Recovery Following Facial Nerve Crush
Sharma N, Moeller CW, Marzo SJ, et al (Loyola Univ Chicago, Maywood, IL;
Loyola Univ Med Ctr, Maywood, IL)
Laryngoscope 120:1523-1530, 2010

Objectives/Hypothesis.—To investigate the effects of various combinatorial treatments, consisting of a tapering dose of prednisone (P), a brief period of nerve electrical stimulation (ES), and systemic testosterone propionate (TP) on improving functional recovery following an intratemporal facial nerve crush injury.

Study Design.—Prospective, controlled animal study.

Methods.—After a right intratemporal facial nerve crush, adult male Sprague-Dawley rats were divided into the following eight treatment groups: 1) no treatment, 2) P only, 3) ES only, 4) ES + P, 5) TP only, 6) TP + P, 7) ES + TP, and 8) ES + TP + P. For each group n = 4–8. Recovery of the eyeblink reflex and vibrissae orientation and movement were assessed. Changes in peak amplitude and latency of evoked response, in response to facial nerve stimulation, was also recorded weekly.

Results.—Brief ES of the proximal nerve stump most effectively accelerated the initiation of functional recovery. Also, ES or TP treatments enhanced recovery of some functional parameters more than P treatment. When administered alone, none of the three treatments improved recovery of complete facial function. Only the combinatorial treatment of ES + TP, regardless of the presence of P, accelerated complete functional recovery and return of normal motor nerve conduction.

Conclusions.—Our findings suggest that a combinatorial treatment strategy of using brief ES and TP together promises to be an effective therapeutic intervention for promoting regeneration following facial nerve injury. Administration of P neither augments nor hinders recovery (Fig 1).

▶ This article is an interesting basic science project examining the effects of electrical stimulation and testosterone both singly and in combination for recovery of facial nerve injury. Comparison is also made to standard therapy of corticosteroid. The rationale behind both electrical stimulation and testosterone is given in good detail and with several references. In short, electrical stimulation's beneficial effects include upregulation of regeneration-associated genes, promoting regrowth, and improving targeting of regrowing axons. Gonadal steroids play both trophic and protective roles in nerve regeneration. Comment is also made on their beneficial effect on muscle helping prevent atrophy and perhaps making muscle fibers more receptive to sprouting axons. These effects are complementary, suggesting the combination would be better than each alone. A review of the literature in its use for both postparotidectomy paresis as well as in idiopathic facial nerve paralysis shows that corticosteroids, on the other hand, only offer anti-inflammatory effects. The authors describe their methodology in good detail and provide several means of analysis to judge effect on nerve recovery from the crush injury. One such analysis is shown in Fig 1 where prednisone alone is marginally better than control, and

A. Onset of Eyeblink Reflex

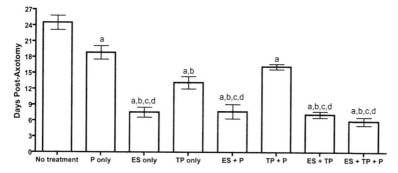

B. Complete Eyeblink Reflex

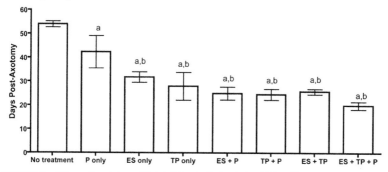

FIGURE 1.—Effects of prednisone (P), brief electrical stimulation (ES), and/or testosterone propionate (TP) on onset and complete return of the eyeblink reflex following an intratemporal facial nerve crush injury (n = 5–8/group). Shown are mean recovery times for the onset of the eyeblink reflex (A) and return of the complete eyeblink reflex (B) following administration of various combinations of P, ES, and TP treatments. As animals were followed for a maximum of 56 dpo, incomplete return of any functional parameter was designated a recovery time of 56 dpo. Vertical lines represent standard error of the mean. a = $P < .05$, relative to no treatment; b = $P < .05$, relative to P only; c = $P < .05$, relative to TP only; d = $P < .05$, relative to TP + P. (Reprinted from Sharma N, Moeller CW, Marzo SJ, et al. Combinatorial treatments enhance recovery following facial nerve crush. *Laryngoscope*. 2010;120:1523-1530, with permission from The American Laryngological, Rhinological and Otological Society, Inc.)

combined electrical stimulation and testosterone are better than either singly. The addition of prednisone did not improve this combination or single effect. One bias in the methodology is that the nerve is decompressed around the injury site to perform the crush and to place the electrical stimulation. This decompression may have limited any benefit from the anti-inflammatory effects of corticosteroids to be seen. However, the beneficial effects of testosterone and electrical stimulation are clear from the data in this model. While not a clinical study, this demonstrates some important basic science approaches to improving facial nerve recovery rates. Proximal electrical stimulation is, however, likely of limited clinical applicability in Bell palsy, given the involvement of the labyrinthine segment and the surgical approaches necessary to obtain access for proximal stimulation. Transcranial magnetic stimulation might provide a noninvasive way to induce the same electrical stimulation and could prove to be the next step in moving this to clinical applicability.

B. J. Balough, CAPT, MC, USN

Direct Nasolabial Lift, a Technique for Palliation of Oncologic Lower-Face Paralysis
Brandt MG, Franklin JH, Moore CC (Univ of Western Ontario, London, Ontario, Canada)
J Otolaryngol Head Neck Surg 39:476-478, 2010

Background.—Facial paralysis can complicate head and neck cancer, either through extension of the malignancy or as an adverse result of surgery. Despite treatment, some patients have advanced oncologic disease or comorbidities that do not permit complex facial reanimation procedures. Static suspension of the lower face unfortunately will allow the lower face to fall with time, causing poor oral competence. Often these patients are too unhealthy or uninterested in having operative techniques that require general anesthesia to resuspend or reanimate the lower face. Office-based techniques are commonly used in such cases to help the patient and limit morbidity. A well-described but seldom used technique in esthetic surgery is direct excision of the skin and subcutaneous tissue at the nasolabial fold. The drawback to the direct nasolabial lift is inconsistent scarring. However, its advantages include ease of performance, control, and minimal morbidity. It was suggested as an adjunct to the functional reconstruction of the lower face.

Method.—A crescent or triangle is outlined at the superior edge of the nasolabial crease. The region is infiltrated with local anesthetic, then the skin and subcutaneous tissues are excised. The edges are reapproximated to ensure adequate lift; if needed, further skin and subcutaneous tissue is excised. Closure is accomplished in two layers using an absorbable-braided suture in an inverted interrupted fashion for the deep layer and an absorbable monofilament suture in a subcuticular fashion for the superficial layer. Antibiotic ointment is applied twice a day for 2 weeks.

Results.—Four patients seeking palliative restoration of oral competence underwent direct nasolabial lifts. All had extensive malignant disease that had required radical parotidectomy. Two patients had undergone static sling procedures initially that failed to restore function to the oral commissure. The other two selected a local office-based procedure. In all cases the patients reported much improved oral function, complete resolution of drooling and buccal mucosal biting, improved mastication, better oral phase swallowing, and less slurred speech. Mouth care and the insertion or removal of dental appliances were not affected. Patients also subjectively felt their quality of life improved.

Conclusions.—Most of the procedures needed to rehabilitate a paralyzed lower face require general anesthesia. The direct nasolabial lift procedure is an outpatient procedure that does not change the overall diameter of the mouth, produces tightening of the buccal soft tissue, and diminishes the occurrence of inadvertent cheek biting. As a result, patients achieve a better quality of life with limited morbidity.

▶ A great deal of attention and literature is rightfully placed on the rehabilitation of the eye after facial paralysis.[1-3] While not as urgent, dysfunction of the oral commissure can adversely affect quality of life to a significant degree. Most techniques to rehabilitate the lower facial function typically require significant operations under general anesthesia (facial sling or muscle transfers), further tissue sacrifice (cheiloplasty), or both (nerve grafting). Often for patients with loss of function after resection for malignancy, further significant surgery or delayed results are not good options. Here the authors describe a simple office procedure that can be used either alone or as a follow-on to prior suspension procedures when the result has been unsatisfactory and which has acceptable cosmetic results. A further advantage is that it can be easily repeated as needed. In the comment, a good discussion is provided of the various quality-of-life measures that have been used to describe the impact of oral function on overall quality of life. These references serve as a useful review for those interested in the topic. Unfortunately, these assessments were not performed on this series of patients pre- and postprocedure, and this is a minor limitation of this article. However, this still proves to be a useful reference for a technique to use in patients with poor oral competency and unwilling or unable to undergo more extensive reconstruction.

B. J. Balough, CAPT, MC, USN

References

1. Hassan SJ, Weymuller EA Jr. Assessment of quality of life in head and neck cancer patients. *Head Neck.* 1993;15:485-496.
2. Bjordal K, Ahlner-Elmqvist M, Tollesson E, et al. Development of a European Organization for Research and Treatment of Cancer (EORTC) questionnaire module to be used in quality of life assessments in head and neck cancer patients: EORTC Quality of Life Study Group. *Acta Oncol.* 1994;33:879-885.
3. Terrell JE, Nanavati KA, Esclamado RM, Bishop JK, Bradford CR, Wolf GT. Head and neck cancer-specific quality of life: instrument validation. *Arch Otolaryngol Head Neck Surg.* 1997;123:1125-1132.

Gamma Knife Surgery of Vestibular Schwannomas: Volumetric Dosimetry Correlations to Hearing Loss Suggest Stria Vascularis Devascularization as the Mechanism of Early Hearing Loss
Wackym PA, Runge-Samuelson CL, Nash JJ, et al (Med College of Wisconsin, Milwaukee)
Otol Neurotol 31:1480-1487, 2010

Objective.—Determine which variables are correlated with early hearing changes after gamma knife surgery of vestibular schwannomas (VSs).

Study Design.—Prospective clinical study of hearing outcomes, radiation dosimetry, conformity, and tumor size of all sporadic unilateral VS patients treated between June 2000 and July 2009.

Setting.—Tertiary referral center.

Patients.—Fifty-nine VS patients with at least 6 months of follow-up data were studied.

Interventions.—Audiometry and imaging were performed to determine auditory thresholds, speech discrimination, and tumor size. Radiation doses to 5 volumes were measured.

Main Outcome Measures.—Pretreatment and posttreatment comparisons were performed with regard to change in tumor size; radiation dose to specific volumes including the internal auditory canal, cochlea, basal turn of the cochlea, and modiolus; and conformity of the treatment.

Results.—The mean follow-up was 63.76 months (standard deviation, ± 29.02 mo; range, 9–109 mo). The median follow-up was 65.5 months. A statistically significant association between maximum radiation dose to the cochlea volume and 3-frequency pure-tone average in patients starting with 50 dB or lesser PTA3 was demonstrated using linear regression analysis.

Conclusion.—Longitudinal changes in hearing occur over time, with the largest changes seen in the first 12 months after treatment. With our study outcomes as basis, limiting the dose of radiation to the cochlea to no more than 4 Gy would likely reduce vascular injury to the stria vascularis and improve hearing outcomes. Shielding the cochlea during the treatment

TABLE 1.—Temporal Bone Volumes Measured, their Radiation-Susceptible Structures, Audiologic Consequences of Injury, and the Radiation Doses Delivered

Volume Measured	Predicted Target	Audiologic Consequence	Maximum Radiation Dose Delivered (Gy)
Cochlea	Stria vascularis, global hair cell loss	Stria vascularis devascularization would result in a strial presbyacusis-like pattern with hearing loss across all frequencies and relative preservation of speech discrimination ability	10.76 (SD, ±5.96)
Basal turn of the cochlea	Hair cell loss in basal turn of the cochlea	Sensory presbyacusis-like pattern with hearing loss affecting the high frequencies and relative preservation of speech discrimination ability	5.22 (SD, ±3.61)
Modiolus	Spiral ganglion neurons, primary afferent dendrites	Neural presbyacusis-like pattern with down-sloping high-frequency hearing loss combined with poor speech discrimination ability	12.26 (SD, ±6.46)
Internal auditory canal	Labyrinthine artery, primary afferent axons, efferent axons	Global loss of hearing and speech discrimination ability	24.21 (SD, ±3.09)

SD indicates standard deviation.

planning process would be one mechanism to accomplish this goal (Table 1).

▶ Stereotactic radiotherapy has become an accepted treatment modality for vestibular schwannomas with efficacy in preventing tumor growth and facial nerve preservation rates comparable to microsurgical resection. This study is significant in that it now attempts to further define modifications to improve hearing preservation in these cases. In this regard, an analogy can be made to the evolution of surgical treatment of these tumors where techniques to preserve facial nerve function followed development of approaches to safely remove the tumors and this in turn was followed by methods to preserve hearing. The authors analyze the data from this prospective cohort in a variety of ways to better understand the factors affecting early hearing loss after radiotherapy. This degree of audiologic evaluation is generally not seen in studies of radiotherapy for vestibular schwannomas. In the discussion, the various theories that account for posttreatment hearing loss are reviewed, compared with the data set, and analyzed to determine if the hearing loss pattern fits with the proposed cause, and these are summarized in Table 1. Given that the radiation tolerance of these structures is unknown, this type of analysis currently is the best available method to localize the cochlear source for the hearing loss. The importance here is to use this information to design different treatment strategies of dose or shielding to improve hearing outcomes or to develop interventions to be given during and after treatment to limit the strial injury.

B. J. Balough, CAPT, MC, USN

Jugular Foramen Tumors: Clinical Characteristics and Treatment Outcomes
Fayad JN, Keles B, Brackmann DE (House Ear Inst and House Ear Clinic, Los Angeles, CA)
Otol Neurotol 31:299-305, 2010

Objective.—To describe the diagnosis, management, and treatment outcome of jugular foramen (JF) tumors.
Study Design.—Retrospective chart review.
Methods.—Charts of the 83 patients diagnosed with JF tumors between January 1997 and May 2008 were reviewed. Presenting symptoms, otologic and neurotologic examination, audiologic thresholds, treatment procedure, surgical technique, tumor size and classification, and postoperative complications were recorded. Facial nerve function was graded using the House-Brackmann scale. Extent of tumor removal was determined at time of surgery, followed by routine radiographic follow-up.
Results.—The mean age of patients with JF tumors was 48.5 years (standard deviation, 16.3 yr), and women (79.5%) outnumbered men (20.5%). Most had glomus jugulare (GJ) tumors (n = 67, 80.7%); 9 patients had lower cranial nerve schwannomas (10.8%), and 7 patients had meningiomas (8.4%). The most frequent initial symptoms included pulsatile tinnitus (84.3%), conductive hearing loss (75.9%), and hoarseness

TABLE 1.—Demographic Characteristics of Patients with JF Tumors by Tumor Type

	GJ, n = 67	Schwannoma, n = 9	Meningioma, n = 7	All, n = 83
Sex, female/male (%)	85.1/14.9	44.4/55.6	71.4/28.6	79.5/20.5
Side, right/left (%)	44.8/52.2	55.6/44.4	71.4/28.6	48.2/49.4
Age, mean yr (SD)	50.2 (16.1)	43.8 (16.1)	39.0 (16.4)	48.5 (16.3)
Tumor size, mean cm (SD)[a]	2.6 (1.2)	3.6 (1.1)	3.5 (1.4)	2.8 (1.2)
PTA, mean dB (SD)	43.5 (31.2)	51.3 (50.0)	17.5 (11.3)	42.6 (32.7)

[a]ANOVA, $p < 0.03$.

TABLE 2.—Symptoms and Findings (% of Patients) for 83 Patients with JF Tumors by Tumor Type

Symptoms	GJ, %	Schwannoma, %	Meningioma, %	All, %
Pulsatile tinnitus	89.6	55.6	71.4	84.3
Hearing loss	80.6	55.6	57.1	75.9
Hoarseness	28.4	55.6	57.1	34.9
Dizziness	20.9	33.3	26.6	22.9
Vertigo	16.4	33.3	0.0	16.9
Headache	16.4	44.4	14.3	19.3
Swallowing problem	13.4	22.2	14.3	14.5
Aural fullness	12.1	0.0	0.0	9.8
Otalgia	10.5	0.0	0.0	8.4
Unsteadiness	7.5	11.1	14.3	8.4
Dysphagia	6.0	1.1	14.3	6.0
Discharge	6.0	22.2	0.0	7.2
Signs				
Retrotympanic mass	91.0	11.1	42.9	78.3
Vocal cord paralysis	11.9	11.1	42.8	13.3
Shoulder weakness	9.0	22.2	28.6	12.0
Absent GAG reflex	7.5	33.3	26.6	12.0
Glossal atrophy	9.0	11.1	28.6	10.8
Facial nerve dysfunction	3.0	0.0	0.0	2.4

(34.9%). Sixty-one patients (73.5%) underwent surgery, 18.1% had radiotherapy, and 8.4% were observed. Total tumor removal was achieved in 81% of surgery cases. New lower cranial nerve (CN) deficits occurred after surgery in 18.9% of GJ, 22.2% of schwannoma, and 50% of the 4 meningiomas. At last follow-up, 88.1% of surgical patients had normal or nearnormal (House-Brackmann I or II) facial function.

Conclusion.—Total resection of GJ tumors, meningiomas, and lower CN schwannomas can be a curative treatment. However, subtotal removal may be required to preserve CN function, vital vascular structures, and the brainstem. Postoperative radiotherapy is used to control residual tumor. When postoperative complications develop in patients, early rehabilitation is important to decrease mortality and morbidity. Therefore, patients should be closely followed (Tables 1 and 2).

▶ Tumors of the jugular foramen are lesions of the cranial base that can have extensive involvement by the time of their diagnosis. This report provides a very large series of these rare tumors and thus provides a valuable reference. The majority were paragangliomas with the minority schwannomas and meningiomas. Table 2 provides a summary of their presenting symptoms and findings. Pulsatile tinnitus was the most common symptom, but glomus lesions nearly matched by hearing loss. Interestingly, though an uncommon symptom, aural fullness was only seen in glomus tumors. Lower cranial nerve involvement (vocal cord paralysis, glossal atrophy, shoulder weakness), though present in all, was more common in meningioma indicating its more aggressive nature. Despite the increased use of stereotactic radiation for other tumors of the skull base, these were primarily treated by surgery alone. Table 5 in the original article demonstrates the approaches used. The infratemporal fossa approach was used for glomus and meningioma tumors but least often used for schwannomas. Facial nerve preservation (House-Brackmann grade 1 or 2) was high initially (> 70%) and improved to nearly 90% by last follow-up. Although few in number, meningiomas did not show this trend but had a worsening facial nerve function over time to only 25% good function by last follow-up. Regarding lower cranial nerve function, the authors emphasize subtotal resection as necessary to preserve function as well as in the elderly. As much as 30% of the entire group developed recurrence. The data and references within this series will likely serve for many years as the primary reference on this topic.

B. J. Balough, CAPT, MC, USN

Management of Complex Cases of Petrous Bone Cholesteatoma

Pandya Y, Piccirillo E, Mancini F, et al (Gruppo Otologico, Casa Di Cura, Piacenza, Italy)

Ann Otol Rhinol Laryngol 119:514-525, 2010

Objectives.—In a retrospective analysis of a quaternary referral neuro-otologic private practice, we identify complex cases of petrous bone cholesteatoma (ie, cases with encasement of vital structures such as the internal carotid artery, jugular bulb, and sigmoid sinus, with further extension to the clivus, sphenoid sinus, or rhinopharynx), review surgical approaches and techniques of management of vital structures, and propose the ideal surgical management.

Methods.—We performed a retrospective case study of 130 cases of petrous bone cholesteatoma submitted to surgery between 1979 and 2009 to identify the complex cases and their classification, approach used, outcomes, and recurrences.

Results.—Of 130 cases, 13 were complex. Facial palsy was the presenting feature in 11 cases, 7 of which presented with grade VI palsy. A long duration of facial palsy (more than 3 years) was seen in 5 cases. Clival involvement was seen in 6 cases; 1 case extended to the sphenoid sinus, and 1 to the rhinopharynx. The internal carotid artery was encased in 11 cases in the vertical and the horizontal parts. The jugular bulb was involved in 7 cases. Modified transcochlear approaches or infratemporal fossa approaches were used in all cases. There were no recurrences.

Conclusions.—Classification is fundamental to choosing the right surgical approach. Transotic and modified transcochlear approaches hold the key to treating complex cases. Infratemporal fossa approach type B has to be used for extension into the clivus, sphenoid sinus, or rhinopharynx. Internal carotid artery, jugular bulb, and sigmoid sinus involvement should be identified before operation (Table 1).

▶ This article covers a 30-year experience with petrous bone cholesteatomas. In particular, the deemed complexes are covered in detail, and a careful discussion of the management details is described. Complex lesions are defined as those that involve vital vascular structures (internal carotid, sigmoid sinus, jugular bulb) or extend into the clivus, sphenoid sinus, or rhinopharynx. The Sanna classification is provided in Table 1 as a reference for understanding the classes of petrous bone cholesteatomas and their extensions. This framework, along with radiologic images, is useful in understanding the subdivisions of the petrous bone as it relates to the important structures that pass through it.

TABLE 1.—Sanna's Classification for Petrous Bone Cholesteatoma

Class	Location	Extension
Class I: supralabyrinthine	Geniculate ganglion of facial nerve	Anterior: horizontal part of ICA Posterior: posterior bony labyrinth Medial: IAC, petrous apex Inferior: basal turn of cochlea
Class II: infralabyrinthine	Hypotympanic and infralabyrinthine cells	Anterior: ICA vertical part, petrous apex, clivus Posterior: dura of posterior cranial fossa and sigmoid sinus Medial: IAC, lower clivus, occipital condyle Inferior: jugular bulb, lower cranial nerves
Class III: infralabyrinthine-apical	Infralabyrinthine compartment, ICA reaching to petrous apex	Anterior: ICA vertical and/or horizontal parts Posterior: posterior fossa through retrofacial air cells Medial: petrous apex, clivus, sphenoid sinus, rhinopharynx Inferior: jugular bulb, lower cranial nerves
Class IV: massive	Entire otic capsule	Anterior: ICA vertical and/or horizontal parts Posterior: posterior fossa dura and IAC Medial: petrous apex, superior and mid-clivus, sphenoid sinus Inferior: infralabyrinthine compartment
Class V: apical	Petrous apex	Anterior: Meckel's cave area and may involve nerve V Posterior: IAC and posterior cranial fossa Medial: superior or midclivus, sphenoid sinus Inferior: infralabyrinthine compartment

ICA — internal carotid artery; IAC — internal auditory canal.

Several case discussions are provided with illustrations and radiographs to better understand this complex anatomy and the requisite surgical approaches for the particular extent of disease. However, the discussion section provides the most important aspects of this article. A small but extremely important point is made that disease of this extent develops slowly over time. Two main factors are thought to be causal for delay in diagnosis: (1) persistent discharge from mastoid cavities that is assumed to be from the cavity itself and not because of continued disease and (2) facial palsy that is assumed to be idiopathic. In both situations, lack of evaluation leads to delay in diagnosis. One example given was a 5-year delay, including facial reanimation procedures, before diagnosis was made. CT is a simple method for identification of disease with confirmation via MRI. Additional valuable information regarding choice of operative approach, techniques for handling dural and vascular involvement, use of endoscopes, and closure of the cavity are provided.

B. J. Balough, CAPT, MC, USN

Outcomes

10-Year Review of Endolymphatic Sac Surgery for Intractable Meniere Disease

Hu A, Parnes LS (Univ of Western Ontario, London, Ontario)
J Otolaryngol Head Neck Surg 39:415-421, 2010

Objective.—To review our 10-year experience of endolymphatic sac surgery (ESS) for intractable Meniere disease (MD).

Design.—Retrospective chart review and survey.

Setting.—Tertiary care centre.

Methods.—Patients presenting for ESS from 1998 to 2007 were reviewed using the 1995 American Academy of Otolaryngology–Head and Neck Surgery (AAO-HNS) guidelines. A quality of life (QOL) questionnaire was mailed out using the Dillman method.

Main Outcome Measures.—(1) 1995 AAO-HNS hearing stage, vertigo class, and functional level; (2) complications and secondary treatments; (3) a 40-question, disease-specific, validated QOL questionnaire (Meniere's Disease Outcome Questionnaire).

Results.—Thirty patients (33 ears) had ESS (63.6% male, mean age 49 years, mean follow-up 30.6 months). Vertigo control was 35.5% class A, 29.0% class B, 6.5% class C, 0% class D, 3.2% class E, and 25.8% class F. If class A and B are considered successful, then 64.5% were successful. Hearing stage improved in 14.8%, remained the same in 51.9%, and worsened in 33.3%. Average preoperative functional level was 4.3 and postoperative level was 3.5 ($p = .0016$). Secondary treatment after ESS was performed in 26%. Three patients (10.0%) had profound sensorineural hearing loss. Twenty-five questionnaire responses (75.8%) were received. There was a significant increase in QOL scores ($p = .000001$), and 80% had an improvement in QOL scores.

Conclusions.—ESS is a surgical option for MD that offers relief from vertigo in selected patients, but patients need to be cautioned about the risk of hearing loss and the requirement for subsequent destructive treatment in a significant proportion of cases (Fig 5).

▶ Surgery of the endolymphatic sac has been among the most studied, longest lasting, and most controversial topics in the otolaryngologic literature. Not infrequently, the debate has reached religious fervor with those who do and those who do not endorse the performance of the procedure. For a disorder that affects as many as 2 per 1000 population (roughly the same rate as asthma), the continuing debate over a procedure that has been around for more than 80 years is always intriguing. One of the many debates centers on the fact that sac procedures offer no better long-term results than the natural history of the disorder. Although retrospective, the study is well controlled and results are carefully examined. As a result, the numbers are small, only 30 patients, which in that context is a minor limitation. One reason for this is that the authors acknowledge that transtympanic gentamicin is their preferred method of second-line therapy. This is an important point, as the results here are from a group not considered to be of the sac camp and can thus be considered unbiased toward favoring a positive outcome. Three main points emerge from the study. First, for those who have previously failed more conservative treatment, a sac procedure provides good to excellent vertigo control in two-thirds. If diet and diuretics can be considered to be effective in a similar number, some 90% of patients with Meniere disease can receive long-term benefit from these 2 nonablative approaches. Second, the importance of treatment impact on quality of life over and above strict vertigo control is presented. This is graphically represented in Fig 5 in which large improvements in all 3 domains (mental, physical, and social) are shown. Third, the authors comment on the risk to

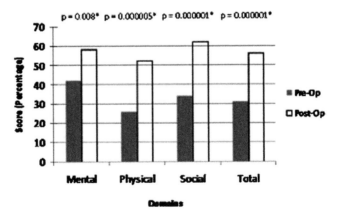

FIGURE 5.—Results of the validated, disease-specific quality of life questionnaire, the Meniere's Disease Outcomes Questionnaire. Forty questions were divided into three domains: mental, physical, and social. There were significant increases in scores in all three domains and in the total score after endolymphatic sac surgery. (Reprinted from Hu A, Parnes LS. 10-Year review of endolymphatic sac surgery for intractable Meniere disease. *J Otolaryngol Head Neck Surg.* 2010;39:415-421, with permission from The Canadian Society of Otolaryngology-Head & Neck Surgery.)

hearing and the need to carefully counsel patients. However, in their methods, they comment that incision and drainage of the sac is their method. Several other large studies have shown equal efficacy with sac-vein decompression rather than incision and drainage and that decompression does not carry the sensorineural hearing loss risk associated with incision and drainage. Thus, this study's results further lend support to sac-vein decompression over drainage in this regard. The bibliography and comparison of their results to other significant studies make this a worthy review article on the topic.

B. J. Balough, CAPT, MC, USN

Long-Term Benefit Perception, Complications, and Device Malfunction Rate of Bone-Anchored Hearing Aid Implantation for Profound Unilateral Sensorineural Hearing Loss
Gluth MB, Eager KM, Eikelboom RH, et al (Univ of Western Australia, Perth, Australia; Ear Science Inst Australia, Perth)
Otol Neurotol 31:1427-1434, 2010

Objective.—To longitudinally evaluate short- and long-term subject satisfaction/benefit perception, device usage rates, complication rates, and external device repair rates of bone-anchored hearing aid (BAHA) implantation on a cohort of adult subjects with profound unilateral sensorineural hearing loss (PUSHL).

Study Design.—Prospective clinical trial.

Setting.—Tertiary referral center.

Patients.—Fifty-six adults with PUSHL, 21 of which underwent BAHA implantation (followed for an average of 3.2 years after implantation; range, 0.8–4.6 yr).

Main Outcome Measures.—Short- and long-term satisfaction/benefit perception outcomes consisting of the Glasgow Hearing Aid Benefit Profile, Abbreviated Profile of Hearing Aid Benefit, and Single-Sided Deafness Questionnaire, including a comparison of results between implanted and nonimplanted subjects. Short- and long-term device usage rates, complications, and device failure issues also were carefully documented.

Results.—There were statistically significant improvements in nearly all measures of benefit perception documented as well as a high rate of long-term device usage (81%). Although satisfaction and benefit perception outcomes generally tended to regress over time when compared with initial short-term outcomes, long-term scores still tended to be significantly improved nevertheless as compared with preoperative levels. Approximately 38% of implants experienced severe local skin reactions (Grade 2 and above) around the implant site at some point throughout the follow-up period, whereas only one (4.8%) required implant removal. 66.7% of subjects required repair of their external sound processor.

Conclusion.—BAHA implantation seems to provide a high level of short- and long-term perceived benefit and satisfaction in subjects with PUSHL and high rate of long-term device usage. Implant site adverse local skin reactions and repairs of the external sound processor were quite common (Table 5).

▶ Use of bone-anchored hearing appliance technologies for the rehabilitation of single-sided deafness has become a common otolaryngology practice. This article is significant in that it examines both short- as well as long-term assessments (average 3.2 years) after implantation. This provides useful information on the continued use and reliability of the devices. In the short-term group,

TABLE 5.—Short- and Long-Term Single-Sided Deafness Questionnaire Results for Implanted Subjects

Question no.	Question	Possible Responses	Short-Term Responses of Respondents n	%	Long-Term Responses of Respondents n	%
1	How many days per week do you use your device?	7 d/wk	6	33	5	38.5
		5–6 d/wk	11	61	6	46.2
		3–4 d/wk	1	6	2	15.4
2	How many hours per day do you use your device?	More than 8	10	55	5	38.5
		Between 4 and 8	7	39	7	53.8
		Between 2 and 4	1	6	1	7.7
3	Has your quality of life improved?	Yes	13	72	9	69.2
		No	1	6	0	0
		Mixed	4	22	4	30.8
4	Try to determine your satisfaction... (10-point rating scale)	Average score	7.8		8.5	
		Range	6–10		6–10	
5.1	Talking to 1 person in a quiet situation	Better	15	83	10	76.9
		No difference	3	17	2	15.4
		Worse	0	0	1	7.7
5.2	Talking to 1 person among a group?	Better	15	83	8	61.5
		No difference	3	17	3	23.1
		Worse	0	0	2	15.4
5.3	Listening to music?	Better	13	72	6	46.2
		No difference	5	28	3	23.1
		Worse	0	0	4	30.8
5.4	Listening to TV/radio?	Better	14	78	7	53.8
		No difference	4	22	3	23.1
		Worse	0	0	2	15.4
		Result missing			1	7.7
5.5	At the dinner table?	Better	16	88	9	69.2
		No difference	1	6	0	0
		Worse	0	0	4	30.8
		Result missing	1	6		
6	Locating where a sound is coming from?	Yes	3	16	0	0
		No	6	33	8	61.5
		Mixed	7	39	4	30.8
		No difference	1	6	1	7.7
		Result missing	1	6		
7	How satisfied are you with the aesthetics? (10-point rating scale)		8.4		7.2	
		Range	4–10		5–10	
8	How do you find the handling of the device?	Very easy	7	39	5	38.5
		Easy	10	55	6	46.2
		Acceptable	1	6	2	15.4

n (%) indicates percentage of subject responses.

some 94% wore their devices > 5 days per week, while in the long-term group, 84% were still using the devices with that degree of frequency. Similar slight declines over time were observed for the other measures studied, and these are represented in Table 5. Noteworthy is that all these patients were highly selected after 2 weeks of test band wear. Local wound complications over time were relatively high and continued throughout the observation period with more than one-third of these occurring after 1 year from implantation. The authors do note that they used the originally described skin flap technique. This rate may be lower with the single-incision technique. There was also a high rate of device failures, requiring repairs. This is of concern as is described in the article that these repairs, unlike those typical for hearing aids, required sending the devices to the manufacturer. The discussion section provides very good commentary on this data set and its implications for shaping patient expectations in the long-term care, maintenance, and expected benefits from this technology; there will be a considerable investment of time, effort, and finances by the patient. It is interesting that this type of study is not provided by the manufacturers in terms of postmarketing surveillance, continued use, device reliability/repair, and satisfaction. Thus, we are dependent on small numbers of patient data from papers such as this.

B. J. Balough, CAPT, MC, USN

Systematic Review of Middle Ear Implants: Do They Improve Hearing as Much as Conventional Hearing Aids?
Tysome JR, Moorthy R, Lee A, et al (St Thomas' Hosp, London, UK)
Otol Neurotol 31:1369-1375, 2010

Objective.—A systematic review to determine whether middle ear implants (MEIs) improve hearing as much as hearing aids.

Data Sources.—Databases included MEDLINE, EMBASE, DARE, and Cochrane searched with no language restrictions from 1950 or the start date of each database.

Study Selection.—Initial search found 644 articles, of which 17 met the inclusion criteria of MEI in adults with a sensorineural hearing loss, where hearing outcomes and patient-reported outcome measures (PROMs) compared MEI with conventional hearing aids (CHAs).

Data Extraction.—Study quality assessment included whether ethical approval was gained, the study was prospective, eligibility criteria specified, a power calculation made and appropriate controls, outcome measures, and analysis performed. Middle ear implant outcome analysis included residual hearing, complications, and comparison to CHA in terms of functional gain, speech perception in quiet and in noise, and validated PROM questionnaires.

Data Synthesis.—Because of heterogeneity of outcome measures, comparisons were made by structured review.

Conclusion.—The quality of studies was moderate to poor with short follow-up. The evidence supports the use of MEI because, overall, they

TABLE 1.—Characteristics of Studies

Study	No. Patients	MEI	Controls	Outcome Measures	Follow-Up/mo	Level of Evidence
Fisch et al. (11)	47	VSB	Own CHA	PTA	3	2b
Fraysse et al. (12)	25	VSB	Own CHA	PTA Bisyllabic word test APHAB	6–22	3b
Lenarz et al. (2)	34	VSB	Own CHA	PTA Freiburger test Göttinger test	36	2b
Luetje et al. (3)	53	VSB	Own CHA	PTA NU-6 R-SPIN PHAP, HDSS and SHACQ	1.5 for VSB D 3 for VSB P	3b
Schmuziger et al. (13)	20	VSB	Own CHA	PTA Freiberger Basler Satz	24	3b
Snik and Cremers (14)	14, although only 5 included	VSB	Own CHA in 5 patients	PTA PS65	Not stated	4
Todt et al. (15)	5	VSB	Own CHA	PTA Freiburger test APHAB	12	2b
Truy et al. (16)	6	VSB	Own CHA	PTA Word/speech recognition tests not specified	3	2b
Uziel et al. (17)	6	VSB	Own CHA	PTA Fournier words APHAB HDSS	Mean 17	3b
Verhaegen et al. (18)	VSB = 22 MET = 10	VSB METS	Matched CHA n = 47	PTA PS65	2	4
Jenkins et al. (19)	282	METS	Own CHA	PTA SRS using CNC words APHAB	12	3b
Jenkins et al. (20)	20	METT	Own CHA	PTA NU-6 CNC APHAB	3	2b
Chen et al. (21)	7	EE	Own CHA	PTA CID-W22 HINT APHAB	10	2b
Hough et al. (1)	103	SOUNDTEC	Own CHA	PTA NU-6 words SPIN APHAB	12	2b
Roland et al. (22)	23	SOUNDTEC	Own CHA	PTA NU-6 SPIN APHAB, HEIP	5	3b
Silverstein et al. (23)	64	SOUNDTEC	Own CHA	PTA NU-6 HINT	3	3b
Kodera et al. (24)	6	Rion	Own CHA	PTA 57-S	Not specified	4

57-S indicates 50 monosyllabic words in Japanese; Basler Satz, SPIN modified in German; CID-W22, 200 monosyllabic words arranged in 4 lists of 50; CNC, Consonant-Nucleus-Consonant (500 monosyllabic words); EE, Esteem Envoy; Fournier word list, disyllabic words in French; Freiburger, monosyllabic words in German; Göttinger, sentences in German; HINT, Hearing in noise test; 250 sentences organized into 25 phonemically balanced lists of 10; METS, Middle Ear Transducer Semi-implantable; METT, Middle Ear Transducer Totally implantable; NU-6, North Western University Auditory Test (200 monosyllabic words); PS65, aided phoneme score in quiet; PTA, Pure-tone audiogram; R-SPIN, Revised speech perception in noise; SPIN, speech perception in noise; VSB D, Vibrant Soundbridge with Digital Processor; VSB P, VSB with Analogue Processor.

Editor's Note: Please refer to original journal article for full references.

TABLE 3.—Audiologic Outcomes of MEI

Study	No. Patients	MEI	Residual Hearing	Functional Gain Versus CHA	Speech Perception in Quiet Versus CHA	Speech Perception in Noise Versus CHA
Fisch et al. (11)	47	VSB	=			
Fraysse et al. (12)	25	VSB	=	+[1]	=	+
Lenarz et al (2)	34	VSB	=	=	+	=
Luetje et al. (3)	53	VSB	=	+ +	+	=
Schmuziger et al. (13)	20	VSB	– –		=	=
Snik and Cremers (14)	5*	VSB	=		– –	
Todt et al. (15)	5	VSB	=	=	=	
Truy et al. (16)	6	VSB	=	+ +	+ +	= =
Uziel et al. (17)	6	VSB		=	+ +	+ +[3]
Verhaegen et al. (18)	22 VSB 10MET	VSB METS	=[4]	=[2]	=	
Jenkins et al. (19)	282	METS	=[4]			
Jenkins et al. (20)	20	METT			=	
Chen et al. (21)	7	EE	=	– –[6]	– –[5]	
Hough et al. (1)	103	SOUNDTEC	=	+	+ +	+
Roland et al. (22)	23	SOUNDTEC	=		+ +	=
Silverstein et al. (23)	64	SOUNDTEC	– –[8]		=	=
Kodera et al. (24)	6	Rion	=[9]	–[7]		+ +

+ + indicates significant positive outcome; – –, significant negative outcome; =, no difference; +, positive outcome (not significant or no significance reported); –, negative outcome (not significant or no significance reported); if no entry, not performed or not reported; METS, MET semi-implantable; METT, MET totally implantable; 1, VSB D; 2, VSB P; 3, signal-to-noise ratio of 10; 4, At 3-mo follow-up; 5, monaural words; 6, up to 2 kHz; 7, at 3 kHz; 8, Center A (n = 37); 9, Center B (n = 31).

Editor's Note: Please refer to original journal article for full references.

*, 14 patients in study but only 5 compared with CHA.

do not decrease residual hearing, result in a functional gain in hearing comparable to CHA, and may improve perception of speech in noise and sound quality. We recommend the publication of long-term results comparing MEI with CHA, reporting a minimum of functional gain, speech perception in quiet and in noise, complications, and a validated PROM to guide the engineering of the new generation of MEI in the future (Tables 1 and 3).

▶ Over the past decade, we have seen the emergence of middle ear implanted hearing devices as a new technology. Several designs and companies are still in their early stages of development, Food and Drug Administration approval, and/or clinical use. And some, such as the SOUNDTEC device, have been brought to market and are now no longer available or supported. In any event, they appear to be here to stay as the technology improves and their role becomes better defined. Thus, this article serves as a useful review of the available literature for those seeking to understand middle ear implanted devices better and become knowledgeable on the subject either to incorporate them into their own practice or to educate patients who inquire. The 2 major competing technical approaches—electromagnetically driven or piezoelectric—are described, as is a brief description of the companies' designs for each. Table 1 lists the studies included in this meta-analysis, and Table 3 provides the corresponding listing of audiologic outcomes. Most have limited periods of follow-up, and none were randomized (although prior hearing aid use was included in nearly all) nor do any compare one device with another. The authors do an excellent job of summarizing the available data on the risks and comparative benefits to conventional hearing aids as well as the limitations of their review.

B. J. Balough, CAPT, MC, USN

Basic and Clinical Research

A Self-Adjusting Ossicular Prosthesis Containing Polyurethane Sponge
Yamada H, Goode RL (Stanford Univ Med Ctr Dept of Otolaryngology–Head and Neck Surgery, CA; Palo Alto Veterans Health Care System, CA)
Otol Neurotol 31:1404-1408, 2010

Hypothesis.—Middle ear ossicular replacement prostheses whose length can adjust in vivo to changes in middle ear dimensions following insertion may have acoustic advantages.

Background.—Optimal tension is an important factor in the acoustic performance of incus-stapes replacement prostheses. Length is the primary determinant of postinsertion tension with conventional prostheses. Postoperative changes in prosthesis tension may occur leading to a worsening of postoperative hearing.

Methods.—Testing of a self-adjusting prosthesis (SAP) containing a polyurethane sponge attached to the head of a titanium partial ossicular replacement prosthesis (PORP) was performed in 5 fresh temporal bones. This SAP was compared with optimal length PORPs at different tensions.

Sound input was 80 dB sound pressure level at 0.1 to 10 khz. Stapes footplate displacement was measured using a laser Doppler vibrometer before and after incus removal and after PORP and SAP insertion between the malleus and stapes. One to 3 glass shims were then inserted between the malleus and optimal length PORP and SAP to change prosthesis tension. Measurement of stapes displacement was repeated with increased prosthesis lengths of 0.15, 0.30, and 0.45 mm.

Results.—There was a clear tendency in the optimal length PORPs for a decrease in footplate displacement below 1.0 kHz, in general proportional to the increasing length. The SAP provided equivalent transmission as the optimal length PORP below 4.0 kHz and better transmission below 1.0 kHz at the varying increased lengths.

Conclusion.—An SAP seems to decrease the effect of changes in prosthesis length between the malleus and stapes at lower frequencies.

▶ Successful ossicular reconstruction depends on many factors. Among these are the correct placement and stiffness of the prosthesis to accurately reconstitute middle ear impedance. This becomes even more challenging during healing where scar contracture and changes in middle ear aeration can alter the tension on the reconstruction from that at the time of surgery. This article represents an interesting approach to begin development of a self-adjusting prosthesis to overcome these limitations. As expected and shown in Fig 3 in the original article, with increasing stiffness, sound transmission in the low frequencies decreases. Fig 4 in the original article shows that the self-adjusting nature of the construct nearly eliminates this effect. It is interesting to note that in both cases they used the malleus in their reconstruction in an assembly technique rather than directly to the tympanic membrane (columella reconstruction). The authors do not mention why they chose this method. It is unclear if the same effect would be seen in going directly to the tympanic membrane, but presumably it would. Our own group's similar research in this area has shown that the ossicular chain is dynamic in its impedance across frequencies. Rather than a static transmission of frequencies across the spectrum, the tympanic membrane and incudomalleolar joint change their vibratory pattern with frequency transmitted. Thus, pursuits of more sophisticated ossicular replacement prostheses that take advantage of these natural properties are a next logical progression in the field. Thus, this study represents a first step along the way.

B. J. Balough, CAPT, MC, USN

Aural Symptoms in Patients With Temporomandibular Joint Disorders: Multiple Frequency Tympanometry Provides Objective Evidence of Changes in Middle Ear Impedance

Riga M, Xenellis J, Peraki E, et al (Demokritos Univ of Thrace, Alexandroupolis, Greece; Natl Univ of Athens, Greece)
Otol Neurotol 31:1359-1364, 2010

Objective.—The association of temporomandibular joint (TMJ) disorders with aural symptoms, such as tinnitus, otic fullness, and subjective decrease of hearing acuity, is a well-established clinical observation. Although several hypotheses have been made about the otic-conductive origin of these complaints, conventional 226-Hz tympanometry has failed to demonstrate any middle ear abnormalities. The aim of this study was to evaluate patients with TMJ disorders with multiple frequency tympanometry (MFT).

Study Design.—Prospective clinical study.

Setting.—Outpatient clinic.

Patients.—The population of this study consisted of 40 patients with unilateral TMJ disorders diagnosed for longer than 1 month.

Interventions.—After verifying that there were no abnormal otoscopic findings, 226-Hz tympanometry, conventional pure-tone audiometry, brainstem auditory evoked potentials, and MFT were performed.

Main Outcome Measure.—Resonant frequency (RF) values.

Results.—With the exception of MFT, no abnormal audiologic findings were revealed. The ear ipsilateral to the lesion demonstrated significantly higher ($p = 0.002$) RF values in comparison to the contralateral ear. The difference in RF values was more obvious in patients aged 45 years or younger.

Conclusion.—The results of this study imply an increase in the stiffness of the middle ear, which has not been detected by conventional tympanometry. This represents the first concrete documentation of minor alterations in the conductive properties of the middle ear and seems to support the various hypotheses on the middle-ear origin of aural complaints in patients with TMJ disorders. Further studies are needed before a clear insight on the presumably multifactorial pathophysiology of these complaints can finally be reached.

▶ Complaints of otalgia are a frequent and often referral to the otolaryngologist. Typically the patients are anxious to understand the underlying cause for their discomfort, and the physical examination is normal and fails to reveal the underlying problem. This creates the dilemma of an extensive and usually nonrewarding series of imaging and other tests or to follow-up and symptomatic treatment. This becomes an even more vexing problem when symptoms of aural fullness, tinnitus, and subjective hearing loss accompany the otalgia. Intuitively, we often know this symptom is the result of a problem in the temporomandibular joint, but can cochlear hydrops be definitively ruled out? Even with normal audiometry and tympanometry, I have seen many patients in referral when pressure equalization tube or nasal steroids have failed to resolve their problem. The middle and external ear represents a complex innervation of 4 different cranial nerves for sensation, which does not include the cochlear nerve, which all map to the spinal nucleus of cranial nerve 5 within the brainstem. This article attempts to provide evidence to make sense of these seemingly unrelated set of auditory and pain symptoms. They are able to correlate abnormal multifrequency tympanometry findings with the symptomatic ears establishing for the first time objective findings of middle ear abnormality to support the subjective symptoms. Furthermore, in their discussion, they provide very supportable theories to explain this relationship between the middle ear and temporomandibular joint, and this too is valuable reading. Thus, for both the novel finding and the common presentation of this problem, this article is included in this year's group of must-reads.

B. J. Balough, CAPT, MC, USN

Biofilms in chronic suppurative otitis media and cholesteatoma: Scanning electron microscopy findings
Saunders J, Murray M, Alleman A (Dartmouth-Hitchcock Med Ctr, Lebanon, NH; Nose and Throat Clinic, San Jose, CA; Univ of Oklahoma Health Science Ctr)
Am J Otolaryngol 32:32-37, 2011

Background.—Biofilms play a role in the pathogenesis of a variety of otorhinolaryngologic diseases, including otitis media and cholesteatoma. Despite this, relatively few studies have undertaken to demonstrate the presence of biofilms tissues from patients with chronic otitis media or infected cholesteatoma.

Objective/Hypothesis.—Our objective is to detect evidence of biofilms human chronic ear infections with scanning electron microscopy (SEM). We hypothesized that bacterial biofilms are present in patients with chronic otitis media.

Study Design.—We performed prospective collection of tissue collected during middle ear surgery from 16 patients undergoing middle ear or mastoid surgery with chronic ear infections.

Methods.—A total of 31 middle and mastoid tissue samples were harvested at the time of surgery and processed with critical point drying for SEM analysis. Samples were then searched for evidence of biofilms.

Results.—Bacterial-shaped objects were identified that displayed both surface binding and the presence of a glycocalyx in 4 patients, findings consistent with bacterial biofilms. Most of these (3 of 4) were in patients with infected cholesteatoma, and biofilms were identified in 60% of cholesteatoma cases (3 of 5). On the other hand, only 1 of 7 cases with chronic suppurative otitis media had evidence of biofilms.

Conclusion.—SEM supports the hypothesis that bacterial biofilms are common in chronic infections associated with cholesteatoma and are present in some cases of chronic suppurative otitis media without cholesteatoma.

▶ The role of biofilms in otitis media with effusion, chronic sinusitis, and dental diseases has been well established. For chronic suppurative otitis, there are still relatively few studies. Thus, this study was selected for review, as it provides an overview of prior studies in this area as well as makes its own contributions. The authors discuss the lack of a standard definition of biofilm and the various imaging techniques that have been used to identify clinical evidence of bacterial biofilms with references to these studies. This provides useful reading for those interested in this emerging aspect of the field. While not surprising that they found evidence of biofilm in cholesteatoma in most samples, it is an interesting finding that in those cases of chronic suppurative otitis media without choles-teatoma they identified biofilm in only 1 specimen. The authors do go on to discuss that this may be because of sampling error caused by the methodology of scanning electron microscopy used that examined only limited areas and thus may be subject to a high false-negative rate and that they used a strict criteria for calling the specimen positive. This is an important discussion point and useful when reviewing other literature regarding the presence or absence of biofilms. This will be the first scientific hurdle for the field to overcome: a uniform definition and diagnostic modality for identification of biofilm within the middle ear. Only after that can their role in the persistence and progression of disease and treatments be evaluated.

B. J. Balough, CAPT, MC, USN

Prevalence of Vestibular and Balance Disorders in Children
O'Reilly RC, Morlet T, Nicholas BD, et al (Alfred I. duPont Hosp for Children, Wilmington, DE; et al)
Otol Neurotol 31:1441-1444, 2010

Objective.—Determine the prevalence of vestibular and balance disorders in children, rate of complaints of imbalance, and odds ratio of related diagnoses.

Patients and Methods.—Retrospective review of pediatric health system during a 4-year period for *International Classification of Diseases, 9th Revision*, codes related to balance disorders. Identified records were searched for chief complaints related to balance and for codes of related otologic and neuro-otologic diagnoses.

Results.—A total of 561,151 distinct patient encounters were found. Unspecified dizziness was diagnosed in 2,283 patients (0.4%). Also, 22% presented with balance complaints. Peripheral disorders were diag-nosed in 159, and central disturbances were diagnosed in 109 (prevalence < 0.0002%). Cumulative prevalence of diagnoses related to balance was 0.45% (2,546/561,151). Of all patients, 5,793 (1.03%) had chief complaint related to balance, and 2,076 (35.84%) were also diagnosed

TABLE 3.—Prevalence of Causes of Dizziness in the Study Population

	n	%
Peripheral causes		
Unspecified peripheral vertigo	77	3
BPPV	42	1.6
Labyrinthitis	15	0.6
Ménière's disease	11	0.4
Vestibular neuritis	7	0.3
Vestibular nystagmus	4	0.2
Unspecified labyrinthine disorder	3	0.1
Total	159	6.2
Central causes		
Central vertigo	71	2.8
Motion sickness	25	1
CVD associated with vertigo	6	0.2
Cervical vertigo	2	0.1
Total	104	4.1
Unspecified dizziness	2,283	89.7

with vestibular disorder. Moreover, 38% with peripheral disturbances and 21% with central disturbances had balance complaints. Odds ratio of syncope was $21\times$ higher than the general pediatric population in patients with unspecified dizziness, and sensorineural hearing loss was 43 times higher in those with peripheral vestibular disorders. In patients with central disorders headache was $16\times$ higher ($p < 0.05$).

Conclusion.—The prevalence of balance disorders in children is low. Children diagnosed with these disorders typically do not present with chief complaint related to balance. Significant associations exist between sensorineural hearing loss, syncope, and headache in children diagnosed with balance disorders (Table 3).

▶ This study represents a large evaluation of the prevalence and distribution of pediatric vestibular disorders from a hospital system dedicated to children; in that regard, it is unique. Some 560 000 patient encounters were screened for balance disorders as a primary complaint, and the distribution of causes is provided in Table 3. It is further unique in that as a search of all patients, it reflects the true prevalence and not just survey data from those reaching the otolaryngologist's or audiologist's office. What these data demonstrate most clearly is that in nearly 90% of cases an identifiable cause for the symptom was not obtained. As the authors discuss, this is because of several factors. First, our diagnostic testing methods are often not suitable for younger children. Devices such as the rotational chair and posturography are not designed for these patient groups. Even caloric testing may be difficult to perform in this group. Second, the awareness and sophistication of primary pediatric providers in evaluating and recognizing balance disorders is low. Third, even subspecialists such as neurotologists or neurologists may have little experience with pediatric balance disorders. Fourth, concurrent symptoms such as hearing loss and headache are frequently associated with those with balance disorders, and these symptoms may receive more attention than the balance disorder. Thus, this article is an important overview of this issue and therefore recommended reading.

B. J. Balough, CAPT, MC, USN

Proteomic analysis of formalin-fixed celloidin-embedded whole cochlear and laser microdissected spiral ganglion tissues
Markaryan A, Nelson EG, Helseth LD, et al (Univ of Chicago, IL; Univ of Illinois at Chicago)
Acta Otolaryngol 130:984-989, 2010

Conclusion.—The results of this study demonstrate that proteomic analysis can be successfully performed on formalin-fixed celloidin-embedded (FFCE) archival human cochlear tissues.

Objective.—To investigate the feasibility of analyzing protein expression in archival cochlear tissues.

Material and Methods.—A new methodology, referred to as Liquid Tissue^{TM}, was used to extract proteins from human cochlear tissue sections and spiral ganglion tissue isolated by laser microdissection (LMD). Protein identification was performed by bioinformatic analysis of high resolution tandem mass spectrometric data from fractionated tryptic peptide samples.

Results.—Twenty-six proteins were identified with a minimum of 2 unique peptides and 450 proteins were identified with 1 unique peptide at a confidence level of 95% in cochlear tissue. Ten proteins were identified with a minimum of 2 unique peptides and 485 proteins were identified with 1 unique peptide at a confidence level of 95% in spiral ganglion tissue.

▶ The fundamental foundation for the study of human disease is pathologic examination. Historically this was done with hematoxylin, eosin staining, and light microscopy. More recently, proteomic and genetic analyses of fresh tissue specimens have rapidly advanced understanding of disease states in a variety of conditions. Unfortunately for the field of otology, the inaccessible location of the inner ear within the dense temporal bone and small delicate nature of the inner ear tissues make live biopsy impossible. Thus, most of our pathologic understanding has been from light microscopic specimens in temporal bone collections. These have been very valuable, but as the authors explain in this article, the fixation technique has made proteomic evaluation of these collections impossible until now. Most disorders of the cochlea and labyrinth are poorly understood at the cellular and molecular level, even those that are quite common such as Meniere disease. As a result, our diagnostic and therapeutic sophistication is limited to indirect approaches to identify and treat these diseases. Thus, this article truly represents a breakthrough in technology to better understand disorders of the inner ear. Many important subsequent studies will come from this technique; therefore, this is an important article for review. Further, with this new advancement, it underscores the need for

physicians to be proactive with their patients to consider temporal bone dona-
tion so that we have robust repositories available for study in both common and
rare conditions. Hopefully this will stir a rebirth in these temporal bone
laboratories.

B. J. Balough, CAPT, MC, USN

**Recreational Noise Exposure Decreases Olivocochlear Efferent Reflex
Strength in Young Adults**
Peng J-H, Wang J-B, Chen J-H (The First Affiliated Hosp of Wenzhou Med
College, Zhejiang, Peoples' Republic of China)
J Otolaryngol Head Neck Surg 39:426-432, 2010

Objective.—To investigate effects of recreational noise exposure on olivocochlear efferent function.

Methods.—Efferent suppression of DPOAEs and acoustic reflexes were
tested in 32 young personal listening device users with normal hearing and
compared with that of healthy, non–noise-exposed young adults.

Results.—The results showed that the efferent suppression of DPOAEs
was mainly at low frequencies (0.75 and 1.0 kHz) in both groups and the
efferent suppression of DPOAEs and acoustic reflexes in the noise exposure group was slightly lower than that in the control group, with no
significant differences.

Conclusions.—Our results revealed that there were no differences in
DPOAE changes or medial olivocochlear bundle function between
normal-hearing subjects exposed to recreational noise and controls and
suggest that recreational noise has different effects on olivocochlear
efferent reflex strength compared with occupational noise exposure.

▶ This article attempts to address an important topic, namely, the contribution
of recreational noise exposures to overall noise-induced hearing loss rates.
Disability compensation from noise-induced hearing loss in the military and
veteran populations (as well as industry, mining, and farming) is climbing
rapidly leading to overall health care costs. During the past 2 decades, personal
music players and headphone use has also increased leading to reports of early
noise-induced hearing loss in teenagers and young adults. Thus, the ability for
early detection of recreational noise-induced hearing loss prior to workplace
noise exposure may influence employment choices or underscore the need
for better protection and increased surveillance. Their approach involves
a variety of common audiologic tests to attempt to detect changes in efferent
outer hair cell and acoustic reflex function. The authors provide a good description of the background information on the topic and the testing methods used.
Unfortunately, the intersubject variability combined with low subject numbers
do not permit any useful conclusions to be drawn from the data. The authors
appropriately acknowledge this point. Similarly, no power calculation was
provided. While a powerful tool, the test-retest and intersubject variability of
otoacoustic emissions make it a limited research modality, and conclusions

drawn from small subject numbers should be viewed with caution. Many investigators are working to overcome these limitations. Thus, the primary value of this selection is in its review of the subject and in the discussion to provide visibility to this topic.

B. J. Balough, CAPT, MC, USN

The future of early disease detection? Applications of electronic nose technology in otolaryngology
Charaklias N, Raja H, Humphreys ML, et al (Gloucestershire Hosps NHS Foundation Trust, Gloucester, UK; et al)
J Laryngol Otol 124:823-827, 2010

Introduction.—Recent advances in electronic nose technology, and successful clinical applications, are facilitating the development of new methods for rapid, bedside diagnosis of disease. There is a real clinical need for such new diagnostic tools in otolaryngology.

Materials and Methods.—We present a critical review of recent advances in electronic nose technology and current applications in otolaryngology.

Results.—The literature reports evidence of accurate diagnosis of common otolaryngological conditions such as sinusitis (acute and chronic), chronic suppurative otitis media, otitis externa and nasal vestibulitis. A significant recent development is the successful identification of biofilm-producing versus non-biofilm-producing pseudomonas and staphylococcus species.

Conclusion.—Electronic nose technology holds significant potential for enabling rapid, non-invasive, bedside diagnosis of otolaryngological disease (Table 1).

▶ The mammalian nose is a precise and sensitive chemical sensor. Dogs and other animals have been used for centuries in a variety of industries to detect

---

TABLE 1.—Published Studies of E-Nose Technology Applications in Otolaryngology

Study	Year	Pts or Specimens Included	Outcome
Shykhon et al.[6]	2004	90 bacterial swabs from 90 pts with ENT infections	88.2% sensitivity for ??*
Thaler & Hanson[7]	2006	11 pts Nasal exhalations sampled	72% sensitivity for sinusitis
Bruno et al.[8]	2008	28 pts (14 CRS, 14 healthy) Nasal swabs taken from middle meatus	≤85% sensitivity for CRS pathological bacteria
Thaler et al.[9]	2008	Biofilm- & non-biofilm-producing mutant strains of pseudomonas & staphylococcus sampled & incubated	72–100% accuracy for biofilm- vs non-biofilm-producing bacteria

E-nose = electronic nose; pts = patients; CRS = chronic rhinosinusitis; ?? = bacterial classification.
Editor's Note: Please refer to original journal article for full references.
*Compared with microbiological culture 'gold standard'.

trace amounts of substances. As an example, specialized trained pigs are used in the harvesting of truffles. Over the past decade, development of similarly sensitive and specific devices to perform the same function has developed in law enforcement, agriculture, and medicine. This article summarizes and reviews those relevant to otolaryngology, and they can be found in Table 1. Current detection of bacterial infections suffers 2 main limitations: delay in diagnosis and detection of only the planktonic form of the bacteria. The goal of electronic nose is to provide rapid bedside diagnostic capability of infecting organisms. Further, the authors discuss at some length how this technology has been shown to also detect organisms forming biofilms—a predominant form of infection in the head and neck. Once this technology is fully realized better, more accurate diagnosis can be envisioned leading to more effective treatment choices. Although short on scientific detail, this article serves as a good overview of the subject and thus is worthy of review.

B. J. Balough, CAPT, MC, USN

Utilization of Fluorescein for Identification and Preservation of the Facial Nerve and Semicircular Canals for Safe Mastoidectomy: A Proof of Concept Laboratory Cadaveric Study

Gragnaniello C, Kamel M, Al-Mefty O (Univ of Arkansas for Med Sciences, Little Rock)
Neurosurgery 66:204-207, 2010

Objective.—Mastoidectomy can be a very challenging procedure for many reasons. The normal anatomy can be distorted because of inflammatory processes and tumors and recurrences. Avoiding injuries to the semicircular canals (SCCs) and facial canal is mandatory, and there is need to find a way to recognize the facial nerve and SCCs for safe performance of mastoidectomy. We describe, as a proof of concept, a novel technique to drill the mastoid while allowing the surgeon to recognize and avoid injuries to vital structures, in the cadaver.

Methods.—Four fresh cadaveric heads (8 sides) were prepared by cannulating the major vessels at the level of the neck. After removal of the mastoid cortex, indocyanine green was injected in the vessels. The sigmoid sinus alongside the facial nerve and SCCs was skeletonized using the drilling guidance provided by the fluorescence. The mucosa covering the air cells of the mastoid is very well vascularized compared with the thick bone representing the outer layer of the SCCs and facial canal. Consequently, after the indocyanine green injection, the mucosa shines whereas the bone does not. The fluorescence guides the drilling displaying air cells that are safe to remove.

Results.—Eight mastoidectomies were performed, resulting in optimal drilling with no injuries to the facial canal and SCCs.

Conclusion.—With this novel technique, it is possible to perfectly skeletonize the facial nerve and the SCCs in the cadaver. We think that this technique can be an adjunct in the armamentarium of trainees that are not familiar with the anatomy of the temporal bone and eventually of neurosurgeons facing lesions that require the removal of various degrees of the mastoid.

▶ This is an interesting article from the neurosurgical literature regarding a proposed technique for intraoperative visualization of the otic capsule structures and fallopian canal within the mastoid cavity. The technique relies upon the relative difference in vascularity of the mucosalized cancellous bone versus the denser and less vascular compact bone surrounding the facial nerve and structures of the inner ear. The material used is indocyanine green, which is routinely used in aneurysm surgery through intravascular injection. Its use in otologic or otolaryngologic surgery is, however, uncommon. This represents a creative and innovative new potential application and thus is worthy of review. The article provides a link to an online digital video that demonstrates the dissection and visualization obtained in the cadaver study. The authors do discuss several limitations, among them the rapid washout of the dye (5-10 minutes), which may require reinjection for longer procedures. The calculations are provided in the article for the dilution and also the maximum dosage, which indicates up to 15 injections can be safely done before the maximum recommended dose is reached. A further consideration is that when inflamed, a mastoid will have increased blood flow enhancing the contrast obtained but with uncertain effects on washout time. This technique will likely never gain much use for routine mastoidectomy in experienced hands. It may have some use in cadaveric training or in complex cases with distorted anatomy. It has been selected for its innovative application and to introduce this material and potential application to the wider audience of otolaryngology.

B. J. Balough, CAPT, MC, USN

Voxel-Based Morphometry Depicts Central Compensation after Vestibular Neuritis
zu Eulenburg P, Stoeter P, Dieterich M (Johannes Gutenberg Univ, Mainz, Germany; Ludwig Maximilians Univ, Munich, Germany)
Ann Neurol 68:241-249, 2010

Objective.—Patients who have had vestibular neuritis (VN) show a remarkable clinical improvement especially in gait and posture >6 months after disease onset.

Methods.—Voxel-based morphometry was used to detect the VN-induced changes in gray and white matter by means of structural magnetic resonance imaging. Twenty-two patients were compared an average 2.5 years after onset of VN to a healthy sex-and age-matched control group.

Results.—Our analysis revealed that all patients had signal intensity increases for gray matter in the medial vestibular nuclei and the right gracile nucleus and for white matter in the area of the pontine commissural vestibular fibers. A relative atrophy was observed in the left posterior hippocampus and the right superior temporal gyrus. Patients with a residual canal paresis also showed an increase of gray matter in middle temporal (MT)/V5 bilaterally.

Interpretation.—These findings indicate that the processes of central compensation after VN seem to occur in 3 different sensory systems. First of all, the vestibular system itself showed a white matter increase in the commissural fibers as a direct consequence of an increased internuclei vestibular crosstalk of the medial vestibular nuclei. Second, to regain postural stability, there was a shift to the somatosensory system due to an elevated processing of proprioceptive information in the right gracile

TABLE.—Listing of All Gray and White Matter Signal Changes in VN Patients Compared to a Group of Healthy Age- and Sex-Matched Controls as Well as the Results of the Correlation Analysis

T-Contrast	Brain Area	BA	x, y, z	Cluster Size	*t* Value
Results of group comparisons					
VN patients vs healthy controls					
Gray matter intensities increase	Medial vestibular nucleus bilaterally		−1, −29, −41	78	4.54
	Right gracile nucleus		4, −44, −56	305	4.47
Gray matter intensities decrease	Right superior frontal gyrus	6	19, −2, 70	171	5.2
	Right superior temporal gyrus	22, 42		33	4.55
	Left posterior hippocampus	29	71, −23, 4	80	4.33
White matter increases	Vestibular commissural fibers		5, −46, −55	400	4.88
White matter decreases	Pontomesencephale haube				
VNR vs VNL patients					
White matter increases	Right middle temporal gyrus (MT/V5)		42, −66, 11	65	4.24
	Left inferior parietal lobule	13	−47, −43, 19	92	4.2
White matter decreases	Left middle temporal gyrus (MT/V5)		−32, −83, 10	72	4.77
VNR patients vs controls					
Gray matter increases	Left middle temporal gyrus (MT/V5)		−35, −79, 9	241	12.89
	Right middle temporal gyrus (MT/V5)		43, −70, 15	141	14.06
White matter decreases	Left precuneus and superior parietal lobule	7	−27, −53, 49	218	7.48
Correlation analysis					
Positive gray matter correlation with duration and degree of canal paresis	Left inferior cerebellar vermis		−8, −55, −56	179	4.67
Negative gray matter correlation with results of dynamic SVV	Left middle temporal gyrus	39	−43, −68, 26	78	4.35
	Right middle temporal and supramarginal gyrus	39, 40	51, −53, 25	198	4.53
	Right posterior cerebellar semilunar lobe		42, −46, −43	312	4.73

p < 0.001; cluster size >15 voxels.

VN = vestibular neuritis; BA = Brodmann area; VNR = VN with lesion on right side; VNL = VN with lesion on left side; SVV = subjective visual vertical.

nucleus. Third, there was a bilateral increase in the area of MT/V5 in VN patients with a residual peripheral vestibular hypofunction. This seems to be the result of an increased importance of visual motion processing (Table).

▶ Vestibular rehabilitation has become the mainstay for treating a variety of balance disorders. However, until this article our understanding of how the central nervous system compensates through neural plasticity–induced changes from vestibular loss has been limited. This study uses voxel-based morphology, which is a new software-based approach, to compare T1-weighted MRI with normalized controls to detect gray and white matter changes. It has advantages over other functional-based imaging technologies particularly for an activity such as balance where traditional functional MRI is not applicable. The Table lists the brain areas identified as changing after unilateral vestibular losses. The authors interpret these changes to reflect the interaction of multiple sensory systems in response to the loss of input. They also note that some association areas decrease in activity, which they feel is reflective for limitations in the ability to compensate. This likely will require further work to validate. While the findings in this article are in themselves unique, the real value is in the introduction of this new technique to evaluate brain changes over time. This methodology provides a tool to potentially determine the effects of varying programs of vestibular rehabilitation or medical therapy. In addition, this tool may also be useful in analyzing auditory disorders including tinnitus.

B. J. Balough, CAPT, MC, USN

5 Pediatric Otolaryngology

Airway

Evaluation of computed tomography virtual bronchoscopy in paediatric tracheobronchial foreign body aspiration

Bhat KV, Hegde JS, Nagalotimath US, et al (Karnataka Inst of Med Sciences, Hubli, India)
J Laryngol Otol 124:875-879, 2010

Objective.—Virtual bronchoscopy is a noninvasive technique which provides an intraluminal view of the tracheobronchial tree. This study aimed to evaluate this technique in comparison with rigid bronchoscopy, in paediatric patients with tracheobronchial foreign bodies undetected by plain chest radiography.

Methods.—Plain chest radiography was initially performed in 40 children with suspected foreign body aspiration. Computed tomography virtual bronchoscopy was performed in the 20 in whom chest radiography appeared normal. Virtual bronchoscopic images were obtained. All patients underwent rigid bronchoscopy performed by an otolaryngologist blinded to the computed tomography virtual bronchoscopy findings, within 24 hours. Virtual bronchoscopic findings were then compared with the results of rigid bronchoscopy.

Results.—In 12 patients, foreign bodies detected by virtual bronchoscopy were confirmed by rigid bronchoscopy. In one case, a mucous plug was perceived as a foreign body on virtual bronchoscopy. In another case, a minute foreign body was missed on virtual bronchoscopy. The following parameters were calculated: sensitivity, 92.3 per cent; specificity, 85.7 per cent; validity, 90 per cent; positive likelihood ratio, 6.45; and negative likelihood ratio, 0.089.

Conclusion.—In the presence of a positive clinical diagnosis and negative chest radiography, computed tomography virtual bronchoscopy must be considered in all cases of tracheobronchial foreign body aspiration, in order to avoid needless rigid bronchoscopy. Computed tomography virtual bronchoscopy is particularly useful in screening cases of

147

occult foreign body aspiration, as it has high sensitivity, specificity and validity.

▶ The availability of a noninvasive technique to locate foreign bodies preoperatively is an attractive option, as it can avoid a general anesthetic in some children with its associated morbidity and mortality. The authors argue that virtual bronchoscopy is such a technique and is particularly useful in locating nonradiopaque foreign bodies missed on plain radiography.

This was a prospective, cross-sectional, comparative study conducted in a tertiary referral hospital in a developing country, over 1 year. Basically 20 children with a possible airway foreign body and normal chest X-ray underwent CT virtual bronchoscopy. All patients underwent rigid bronchoscopic evaluation performed by an otolaryngologist blinded to the CT virtual bronchoscopy findings, within 24 hours. Virtual bronchoscopy has a high sensitivity and specificity but neither is 100%. The authors argue for a greater role in developing countries, but what is missing in the study is an algorithm that will indicate when rigid bronchoscopies can be safely avoided using this technique. This is clearly for future research.

R. B. Mitchell, MD

Propranolol in the Management of Airway Infantile Hemangiomas
Rosbe KW, Suh K-Y, Meyer AK, et al (Univ of California, San Francisco)
Arch Otolaryngol Head Neck Surg 136:658-665, 2010

Objective.—To report our experience with propranolol in managing airway infantile hemangiomas.

Design.—Case series of 3 consecutive patients who had extensive, symptomatic airway infantile hemangiomas treated with propranolol.

Setting.—Tertiary academic medical center.

Patients.—Three infants with facial cutaneous hemangiomas who developed stridor that progressed to respiratory distress, which according to laryngoscopic examination results was confirmed to be caused by extensive subglottic hemangiomas. These patients underwent follow-up during their course of therapy, ranging from 3 weeks to 15 months.

Results.—Patient 1 failed to respond to systemic corticosteroids, laser ablation, and intravenous vincristine for her airway hemangioma and had to undergo tracheotomy. She was given propranolol after her tracheotomy and had a significant reduction in her subglottic airway obstruction. Patient 2 developed progressive stridor secondary to airway hemangioma at age $6\frac{1}{2}$ months following tapering of systemic corticosteroids prescribed for her periorbital hemangioma. Systemic corticosteroids were restarted with the addition of propranolol. The stridor improved within 24 hours, and she was able to be weaned off corticosteroids. Patient 3 was also treated with initial combined therapy of systemic corticosteroids and propranolol.

He had a significant reduction in stridor within 24 hours and was weaned off corticosteroids.

Conclusions.—Our 3 patients had severe respiratory symptoms related to their airway infantile hemangiomas. In the first patient, propranolol was used when other treatments were ineffective or associated with intolerable adverse effects. In the second and third patients, propranolol was part of a dual regimen that resulted in rapid resolution of airway symptoms and allowed for quicker weaning of corticosteroids.

▶ Over the last 5 years, there have been several reports of the use of propranolol for head and neck hemangiomas. Propranolol is an attractive therapeutic alternative to systemic steroids because it can avoid the common adverse effects of prolonged high-dose steroid use, but it is not without its own potential risks, including bradycardia, hypotension, and hypoglycemia. Several articles in the literature now report the use of propranolol in the management of airway infantile hemangiomas, including the use of propranolol as the initial and sole therapy. This is a small case series with a good review of the current literature and good clinical photographs of the response to treatment over time. It is still too early to recommend the sole use of propranolol in the management of symptomatic airway infantile hemangiomas. There is also debate about the degree of monitoring and workup prior to starting the infant on propranolol. I agree with the authors that this is an exciting development, but controlled trials and long-term follow-up are warranted to assess efficacy and potential toxic effects of propranolol before it can be considered a safe and an effective alternative for first-line treatment for airway infantile hemangioma.

R. B. Mitchell, MD

Basic and Clinical Research

Posterior Hyoid Space as Related to Excision of the Thyroglossal Duct Cyst

Maddalozzo J, Alderfer J, Modi V (Children's Memorial Hosp, Chicago, IL)
Laryngoscope 120:1773-1778, 2010

Objectives/Hypothesis.—The anatomy of the anterior neck in the area of the hyoid, thyrohyoid membrane, and epiglottis is herein redescribed and compared to its classical depiction. The concept of the posterior hyoid space (PHS) is defined and substantiated through review of archived tissue and cadaver larynx dissection as well as by observation at many surgical dissections. The true anatomy of these relationships provides an insight into the effectiveness of the Sistrunk procedure. The author believes that recurrence of thyroglossal duct cysts (TGDC) occurs as a consequence of incomplete resection of: 1) microscopic suprahyoid ductules and/or 2) infra- and perihyoid tissue.

Study Design.—The senior author has been using the concept of the posterior hyoid space as applied to the Sistrunk procedure for more than 20 years. A retrospective study was done on cases from April 2003 to

August 2008, and outcome was reviewed and compared to historical controls to determine the impact of applying this anatomic concept.

Methods.—A retrospective chart review was undertaken on 60 surgical cases performed for a 5-year period with clinical follow-up extended to an additional 7 months. Data collected included age at surgery, presenting symptoms, imaging characteristics, thyroid status, pathology results, and postoperative complications. All 60 were under the age of 18 who underwent a modified Sistrunk procedure and had a postoperative diagnosis of TGDC. Each patient had a minimum follow-up period of 4 months to check for recurrences. No revision was included in this study.

Results.—Sixty patients met criteria for the study. There was one recurrence (1.67%); a complication rate of 6.67%. Complications were minor and wound related. Mean follow-up was 17 months.

Conclusions.—The technique of applying the concept of a PHS to ensure the complete resection of the middle third of the hyoid bone and offending tissues is believed to decrease recurrence of TGDC secondary to incomplete resection in the perihyoid area.

▶ Sistrunk procedure is the choice method of surgical excision of a thyroglossal cyst because of the low rate of recurrence when it is used. This article introduces the concept of posterior hyoid space (PHS) that the authors believe is important to identify to minimize recurrence of the cyst. Basically, the thyrohyoid membrane is identified and used as a conduit to locate the posterior aspect of the hyoid bone. The authors argue that identification of the PHS allows surgeons to accurately assess the dimensions of the hyoid in both its inferior to superior and anterior to posterior aspects and thus to facilitate complete resection of the hyoid (Fig 2). The study reports a single recurrence

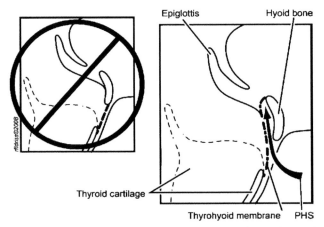

FIGURE 2.—Schematic drawing of the base of the tongue and upper laryngeal area. The dotted line demonstrates the thyrohyoid membrane's (THM) primary insertion on the preepiglottic tissues and its reflection and attachment on the superior rim of the hyoid. Arrow indicates PHS. (Reprinted from Maddalozzo J, Alderfer J, Modi V. Posterior hyoid space as related to excision of the thyroglossal duct cyst. *Laryngoscope.* 2010;120:1773-1778, with permission from The American Laryngological, Rhinological and Otological Society, Inc.)

out of 60 children, a recurrence rate of 1.67% that compares favorably to published case series. This is an interesting and comprehensive study of thyroglossal duct cysts. The concept and importance of PHS cannot be validated using this study. However, the surgical approach makes sense anatomically and may lead to a reduction in the recurrence rate of thyroglossal duct cysts.

R. B. Mitchell, MD

General

A Randomized Clinical Trial of the Efficacy of Scheduled Dosing of Acetaminophen and Hydrocodone for the Management of Postoperative Pain in Children After Tonsillectomy

Sutters KA, Miaskowski C, Holdridge-Zeuner D, et al (Children's Hosp Central California, Madera; Univ of California, San Francisco; et al)

Clin J Pain 26:95-103, 2010

Objectives.—To determine the effectiveness of around-the-clock (ATC) analgesic administration, with or without nurse coaching, compared with standard care with as needed (PRN) dosing in children undergoing outpatient tonsillectomy.

Methods.—Children 6 to 15 years of age were randomized to receive acetaminophen and hydrocodone (167 mg/2.5 mg/5 mL) for 3 days after surgery: Group A (N = 39)—every 4 hours PRN, with standard postoperative instructions; Group B (N = 34)—every 4 hours ATC, with standard postoperative instructions, without nurse coaching; and Group C (N = 40)—every 4 hours ATC, with standard postoperative instructions, with coaching. Parents completed a medication log, and recorded the presence and severity of opioid-related adverse effects and children's reports of pain intensity using a 0 to 10 numeric rating scale.

Results.—No differences were found in analgesic administration or pain intensity scores between the 2 ATC groups. Therefore, they were combined for comparison with the PRN group. Children in the ATC group received more analgesic than those in the PRN group ($P < 0.0001$). Children in the PRN group had higher pain intensity scores compared to children in the ATC group, both at rest ($P = 0.017$) and with swallowing ($P = 0.017$). Pain intensity scores for both groups were higher in the morning compared with the evening ($P < 0.0001$). With the exception of constipation, scheduled analgesic dosing did not increase the frequency or severity of opioid-related adverse effects.

Discussion.—Scheduled dosing of acetaminophen and hydrocodone is more effective than PRN dosing in reducing pain intensity in children after tonsillectomy. Nurse coaching does not impact parent's adherence to ATC dosing.

▶ This is an interesting study that should be read by otolaryngologists who perform tonsillectomy in children. Postoperative pain after tonsillectomy is a common problem that can lead to dehydration and secondary bleeding. It also has predictable characteristics (eg, prolonged duration, relatively constant in nature, moderate to severe intensity). Clearly, scheduled dosing regimens may be beneficial. The authors review previous randomized controlled trials that have reported mixed results and make a good argument for further research. Findings from this study suggest that regular dosing of acetaminophen with hydrocodone was more effective than PRN dosing in reducing children's pain in the first 3 days after tonsillectomy. The differences beyond the early postoperative period were relatively small and of modest clinical significance. With the exception of constipation, scheduled analgesic dosing did not increase the frequency or severity of opioid-related adverse effects. Written instructions are sufficient interventions to promote adherence to a prescribed scheduled analgesic dosing regimen. In conclusion, scheduled dosing of analgesics should be considered during the first 48 hours after tonsillectomy with transition to an as needed approach as the child's pain intensity and analgesic requirements decrease. Written instructions are sufficient, and concern about adverse events related to opioid overuse is overstated.

R. B. Mitchell, MD

Ankyloglossia, Exclusive Breastfeeding, and Failure to Thrive
Forlenza GP, Paradise Black NM, McNamara EG, et al (Univ of Florida, Gainesville; Shands Hosp at Univ of Florida, Gainesville)
Pediatrics 125:e1500-e1504, 2010

A 6-month-old term boy was hospitalized to evaluate the cause of his failure to thrive, mandated as part of an investigation by the Department of Children and Families after an allegation of medical neglect was made. On admission the patient was below birth weight, and a medical workup for failure to thrive was pursued; however, he was noted to have severe ankyloglossia and was an exclusively breastfed infant. The only interventions during his hospitalization were frenotomy and assistance to the mother to increase her milk supply. The infant immediately experienced weight gain and has continued to show slow, but steady, weight gain as an outpatient. We illustrate here many of the controversies concerning ankyloglossia.

▶ Ankyloglossia, or tongue tie, is a common problem seen by otolaryngologists. It can present in the newborn with feeding difficulty or in an older child with speech problems. There is a reported incidence of 1% to 10%. Both the diagnosis and treatment of ankyloglossia are controversial. This is an interesting report of the consequences of untreated clinically significant ankyloglossia in a breastfed infant. The Academy of Breastfeeding Medicine defines ankyloglossia as "the presence of a sublingual frenulum which changes the appearance and/or function of the tongue because of decreased length, lack of elasticity, or attachment too distal beneath the tongue or too close to the gingival ridge." This report is a good review of the current literature. It includes the assessment of ankyloglossia using the Hazelbaker scale (Table 1), which

TABLE 1.—Hazelbaker Assessment Tool for Lingual Frenulum Function

Assessment Tool for Lingual Frenulum Function (ATLFF) © Alison K. Hazelbaker, PhD, IBCLC March 1, 2009	Mothers name: _____ Baby's name: _____ Baby's age: _____ Date of assessment: _____

FUNCTION ITEMS

Lateralization 2 Complete 1 Body of tongue but not tongue tip 0 None	**Cupping of tongue** 2 Entire edge, firm cup 1 Side edges only, moderate cup 0 Poor **OR** no cup
Lift of tongue 2 Tip to mid-mouth 1 Only edges to mid mouth 0 Tip stays at alveolar ridge **OR** tip rises only to mid-mouth with jaw closure **AND/OR** mid-tongue dimples	**Peristalsis** 2 Complete anterior to posterior (originates at tip) 1 Partial: originating posterior to tip 0 None **OR** Reverse peristalsis
Extension of tongue 2 Tip over lower lip 1 Tip over lower gum only 0 Neither of the above **OR** anterior or mid-tongue humps and/or dimples	**Snap back** 2 None 1 Periodic 0 Frequent **OR** with each suck
Spread of anterior tongue 2 Complete 1 Moderate **OR** partial 0 Little **OR** none	

APPEARANCE ITEMS

Appearance of tongue when lifted 2 Round **OR** square 1 Slight cleft in tip apparent 0 Heart shaped	**Elasticity of lingual frenulum** 2 Very elastic (excellent) 1 Moderately elastic 0 Little **OR** no elasticity
Length of lingual frenulum when tongue lifted 2 More than 1 cm **OR** absent frenulum 1 1 cm 0 Less than 1 cm	**Attachment of lingual frenulum to tongue** 2 Posterior to tip 1 At tip 0 Notched **OR** under the mucosa at the tongue base
Attachment of lingual frenulum to inferior alveolar ridge 2 Attached to floor of mouth **OR** well below ridge 1 Attached just below ridge 0 Attached to ridge	

SCORING

Function Item score: _____ Appearance Item score: _____	Combined Score: _____ / _____

Treatment Recommendations Based on Scoring

14 = Perfect Function score regardless of Appearance Item score. Surgical treatment not recommended.

11 = Acceptable Function score only if Appearance Item score is 10.

<11 = Function Score indicates function impaired. Frenotomy should be considered if management fails. Frenotomy necessary if Appearance Item score is < 8.

TABLE 2.—Frenotomy Decision Rule for Breastfeeding Infants

Mother with nipple pain or trauma while breastfeeding
AND/OR
inability to maintain latch
AND/OR
poor weight gain in the infant (<15 g/d)
AND
a visible membrane anterior to the base of the tongue, which restricts tongue movement, leading to:
inability to touch the roof of the mouth
OR
inability to cup an examining finger
OR
inability to protrude the tongue past the gum line

quantifies aspects of lingual appearance and function, and the frenotomy decision rule for breastfeeding infants (Table 2), which uses signs and symptoms. Both can be useful in decision making. There is also a good review of studies that look at outcomes that are generally favorable. The report illustrates how crucial tongue mobility is for successful breastfeeding and how important it is to take seriously maternal concerns regarding breastfeeding pain and difficulty.

R. B. Mitchell, MD

Balloon Catheter Sinuplasty and Adenoidectomy in Children With Chronic Rhinosinusitis

Ramadan HH, Terrell AM (West Virginia Univ School of Medicine, Morgantown)
Ann Otol Rhinol Laryngol 119:578-582, 2010

Objectives.—Adenoidectomy is the first step in the surgical management of children with chronic rhinosinusitis (CRS). Adenoidectomy, however, is only effective in half of these children. Although endoscopic sinus surgery is effective for CRS, there is concern for facial growth retardation and major complications. We propose that balloon catheter sinuplasty (BCS) is a minimally invasive, effective procedure in the treatment of pediatric CRS.

Methods.—We undertook a nonrandomized, controlled, prospective review of children with failed medical management of CRS who underwent BCS or adenoidectomy. Outcomes were assessed at 1 year of follow-up and were based on SN-5 scores and the need for revision surgery.

Results.—Forty-nine children who satisfied the inclusion criteria were reviewed. Thirty of the children had BCS. The age range was 4 to 11 years (mean, 7.7 years), and the mean computed tomography score (Lund-Mackay system) was 7.5. Twenty-four of the 30 patients (80%) who underwent BCS showed improvement of their symptoms after 12 months of follow-up, compared with 10 of the 19 patients (52.6%) who underwent adenoidectomy ($p < 0.05$). A multivariate analysis using logistic regression analysis with age, sex, asthma, and computed tomography score as covariables showed that BCS was also more effective than adenoidectomy in older children. None of the other variables showed statistical significance.

Conclusions.—Balloon catheter sinuplasty offers a procedure that is more effective than adenoidectomy and less invasive than endoscopic sinus surgery in the treatment of pediatric CRS.

▶ Balloon catheter sinuplasty (BCS) has evolved as a surgical option in adults undergoing functional endoscopic sinus surgery (FESS), specifically as a means of promoting drainage from the maxillary and frontal sinuses. BCS not only has its enthusiasts but also a large number of critics. This study argues that BCS can be an option in pediatric sinus surgery before considering FESS. BCS has been shown to be safe and effective in children. This study argues that BCS (in addition to adenoidectomy) is more effective than adenoidectomy alone in the treatment of chronic pediatric sinusitis and could be offered before FESS. The study has significant methodological problems. The patients were not randomized. The single surgeon is enthusiastic about the new technology, and no child underwent BCS without an adenoidectomy. The authors offer no rationale for why BCS may have a role in children. There was also no power analysis at the start of the study. The differences between the 2 groups could have been the result of a small study population and not a significant outcomes difference. Nonetheless, this is a new procedure that requires further study and may find a future role in pediatric sinus surgery.

R. B. Mitchell, MD

Balloon Dilation Eustachian Tuboplasty: A Feasibility Study
Ockermann T, Reineke U, Upile T, et al (Bielefeld Academic Teaching Hosp, Germany; Chase Farm and Barnet Hosps, London, UK)
Otol Neurotol 31:1100-1103, 2010

Objective.—To assess the feasibility and safety of balloon dilation Eustachian tuboplasty (BET) as an option for treatment of patients with Eustachian tube dysfunction.

Patients and Interventions.—A cadaveric study of 5 temporal human bones was performed. Each bone underwent transnasal balloon dilation Eustachian tuboplasty (BET) with computed tomography and post-dilation histology. The procedure involved the dilation of the cartilaginous and bony portion of the Eustachian tube with a balloon catheter.

Results.—BET is technically easy to perform. No damage to essential structures, particularly the carotid canal, was found.

Conclusion.—This newly introduced method seems to be a feasible and safe procedure to dilate the Eustachian tube.

▶ A large proportion of children develop at least a temporary dysfunction of the Eustachian tube (ET). This has made insertion of tympanostomy tubes one of the most common pediatric surgeries. In a small percentage of children, multiple sets of tubes are inserted, and the problem can continue to adulthood. Dilatation of the ET, in these children, becomes an interesting alternative to solve a complex problem. The proximity of the internal carotid artery is of clinical importance to avoid the catastrophic injuries and deaths that have been anecdotally reported in the past during patulous ET injection procedures. This is a well-written and interesting study that may have future clinical implications. The authors present a novel technique to perform minimally invasive surgery on the cartilaginous and bony ET. They use a balloon catheter with a newly designed endoscope to widen the cartilage and bony lumen. This technique was easily performed in the human cadaveric study. Complications as investigated by high-resolution imaging and histology were minimal. This method seems safe and feasible but clearly needs further study.

R. B. Mitchell, MD

Balloon Dilation for Recurrent Stenosis After Pediatric Laryngotracheoplasty
Bent JP, Shah MB, Nord R, et al (Children's Hosp at Montefiore, Bronx, NY)
Ann Otol Rhinol Laryngol 119:619-627, 2010

Objectives.—We assessed the safety and efficacy of balloon dilation as treatment for recurrent stenosis after pediatric laryngotracheoplasty.

Methods.—We studied a retrospective case series at an academic tertiary care children's hospital. We included all patients under the age of 18 years with subglottic or tracheal stenosis treated at our institution with balloon dilation between June 2007 and April 2009. The records were analyzed for patient demographics, presenting symptoms, surgical technique, and airway description. The outcome measures were airway diameter, postoperative symptoms, tracheotomy status, and complications.

Results.—Ten patients (9 with subglottic stenosis and 1 with tracheal stenosis) underwent 20 balloon dilation procedures without complication. The average age at the time of the procedure was 17 months (range, 3 months to 9 years). The patient presenting symptoms were stridor in 7 cases and tracheotomy in 3 cases. Vascular balloons (diameter range, 6 to 12 mm; length, 20 mm) were inflated to 10 to 12 cm H_2O pressure for an average of 40 seconds (range, 10 to 120 seconds). Each procedure consisted of 1 to 3 dilation cycles. The immediate postdilation airway area increased by an average factor of 4.9 (range, 1.9 to 9). Six patients had repeat procedures with an average interval between dilations of 67 days (range, 6 to 337 days). Stridor was eliminated or greatly improved in all patients on the first postoperative day; 7 patients sustained this benefit, with an average followup time of 10 months (range, 4 to 23 months). Six of the 10 patients had undergone previous laryngeal reconstruction (age range, 3 months to 4 years). Of these 6, 3 have no tracheotomy, with a mean followup of 12.5 months. The 3 children who benefited the least from dilation were noted to have more diffuse and chronic inflammation of the larynx in comparison to the responders.

Conclusions.—This case series suggests that balloon dilation is a relatively safe and effective procedure. It may be particularly well suited to recent stenosis after laryngotracheal reconstruction.

▶ Over the last few years, pediatric otolaryngologists have had a renewed interest in balloon dilation as an alternative to open laryngotracheoplasty (LTP). Balloon laryngoplasty offers an alternative to LTP and contemporary endoscopic approaches to subglottic stenosis. The balloon imparts radial forces, rather than the shearing forces associated with rigid dilation, and this variation in technique should theoretically create less trauma and therefore less recurrent stenosis. The authors present 10 children with a mean age of 24.5 months at the time of the initial procedure, who underwent balloon dilations on 20 separate occasions without complication. Balloon laryngoplasty provides another option for treating subglottic stenosis. This report suggests that the technique is relatively safe and effective. It may have its greatest role in restenosis after LTP. The authors also correctly point out that balloon dilation has been discussed extensively and often quite favorably at many recent national meetings, but surprisingly, this trend is not reflected in the otolaryngology literature, which scarcely addresses pediatric balloon laryngoplasty.

R. B. Mitchell, MD

Outcomes

A prospective evaluation of psychosocial outcomes following ear reconstruction with rib cartilage in microtia

Steffen A, Wollenberg B, König IR, et al (Univ of Lübeck, Germany)
J Plast Reconstr Aesthet Surg 63:1466-1473, 2010

Little is known about the psychosocial improvement of microtic patients following reconstruction with rib cartilage. Furthermore, no data exist on detailed follow-ups of patients who refused ear repair. To the best of our knowledge, this is the first report of a prospective evaluation of psychosocial outcomes with a validated instrument in ear reconstruction with rib cartilage.

Twenty-one patients, who had undergone rib-cartilage reconstruction to treat a congenital auricular defect, were evaluated prospectively for psychosocial changes using a clinically validated questionnaire. In addition, patients were asked to judge the new auricle and thoracic scar. Twenty-three patients, who decided against an ear reconstruction following consultation, were analysed for the reasons behind their refusal.

Almost 66% of the treated patients were able to integrate the new ear into their body concept. If faced with the same surgery decision again, 88% would still choose to undergo ear reconstruction with rib cartilage. There were strong postoperative improvements in psychosocial attitude ($p = 0.02$). In our sample, patients who declined ear repair showed higher values of psychosocial attitude ($p = 0.006$) compared with the preoperative results in treated patients.

Our study shows that the clinically known improvement of psychosocial aspects can be documented by a validated psychological test. The patient's expectations and surgical limits of the reconstruction with rib cartilage need detailed discussion prior to surgery to prevent dissatisfaction despite surgical success. Our data help to accept a child's denial as these patients have a good psychosocial standing even with an unrepaired microtia.

▶ This is an interesting study looking at the psychological outcomes of a surgical procedure that can affect the appearance of a child significantly. Ear reconstruction with autologous rib cartilage is currently the most accepted method for the repair of auricular defects. And alternatives include using a prosthesis or refusing any intervention. This study examined patients, using a psychometric questionnaire, before and following ear reconstruction with rib cartilage in a prospective manner and compared these results with those from patients who declined ear reconstruction. This approach is likely to yield helpful insights that could aid in advising patients and their families and in discussing their expectations prior to surgery. The survey return rate was 76%, which is very good. Interestingly, patients with microtic ears who decide against ear repair tend to have higher preoperative self-esteem and a better psychosocial attitude than those who opt for surgery. This study underscores the very high rates of acceptance of and satisfaction with ear reconstruction with autologous rib cartilage. Patients appear to experience improved psychological well-being following ear reconstruction. The thoracic scar is not the most stressful part of the reconstructive process and is well accepted as part of the surgical technique. There are obvious limitations of this study including selection bias and a small study population. Nonetheless, this is an approach to studying surgical outcomes that should be used more extensively.

R. B. Mitchell, MD

Childhood tonsillectomy: who is referred and what treatment choices are made? Baseline findings from the North of England and Scotland Study of Tonsillectomy and Adenotonsillectomy in Children (NESSTAC)

Lock C, Wilson J, Steen N, et al (Newcastle Univ, Newcastle upon Tyne, UK; et al)

Arch Dis Child 95:203-208, 2010

Background.—Tonsillectomies are frequently performed, yet variations exist in tonsillectomy rates. Clinicians use guidelines, but complex psychosocial influences on childhood tonsillectomy include anecdotal evidence of parental enthusiasm. Studies indicate that undergoing preferred treatment improves outcome. Despite the enthusiasm with which tonsillectomy is offered and sought, there is little evidence of efficacy. This resulted in a randomised controlled trial to evaluate the cost-effectiveness of (adeno)-tonsillectomy in children with recurrent sore throats.

Objective.—To compare characteristics of children entering the randomised trial with those recruited to a parallel, non-randomised study, to establish trends in referral and patient preferences for treatment.

Design.—Baseline data from a randomised controlled trial with parallel non-randomised preference study, comparing surgical intervention with medical treatment in children aged 4–15 years with recurrent sore throat referred to five secondary care otolaryngology departments located in the north of England or west central Scotland.

Results.—Centres assessed 1546 children; 21% were not eligible for tonsillectomy. Among older children (8–15 years), girls were significantly more likely to be referred to secondary care. Of 1015 eligible children, 268 (28.2%) agreed to be randomised, while 461 (45.4%) agreed to the parallel, non-randomised preference study, with a strong preference for tonsillectomy. Participants reporting that progress at school had been impeded or with more experience of persistent sore throat were more likely to seek tonsillectomy. Referred boys were more likely than girls to opt for medical treatment. Socio-economic data showed no effect.

Conclusion.—Preference for tonsillectomy reflects educational impact and recent experience, rather than age or socio-economic status.

▶ This is an interesting report that highlights the difficulties in performing randomized controlled trials looking at outcomes of surgical versus medical/observational therapies. The data reported are from a randomized controlled trial in the United Kingdom to evaluate the cost-effectiveness of (adeno)tonsillectomy in children with recurrent sore throats (North of England and Scotland Study of Tonsillectomy and Adenotonsillectomy in Children). Surgical intervention was compared with medical treatment in children with recurrent sore throat (trial group). Eligible subjects who declined randomization received their preferred treatment and were offered enrollment in a parallel nonrandomized preference study (preference group). Trial and preference subjects completed identical outcome measures at each data collection point. This article compares baseline characteristics of children and parents entering the trial, with those entering the preference study, for trends in referral and patient preferences for treatment. It is interesting that the majority of parents (63%) who agreed to participate opted for the preference option and mostly (84%) for tonsillectomy. Standard randomized controlled trials were used where there are strong preferences, experiences of high nonparticipation (refusal) rates, and consequently decreased generalizability. This study is worth reading if a randomized controlled trial of surgical outcomes is being considered.

R. B. Mitchell, MD

Outcome of Adenotonsillectomy for Obstructive Sleep Apnea Syndrome in Children

Ye J, Liu H, Zhang G-H, et al (Third Affiliated Hosp of Sun Yat-sen Univ, Guangzhou, China)
Ann Otol Rhinol Laryngol 119:506-513, 2010

Objectives.—We evaluated the outcome of adenotonsillectomy for obstructive sleep apnea syndrome (OSAS) in children using polysomnography (PSG) data and a quality-of-life (QOL) instrument.

Methods.—We enrolled children (4 to 14 years of age) who had OSAS diagnosed by overnight PSG and who underwent both adenoidectomy and tonsillectomy between January 2003 and February 2008. All of them had completed postoperative PSG and a paired Obstructive Sleep Apnea 18-Item Quality-of-Life Questionnaire (OSA-18) survey. The statistical analyses were performed with a statistical software package.

Results.—The study included 84 children with a mean age of 7.1 years. The mean preoperative apnea-hypopnea index (AHI) for the study population was 24.6, and the mean postoperative AHI was 3.8 episodes per hour. The percentage of children who had normal PSG parameters after adenotonsillectomy ranged from 69.0% to 86.9% because of fluctuation of the criteria used to define OSAS. Nine children (30%) with severe preoperative OSAS had persistent OSAS (an AHI of at least 5) after surgery. Improvements in QOL were comparable in the cured and not-cured groups ($p > 0.05$). Risk factors for persistent OSAS were obesity and a high preoperative AHI, on multiple logistic regression analysis.

Conclusions.—Adenotonsillectomy is associated with improvements in PSG, behavior, and QOL in children with OSAS. However, it may not resolve OSAS in all children. The efficacy and role of additional therapeutic options require more study.

▶ There have been several outcome studies including 2 meta-analyses that have shown that time and attendance (T&A) for pediatric obstructive sleep apnea (OSA) improves but does not cure the sleep disorder in all children. This study from Sun Yat-sen University, Guangzhou, China reports no new data but is interesting in that it shows that pediatric OSA is a global problem. The goal of this study was to report surgical outcomes and to identify variables that predispose children to persistent OSA after surgery. They conclude that although T&A for OSA successfully improves the polysomnography parameters in most children, obesity and severity of OSA may increase the risk of residual OSA after surgery. The change of OSA-18 quality-of-life scores was not correlated with either the preoperative apnea-hypopnea index (AHI) score or the reduction of AHI scores. With obesity becoming an increasing global problem, the efficacy and role of additional therapeutic options for children with residual OSA requires more study.

R. B. Mitchell, MD

Percutaneous versus Open Tracheostomy in the Pediatric Trauma Population
Raju A, Joseph D'AK, Diarra C, et al (Cooper Univ Hosp and UMDNJ–Robert Wood Johnson Med School, Camden, NJ)
Am Surg 76:276-278, 2010

The purpose of this study was to determine the safety and efficacy of percutaneous *versus* open tracheostomy in the pediatric trauma population.

A retrospective chart review was conducted of all tracheostomies performed on trauma patients younger than 18 years for an 8-year period. There was no difference in the incidence of brain, chest, or facial injury between the open and percutaneous tracheostomy groups. However, the open group had a significantly lower age (14.2 *vs.* 15.5 years; $P < 0.01$) and higher injury severity score (26 *vs.* 21; $P = 0.015$). Mean time from injury to tracheostomy was 9.1 days (range, 0 to 16 days) and was not different between the two methods. The majority of open tracheostomies were performed in the operating room and, of percutaneous tracheostomies, at the bedside. Concomitant feeding tube placement did not affect complication rates. There was not a significant difference between complication rates between the two methods of tracheostomy (percutaneous one of 29; open three of 20). Percutaneous tracheostomy can be safely performed in the injured older child.

▶ Percutaneous dilatational tracheostomy has not been used in airway management of children because the small and mobile characteristics of the trachea are thought to make them dangerous in this population. Previous research has shown percutaneous dilatational tracheostomy to be safe as an alternative to open tracheostomy, but study populations have been small. This study suggests that a percutaneous dilatational tracheostomy may have a role in some pediatric trauma patients and may be underutilized, especially in injured children older than 10 years of age. Percutaneous tracheostomy has several advantages over open tracheostomy. It can be done quickly in the intensive care unit setting without the need for special lighting, additional operating room personnel, or additional monetary costs. The complication rates are not higher than that of open tracheostomy. Patient selection is clearly key and must take into account the surgeon's comfort with the technique. The surgeon must be prepared to convert to open tracheostomy immediately should technical problems preclude safe percutaneous placement of the tracheostomy tube. This is an interesting option in a select group of older children.

R. B. Mitchell, MD

Topical Ciprofloxacin Is Superior to Topical Saline and Systemic Antibiotics in the Treatment of Tympanostomy Tube Otorrhea in Children: The Results of a Randomized Clinical Trial

Heslop A, Lildholdt T, Gammelgaard N, et al (Aarhus Univ Hosp, Denmark; The ENT Clinic, Horsens, Denmark)
Laryngoscope 120:2516-2520, 2010

Objectives/Hypothesis.—To compare the clinical failure rates among children with otorrhea through tympanostomy tubes treated with topical or systemic antibiotics versus topical saline.

Study Design.—Randomized, double-blind, controlled patient study.

Methods.—A three-armed randomized clinical trial using topical ciprofloxacin or oral amoxicillin or topical saline. The primary outcome was treatment failure defined as presence of otorrhea in at least one ear after 7 days of treatment.

Results.—The treatment failure rates were 23% and 70% in the group treated with topical ciprofloxacin and oral amoxicillin, respectively. Treatment failures were seen in 58% of children treated with topical saline. Thus, topical ciprofloxacin significantly reduced treatment failures compared to both oral amoxicillin and topical saline. The most frequent bacteria isolated from treatment failures in general were streptococci and *Moraxella catarrhalis.*

Conclusions.—The significant effect of topical ciprofloxacin is probably related to a higher local concentration of antibiotics in the middle ear rather than the result of mechanical rinsing and dissolution of the bacterial load.

▶ Early postoperative tube otorrhea has been reported in up to 20% of children after tympanostomy tube (TT) insertion, whereas delayed otorrhea occurs in as many as 68% of children. Clearly, this is a problem that most otolaryngologists see in their practice. The objective of this study was to conduct a 3-arm randomized double-blind trial to assess the outcome of systemic antibiotics or topical ciprofloxacin or saline rinsing of the external ear canal in children with TT otorrhea. This study supports the superiority of topical treatment with ciprofloxacin in cases of TT otorrhea in terms of clinical effectiveness. However, the 3 groups might differ regarding compliance. This was not analyzed in the study, but one might suspect that a higher compliance was obtained among the children receiving local treatment versus the amoxicillin group, in which the failure rates were the highest. The study also lacks a fourth arm of the spontaneous course of TT otorrhea for comparison.

R. B. Mitchell, MD

Surgical Technique

Injection Pharyngoplasty With Calcium Hydroxylapatite for Velopharyngeal Insufficiency: Patient Selection and Technique
Brigger MT, Ashland JE, Hartnick CJ (Naval Med Ctr San Diego, CA; Massachusetts General Hosp, Boston; Harvard Med School, Boston, MA)
Arch Otolaryngol Head Neck Surg 136:666-670, 2010

Objective.—To identify children who may benefit from calcium hydroxylapatite (CaHA) injection pharyngoplasty for symptomatic velopharyngeal insufficiency (VPI).

Design.—Retrospective review of children with VPI who underwent injection pharyngoplasty with CaHA.

Setting.—Multidisciplinary pediatric aerodigestive center.

Patients.—Children with symptomatic VPI as defined by abnormal speech associated with subjective and objective measures of hypernasality.

Intervention.—Posterior pharyngeal wall augmentation with injectable CaHA.

Main Outcome Measure.—Nasalence scores recorded as number of standard deviations (SDs) from normalized scores, and perceptual scoring recorded as standardized weighted score and caretaker satisfaction from direct report.

Results.—Twelve children who had undergone injection pharyngoplasty with CaHA were identified. Of the 12 children, 8 demonstrated success at 3 months as defined by nasalence (<1 SD above normal nasalance scores), perceptual scoring (decrease in weighted score), and overall caretaker satisfaction. Four children were followed up for more than 24 months and continued to demonstrate stable success. The 4 children who failed the procedure all failed before the 3-month evaluation and demonstrated increased baseline severity of VPI as defined by increased preoperative nasalence scores (5.25 SD vs 2.4 SD above normalized scores), perceptual scores (weighted score, 4.25 vs 3.85), and characteristic nasendoscopy findings of a broad-based velopharyngeal gap or unilateral adynamism. Three of the 4 treatment failures occurred early in the senior author's (C.J.H.) experience with the technique.

Conclusions.—Injection pharyngoplasty with CaHA is a useful adjunct in the treatment of children with mild VPI. Efficacy and safety have been demonstrated more than 24 months after injection. Patient selection and operative technique are critical to the success of the procedure. Success is seen most often in children with mild VPI and small well-defined velopharyngeal gaps consistent with touch closure.

▶ The primary surgical procedures used to correct moderate to severe velopharyngeal insufficiency are the sphincter pharyngoplasty and the posterior pharyngeal flap. Both provide an increase in tissue bulk to the nasopharynx, although the sphincter pharyngoplasty has been postulated to provide some degree of dynamic muscle action. However, both procedures are relatively invasive and are associated with a difficult postoperative recovery period. Posterior pharyngeal wall augmentation is a third option that can be performed using cartilage, fat, fascia, paraffin, silicone, acellular dermis, polytetrafluoroethylene, and injectable calcium hydroxylapatite (CaHA). Patient selection for posterior pharyngeal wall augmentation is a challenge and is the subject of this retrospective review of 12 children who had undergone injection pharyngoplasty with CaHA. They conclude that CaHA injection pharyngoplasty is a safe, easily performed procedure with low morbidity in selected children with clear indications. It can serve as a valuable adjunct to speech therapy and does not preclude the child from undergoing more invasive procedures. Larger study populations and longer follow-up periods are needed in future studies.

R. B. Mitchell, MD

Neonatal vs Delayed-Onset Fourth Branchial Pouch Anomalies: Therapeutic Implications

Leboulanger N, Ruellan K, Nevoux J, et al (Université Pierre et Marie Curie, Paris, France; Armand-Trousseau Children's Hosp, Paris, France)

Arch Otolaryngol Head Neck Surg 136:885-890, 2010

Objectives.—To determine the presentation of third or fourth branchial pouch anomalies in various age groups of children and evaluate endoscopic cauterization as a treatment technique.

Design.—Retrospective study of patients treated from 2000 to 2009.

Setting.—Tertiary care children's hospital.

Patients.—Pediatric patients aged 0 to 18 years (mean age, 5.5 years), including 5 neonates.

Interventions.—Endoscopic and/or open surgical management of third and fourth branchial pouch anomalies; clinical and endoscopic follow-up.

Main Outcome Measures.—Absence of clinical recurrence; closure of the sinus tract.

Results.—Two forms of presentation were identified: a neonatal form, characterized by a voluminous and compressive cervical mass (5 of 20 [25%]) and a childhood form, presenting as a cervical abscess (15 of 20 [75%]). The vast majority of our patients regardless of presentation were treated endoscopically (n = 19), with a success rate of 68% (13 of 19) after 1 procedure, 79% (15 of 19) after 2 procedures, and 89% (17 of 19) after 3 procedures. Neonatal and adult presentations require slightly different therapeutic approaches.

Conclusions.—Third and fourth branchial pouch anomalies can present in 2 distinct forms: a neonatal form and a childhood form. The endoscopic technique should be the favored approach for both forms: whenever possible, in view of its simplicity, rapidity, and the lack of serious postoperative complications. Recurrences can be treated by repeated cauterization using the same technique, with good long-term outcomes. An age-based management algorithm has been developed.

▶ This is a case series and a good review of the current management on third and fourth branchial pouch anomalies. The distinction between third and fourth branchial pouch abnormalities can only be established at the time of dissection because their clinical presentations are similar. From a practical point of view, the anatomic differences between these 2 lesions are of little significance because their clinical presentations and management strategies are often the same. From 90% to 100% of these sinus tracts are situated on the left side of the neck. In older children, they often present as abscesses, cervical masses, or rapidly relapsing thyroiditis. In the neonatal period, the presentation is usually of a cystic mass or an abscess, which may lead to dyspnea with stridor, dysphagia, and feeding difficulties. Although cervical excision is the classical approach, in the last 15 years a less-invasive treatment has evolved, namely, endoscopic cauterization limited to the sinus tract orifice. A therapeutic algorithm, taking into account the age of the patient and the clinical presentation, is included (Fig 5 in the original article). This study describes 2 forms of fourth branchial pouch anomalies: (1) a neonatal form that presents with a voluminous cervical mass containing air and possibly requiring a cervicotomy and (2) a late-onset form in children that presents with abscess formation and for which an endoscopic approach is indicated. The study provides a logical and practical approach to the management of these congenital anomalies.

R. B. Mitchell, MD

Adenotonsillectomy Outcomes in Treatment of Obstructive Sleep Apnea in Children: A Multicenter Retrospective Study
Bhattacharjee R, Kheirandish-Gozal L, Spruyt K, et al (Univ of Louisville, KY; et al)
Am J Respir Crit Care Med 182:676-683, 2010

Rationale.—The overall efficacy of adenotonsillectomy (AT) in treatment of obstructive sleep apnea syndrome (OSAS) in children is unknown. Although success rates are likely lower than previously estimated, factors that promote incomplete resolution of OSAS after AT remain undefined.

Objectives.—To quantify the effect of demographic and clinical confounders known to impact the success of AT in treating OSAS.

Methods.—A multicenter collaborative retrospective review of all nocturnal polysomnograms performed both preoperatively and postoperatively on otherwise healthy children undergoing AT for the diagnosis of OSAS was conducted at six pediatric sleep centers in the United States and two in Europe. Multivariate generalized linear modeling was used to assess contributions of specific demographic factors on the post-AT obstructive apnea-hypopnea index (AHI).

Measurements and Main Results.—Data from 578 children (mean age, 6.9 ± 3.8 yr) were analyzed, of which approximately 50% of included children were obese. AT resulted in a significant AHI reduction from 18.2 ± 21.4 to 4.1 ± 6.4/hour total sleep time ($P < 0.001$). Of the 578 children, only 157 (27.2%) had complete resolution of OSAS (i.e., post-AT AHI <1/h total sleep time). Age and body mass index z-score emerged as the two principal factors contributing to post-AT AHI ($P < 0.001$), with modest contributions by the presence of asthma and magnitude of pre-AT AHI ($P < 0.05$) among nonobese children.

Conclusions.—AT leads to significant improvements in indices of sleep-disordered breathing in children. However, residual disease is present in a large proportion of children after AT, particularly among older (>7 yr) or obese children. In addition, the presence of severe OSAS in nonobese children or of chronic asthma warrants post-AT nocturnal polysomnography, in view of the higher risk for residual OSAS.

▶ Adenotonsillectomy (AT) has been shown to lead to significant improvements in most cases of obstructive sleep apnea syndrome (OSAS) in children, as reported from several meta-analysis studies. This report is a multicenter collaborative study from several centers in and outside the United States that aimed to delineate factors that may assist in the prediction of the clinical response to AT in children with OSAS through available demographic and polysomnographic information on children who underwent overnight polysomnograms (PSGs) before and after AT. The findings on 578 children provide evidence that AT is not uniformly effective in curing OSAS in children and that in the context of increasing obesity rates in children, the ability of AT to normalize OSAS needs to be viewed with great skepticism. Older children and obese children were least likely to respond to AT. Previous studies have shown that the severity of underlying OSAS, as determined by the pre-AT apnea-hypopnea index (AHI), affected the surgical response. In this study, the effect of pre-AT AHI was remarkably small compared with that of age and body mass index z-score and was applicable only to the nonobese children. In addition, this study shows that the presence of asthma contributes to an increased risk of persistent OSAS after AT, particularly among nonobese children. This study provides important data that can direct future criteria for use of postoperative PSG in children after AT for OSAS.

R. B. Mitchell, MD

Changes and consistencies in the epidemiology of pediatric adenotonsillar surgery, 1996-2006
Bhattacharyya N, Lin HW (Brigham and Women's Hosp, Boston, MA; Harvard Med School, Boston, MA)
Otolaryngol Head Neck Surg 143:680-684, 2010

Objective.—Determine changes in rates for pediatric adenotonsillar procedures over time with attention to infectious indications.
Study Design.—Historical cohort study.
Setting.—Academic medical center.
Subjects and Methods.—The National Survey of Ambulatory Surgery and the National Hospital Discharge Survey 1996 and 2006 releases were examined, extracting all cases of pediatric tonsillectomy, adenotonsillectomy, and adenoidectomy. The aggregate numbers and rates of adenotonsillar procedures performed overall and specifically for chronic infectious etiologies were determined. These procedure rates were then compared to determine differences in performance rates between 1996 and 2006.
Results.—In 1996, an estimated 441,870 ± 23,315 children underwent some form of adenotonsillar surgery in the ambulatory and inpatient settings (60,034 ± 6994 tonsillectomies, 255,217 ± 18,960 adenotonsillectomies, and 126,619 ± 11,627 adenoidectomies), while in 2006, the total rose to 695,029 ± 36,979 children (58,111 ± 9645 tonsillectomies, 506,778 ± 32,054 adenotonsillectomies, and 129,540 ± 15,714 adenoidectomies). However, when examined according to infectious indications, a notable decline in the population rate of tonsillectomy from 0.62 per

1000 children in 1996 to 0.53 per 1000 in 2006 was found ($P = 0.252$). Moreover, the larger decline in the rate of adenotonsillectomy for infectious indications from 2.20 per 1000 to 1.46 per 1000 was significant ($P = 0.003$). There was no significant change adenoidectomy rates for chronic infectious etiologies (0.25 versus 0.21 per 1000, $P = 0.326$).

Conclusion.—Although there was an overall increase in the rate of performance of adenotonsillar surgery, population adjusted performance rates of these procedures specifically for infectious indications declined from 1996 to 2006.

▶ This study reports data from the 1996 and 2006 releases of the National Hospital Discharge Survey (NHDS) and National Survey of Ambulatory Surgery (NSAS) looking at the indications and incidence of the various tonsil and adenoid procedures on a national level in both the inpatient and outpatient surgical settings. In 1996, an estimated 417 043 and 24 827 children underwent tonsillectomy, adenotonsillectomy, or adenoidectomy in the ambulatory and inpatient settings, respectively. The mean ages for ambulatory patients and inpatients were 6.8 and 6.1 years, respectively, and sex distributions were 49.8% men and 58.3% men, respectively. In 2006, an estimated 682 598 and 34 573 children underwent tonsillectomy, adenotonsillectomy, or adenoidectomy in the ambulatory and inpatient settings, respectively. The mean ages were 6.3 and 7.3 years, respectively. Sex distributions were 51.8% men and 65.8% men. Although there was an overall increase in the rate of performance of tonsil and adenoid procedures overall, the population-adjusted rates of performance of these procedures for infectious indications declined from 1996 to 2006. The inclusion of both NSAS and NHDS data in the current study not only provides the most recent information on several of the most frequently performed otolaryngologic procedures on a national level but also incorporates both inpatient and outpatient data sets, which has not been previously reported for adenotonsillar surgery. In contrast to the relative stability of the incidence of tonsillectomy from 1996 to 2006, they report that pediatric adenotonsillectomy incidence nearly doubled. This is likely in large part because of the recent recognition of the morbidity of obstructive sleep apnea and sleep-disordered breathing. These data argue against assertions that care providers are less inclined to pursue medical therapeutic options for chronic tonsillitis and/or adenoiditis in favor of potentially more lucrative surgical interventions. The authors mention a well-publicized presidential comment on possible financial motivations for tonsillectomy during the recent health care debate. The American Academy of Otolaryngology–Head and Neck Surgery are due to publish an evidence-based guideline on tonsillectomy in children in January 2011 that will provide further information on this commonly performed surgical procedure.

R. B. Mitchell, MD

Cost and Outcomes After Cold and Mixed Adenotonsillectomy in Children

Ferreira RF, Serapiao CJ, Ferreira APRB, et al (Univille, Joinville, Brazil; et al)
Laryngoscope 120:2301-2305, 2010

Objective/Hypothesis.—To compare cold and mixed (electrocautery tonsillectomy with curettage adenoidectomy) adenotonsillectomies in children in terms of hospital medications' and materials' costs, surgical time, aspirated blood volume, and postoperative pain.

Study Design.—Randomized clinical trial in community hospitals.

Methods.—Seventy-two patients aged 3 to 12 years, undergoing adenotonsillectomy, were randomized in two groups through sealed envelopes that were opened just prior to the procedure. Surgical time and aspirated blood volume were measured by a staff nurse. Hospital medication and material costs were supplied by the hospital's accounting department. A validated facial pain scale was used from the day of surgery to the 10th postoperative day to quantify pain.

Results.—Bicaudal *t* test showed that materials' cost was lower in the mixed technique. Surgical time and aspirated blood volume were also lower with the mixed technique. The postoperative pain was more intense in the cold technique on the day of surgery, but was more intense in the mixed technique from the 4th day to the 6th day. Linear regression showed a weak association between materials' cost and aspirated blood volume.

Conclusions.—Mixed technique reduces the costs of materials while offering the patient and the surgeon a safer and faster method to perform adenotonsillectomy, although it is slightly more painful than the cold technique in the latter part of the postoperative period.

▶ This study looked at 2 methods of performing adenotonsillectomy (T&A) using a variety of outcomes measures. The objective was to conduct a parallel, single-blind, randomized trial in children, comparing cold technique T&A with mixed technique T&A (cold adenoidectomy and electrocautery tonsillectomy) in terms of hospital medications and material costs, surgical time, aspirated blood volume, and postoperative pain. Although the study population was relatively small, the methodology was good and minimized bias. The results and conclusions are interesting. The material costs were lower in the mixed technique group. Aspirated blood volume and surgical time were also significantly lower in the mixed technique group. The postoperative pain was more intense in the cold technique group on the day of surgery and was more intense in the mixed technique group from the fourth to sixth days. Unfortunately, the small study population made the assessment of postoperative bleeding impossible. This study highlights the reasons why there has been a move away from a cold technique; the mixed technique is a good alternative to the cold technique, offering the patient and surgeon a method with lower material costs that is safe and fast, and with less bleeding, although slightly more painful than the cold technique.

R. B. Mitchell, MD

Dental caries as a side effect of infantile hemangioma treatment with propranolol solution

Girón-Vallejo O, López-Gutiérrez JC, Fernández-Pineda I, et al (Virgen de la Arrixaca Children's Hosp, Murcia, Spain; La Paz Children's Hosp, Madrid, Spain; Virgen del Rocío Children's Hosp, Sevilla, Spain)
Pediatr Dermatol 27:672-673, 2010

We report the case of an 18-month-old boy who presented with caries in the upper central incisors associated with the use of propranolol solution for the treatment of an infantile hemangioma. This side effect of propranolol solution has not been reported before, and it may result from a sucrose-based excipient of the solution, or decreased salivation caused by beta-adrenergic antagonist effect of propranolol.

▶ This is an interesting case report that is of interest to otolaryngologists who are increasingly using propranolol, often as first-line treatment of hemangioma. Infantile hemangioma (IH) is the most common benign tumor in children and has a distinctive life cycle, characterized by a proliferative phase in early infancy followed by an involutional phase. The response of IH to propranolol therapy was reported initially in 2008. Potential significant adverse effects can include bradycardia, hypotension, hypoglycemia, and bronchospasm. The child in this report presented with dental caries that developed a few weeks after the treatment with oral propranolol solution therapy. Two hypotheses are proposed: (1) the liquid solution includes sugar in its formulation. Accumulating evidence exists on a clinical and experimental basis, which shows a significant association between the intake of sucrose-based medication and an increased incidence of dental caries and (2) propranolol as a beta-adrenergic antagonist can affect salivary gland function, enhancing susceptibility to caries by decreasing proline-rich proteins and causing decreased salivation resulting in tooth decay. In conclusion, they recommend that physicians should be aware of potential adverse effects related to the use of propranolol, including dental caries.

R. B. Mitchell, MD

Exploring the Critical Distance and Position Relationships Between the Eustachian Tube and the Internal Carotid Artery

Bergin M, Bird P, Cowan I, et al (Christchurch Hosp, New Zealand; Univ of Otago, Christchurch, New Zealand)
Otol Neurotol 31:1511-1515, 2010

Objective.—Endoscopic surgery to the nasopharyngeal portion of the Eustachian tube (ET) has been advocated for ET dysfunction. It is therefore essential to understand the relationship between the ET and the internal carotid artery (ICA) from an endoscopic perspective.
Study Design.—Retrospective database review.

Setting.—Tertiary and University Hospital.

Patients.—General population undergoing cervical CT scanning.

Intervention(s).—397 sides were reviewed in 200 CT scans.

Main Outcome Measure(s).—Measurements were taken from the anterosuperior ET torus to the ICA and from the fossa of Rosenmüller (FR) to the ICA. The data were analyzed for any minimum "safe distance." The ICA variability was further investigated by its distance from the midline, and the angle the midline makes with a line drawn from the ET to the ICA. The artery was assessed for an aberrant path.

Results.—The minimum distance from ET to ICA was 10.4 mm (average 23.5 mm). The predicted "safe distance" decreases with age from 8.0 mm to 5.4 mm in females and 10.2 to 7.8 mm in males. FR to ICA distance was very small in some patients (minimum 0.2 mm). The ICA was an average 23.7 mm from the midline (minimum 11.5 mm). The ET/ICA/midline angle varied from 17.0- to 53.6- (average 37.7-). 36% have at least 1 aberrant ICA. These patients have significantly shorter ET/ICA distances (95% CI 0.4 Y 2.2 mm, $p = 0.004$).

Conclusion.—The distance from ICA to ET varies between males and females. There is no safe distance from FR to ICA. Patients with an aberrant ICA have shorter distances, so contrast CT scanning is advised prior to surgery so that each patient's own carotid anatomy may be known.

▶ Endoscopic surgery to the nasopharyngeal portion of the eustachian tube (ET) has been demonstrated to be successful for treatment of middle ear disease because of a dysfunctional ET that is refractory to medical management and conventional transtympanic ventilation tube insertion. Successful techniques have used both laser and microdebrider techniques and have generally been considered safe. Surgery on the nasopharyngeal portion of the ET should in particular be mindful of the internal carotid artery (ICA) to avoid catastrophic complications. We note the frequent intimate association between the fossa of Rosenmüller and the ICA. This distance can be as little as 0.2 mm. It is important that ET dissection does not mistakenly commence in the fossa. This position needs to be carefully identified endoscopically to avoid confusion. If the endoscope is sited posteriorly in the nasopharynx, the fossa may become confused with the ET. This article has a series of interesting CT scans and should be read by any otolaryngologist contemplating surgery on the ET. The simple message is: other than for minor surgery to the nasopharyngeal ET, get a prior contrast-enhanced CT scan.

R. B. Mitchell, MD

6 Rhinology and Skull Base Surgery

Basic and Clinical Research

Different Biofilms, Different Disease? A Clinical Outcomes Study

Foreman A, Wormald P-J (Univ of Adelaide and Flinders Univ, Australia)
Laryngoscope 120:1701-1706, 2010

Objectives/Hypothesis.—A potential role for biofilms in Chronic Rhinosinusitis (CRS) has been proposed, and the adverse impact they have on disease severity and postoperative outcomes has also been well described. Recent advances have allowed the species within the biofilms of CRS patients to be clearly characterized. This study investigates whether different biofilm species have different disease outcomes.

Study Design.—Retrospective review.

Methods.—Twenty-four patients with medically recalcitrant CRS undergoing Endoscopic Sinus Surgery (ESS), in whom we had previously characterized their biofilms using fluorescence in situ hybridization (FISH), were reviewed a median of 11 months after their surgery. They were evaluated for preoperative disease markers and evidence of ongoing disease in the postoperative period.

Results.—Thirty-seven biofilms were identified in the 24 patients. Almost half had polymicrobial biofilms. The presence of polymicrobial, rather than single-species biofilms adversely affected preoperative disease severity but did not alter postsurgical outcome. Patients with single organism *Haemophilus influenzae* biofilms presented with mild disease symptomatically and radiologically and achieved normal mucosa a short time after their surgery. Conversely, patients with *Staphlococcus aureus* in their biofilm makeup had more severe disease and a more complicated postoperative course. The effect of *Pseudomonas aeruginosa* and fungal biofilms is less clear.

Conclusions.—Different biofilm species are associated with different disease phenotypes. *H. influenzae* biofilms are typically found in patients with mild disease, whereas *S. aureus* is associated with a more severe, surgically recalcitrant pattern.

▶ Biofilms have been consistently demonstrated on the mucosal surface of patients with chronic rhinosinusitis (CRS) by a number of recent studies. The

171

presence of biofilms has also been associated with more severe disease preoperatively and poorer evolution following Endoscopic Sinus Surgery (ESS), albeit in a few limited studies. This retrospective study of patients with CRS builds upon our inquiry into biofilms and their potential role in CRS by examining whether different biofilm species have different disease outcomes. Twenty-four patients with medically recalcitrant CRS undergoing ESS (in whom biofilms had been previously characterized) were reviewed about 1 year postoperatively. Thirty-seven biofilms were identified and almost half had polymicrobial biofilms. Patients with single organism *Haemophilus influenzae* biofilms presented with mild disease symptomatically and radiologically and achieved normal mucosa in a short time after their surgery. Conversely, patients with *Staphylococcus aureus* biofilm had more severe disease and a more complicated postoperative course. The authors concluded that different biofilm species are associated with different CRS phenotypes with *S aureus* biofilms being associated with a more severe surgically recalcitrant course. The concept of this study is very intriguing, and certainly it offers 1 hypothesis attempting to explain the spectrum of disease severity that we all see in CRS. However, I think the conclusions are a little too strong given the small numbers, lack of meaningful data on some organisms (specifically pseudomonas and fungus), and a few of the other methodological limitations. Most notably, in addition to the fact that this is a retrospective study of only 24 patients, a glaring shortcoming is that disease severity in this article was measured only using objective criteria (presence of infections, endoscopic appearance of mucosa) and there was no consideration or measurement of patient symptoms using validated surveys. Nevertheless, this study highlights some novel concepts in the area of biofilm research. Many of us suspect that biofilms may be playing a role in (some forms of?) CRS, but exactly what role and through which mechanisms remains unclear.

R. Sindwani, MD

Presence of Olfactory Event-Related Potentials Predicts Recovery in Patients with Olfactory Loss Following Upper Respiratory Tract Infection
Rombaux P, Huart C, Collet S, et al (Université Catholique de Louvain, Brussels, Belgium; et al)
Laryngoscope 120:2115-2118, 2010

Objectives/Hypothesis.—The aim of the present study was to evaluate the course of olfactory dysfunction in patients with olfactory loss following infections of the upper respiratory tract.

Study Design.—Prospective cohort.

Methods.—A total of 27 patients were included; each patient was evaluated twice. Psychophysical testing of olfactory function was performed with the Sniffin' Sticks test and chemosensory functions with event-related potential (ERP).

Results.—At T1, 15 patients were considered hyposmic, 12 as anosmic. Accordingly, nine and 27 patients demonstrated olfactory ERP. At T2, 16 and 11 patients were considered as hyposmic and anosmic, and 11 demonstrated olfactory ERP. Analysis of variance did not show significant differences for any parameters between T1 and T2: threshold, discrimination, identification (TDI) scores at the Sniffin' Sticks and amplitudes and latencies of N1 and P2 in the ERP. However, seven patients demonstrated an increase of more or equal to six points at the TDI score, indicating significant improvement. Four of the seven patients had olfactory ERP at T1 (57%); of those patients who did not show improvement, five of 20 (25%) exhibited olfactory ERP. Thus, the presence of olfactory ERP predicts a positive evolution of olfactory function with a relatively high specificity of 83%.

Conclusions.—The current findings clearly confirm earlier results on recovery rate of postinfectious olfactory loss. The new finding is that the presence of olfactory ERP at the first consultation is also a positive predictive factor of a favorable outcome in this disease.

▶ Postinfectious olfactory loss is characterized by a sudden loss of olfactory function following an infection of the upper respiratory tract (URTI). Treatment options are extremely poor and prognostic tests for counseling would be beneficial but do not exist. Olfactory function may be assessed in the clinic with psychophysical methods (validated smell identification tests) and increasingly with electrophysiological recordings (event-related potentials [ERPs]) following both olfactory and trigeminal stimulation[1] in specialized centers. This study evaluated the course of olfactory dysfunction in 27 patients with olfactory loss following URTI. Psychophysical testing of olfactory function was performed with the Sniffin' Sticks test and chemosensory functions with ERP twice. The study found that at T1, 15 patients were considered hyposmic, 12 as anosmic. Accordingly, 9 and 27 patients demonstrated olfactory ERP. At T2, 16 and 11 patients were considered as hyposmic and anosmic and 11 demonstrated olfactory ERP. Four of the 7 patients had olfactory ERP at T1 (57%); of those patients who did not show improvement, 5 of 20 (25%) exhibited olfactory ERP. Analysis showed that the presence of olfactory ERP predicted a positive evolution of olfactory function with a relatively high specificity of 83%. This study found that on an individual basis, there is a significant improvement of olfactory function in patients with postinfectious olfactory loss in 7/27 (26%) of patients over a period of approximately 9 months, although recovery to normosmia was very rare (only 4% of patients). Importantly, hyposmia in combination with olfactory ERP at T1 seemed to be related to a higher chance of olfactory recovery. Postinfectious olfactory loss is believed to be because of damage of olfactory receptor neurons.[2] Pathophysiology of the disorder is not yet understood, but it might be related to either a toxic attack of the neuroepithelium from the viruses or dysfunction of perireceptor events. Ongoing research into the clinical significance, validation, and nuances of ERP in smell disorders is needed.

R. Sindwani, MD

References

1. Rombaux P, Weitz H, Mouraux A, et al. Olfactory function assessed with orthonasal and retronasal testing, olfactory bulb volume and chemosensory event related potentials. *Arch Otolaryngol Head Neck Surg.* 2006;132:1346-1351.

2. Yamagishi M, Fujiwara M, Nakamura H. Olfactory mucosal findings and clinical course in patients with olfactory disorders following upper respiratory viral infection. *Rhinology.* 1994;32:113-118.

Radiographic and Anatomic Characterization of the Nasal Septal Swell Body

Costa DJ, Sanford T, Janney C, et al (Saint Louis Univ School of Medicine, MO; Saint John's Mercy Med Ctr, Saint Louis, MO)
Arch Otolaryngol Head Neck Surg 136:1107-1110, 2010

Objective.—To analyze the radiographic, anatomic, and histologic characteristics of the nasal septal swell body.

Design.—Computer-aided analysis of magnetic resonance images (MRIs) and histologic examination of cadaveric nasal septa.

Setting.—Tertiary medical center.

Patients.—Fifty-four head MRI studies were performed on adult live patients; we also used 10 cadaveric nasal septa.

Main Outcome Measures.—Radiographic dimensions of the swell body and distances to other nasal landmarks were measured. Nasal septa and swell body histologic characteristics were evaluated using light microscopy. Relative proportions of vascular, connective, and glandular tissues within the swell body and the adjacent septum were compared.

Results.—The swell body was fusiform shaped and located anterior to the middle turbinate, with mean (SD) width of 12.4 (1.9) mm; height, 19.6 (3.2) mm; and length, 28.4 (3.5) mm. The epicenter was 24.8 (2.9) mm from the nasal floor, 43.9 (4.1) mm from the nasal tip, and 39.0 (4.6) mm from the sphenoid face. Histologic analyses revealed that, compared with adjacent septal mucosa, the swell body contained significantly more venous sinusoids (37% vs 16%, $P < .001$) and fewer glandular elements (28% vs 41%, $P < .001$).

Conclusions.—The swell body is a conserved region of the septum located anterior to the middle turbinate approximately 2.5 cm above the nasal floor. The high proportion of venous sinusoids within the swell body suggests the capacity to alter nasal airflow. Additional study is required before these findings are used in a clinical setting.

▶ The septal swell body (SB) is a widened region of the anterior nasal septum. This mucosal-lined swelling is readily identifiable on anterior rhinoscopy, nasal endoscopy, and sinonasal imaging studies. Little is known about its structure or function. This study analyzed the radiographic, anatomic, and histologic characteristics of the SB. Radiographic dimensions of the SB and distances to other nasal landmarks were measured. Nasal septa and SB histologic characteristics were evaluated using light microscopy. Relative proportions of vascular, connective, and glandular tissues within the SB and the adjacent septum were compared. The study found that the SB was fusiform shaped and located anterior to the middle turbinate, with the dimensions of 12 mm × 20 mm × 28 mm with its epicenter 25 mm from the nasal floor, 44 mm from the nasal tip, and 39 mm from the sphenoid face. Histologically, compared with adjacent septal mucosa, the SB demonstrated significantly more venous sinusoids (37% vs 16%, P < .001) and fewer glandular elements (28% vs 41%, P < .001), suggesting the capacity of this structure to alter nasal airflow. The anatomy and histologic characteristics of the SB may provide clues to the potential function of this poorly understood structure. Nasal airflow is regulated predominantly by the nasal turbinates. However, the observation that the SB contains significant vasoerectile tissue has prompted suggestions that it may also influence nasal airflow. The anatomic location of the SB would appear supportive of this, as it occupies the space anterior to the middle turbinate and superior to the anterior portion of the inferior turbinate, approaching the region of the internal nasal valve. The article stresses that (1) this structure should not be confused with a septal deviation (a question easily answered with pre- and postdecongestion examinations) and (2) with further research, targeting this structure in the treatment of nasal obstruction may be a possibility.

R. Sindwani, MD

General

A History of Cigarette Smoking Is Associated With the Development of Cranial Autonomic Symptoms With Migraine Headaches
Rozen TD (Geisinger Wyoming Valley, Wilkes-Barre, PA)
Headache 51:85-91, 2011

Objective.—To look at the smoking history of migraine patients and to determine if a history of cigarette smoking is associated with the development of cranial autonomic symptoms with migraine headaches.

Background.—It has recently been noted that a significant number of migraine patients may develop autonomic symptoms during their attacks of headache. Why some headache patients activate the trigeminal autonomic reflex and develop cranial autonomic symptoms while others do not is unknown. Cluster headache occurs more often in patients with a history of cigarette smoking, suggesting a link between tobacco exposure and cluster headache pathogenesis. Could cigarette smoking in some manner lead to activation of the trigeminal-autonomic reflex in headache patients? If cigarette smoking does lower the threshold for activation of the trigeminal autonomic reflex then do migraine patients who have a history of cigarette smoking more often develop cranial autonomic symptoms than migraineurs who have never smoked?

Methods.—Consecutive patients diagnosed with migraine (episodic or chronic) who were seen over a 7-month time period at a newly established headache center were asked about the presence of cranial autonomic symptoms during an attack of head pain. Patients were deemed to have positive autonomic symptoms along with headache if they experienced at least one of the following symptoms: eyelid ptosis or droop, eyelid or orbital swelling, conjunctival injection, lacrimation, or nasal congestion/ rhinorrhea. A smoking history was determined for each patient including was the patient a current smoker, past smoker, or had never smoked. Patients were deemed to have a positive history of cigarette smoking if they had smoked continuously during their lifetime for at least at 1 year.

Results.—A total of 117 migraine patients were included in the analysis (96 female, 21 male). Forty-six patients had a positive smoking history, while 71 patients had no smoking history. Some 70% (32/46) of migraineurs with a positive history of cigarette smoking had cranial autonomic symptoms along with their headaches, while only 42% (30/71) of the nonsmoking patients experienced at least 1 autonomic symptom along with headaches and this was a statistically significant difference ($P < .005$). In total, 74% of current smokers had autonomic symptoms with their headaches compared with 61% of past smokers and this was not a statistically significant difference. There was a statistically significant difference between the number of current smokers who had autonomic symptoms with their headaches compared with the number of patients who never smoked and had autonomic symptoms ($P < .05$). Overall, 52% of the studied migraineurs had autonomic symptoms. There was a statistically significant difference between autonomic symptom occurrence in male and female smokers vs male and female nonsmokers. Each subtype of cranial autonomic symptoms was all more frequent in smokers.

Conclusion.—A history of cigarette smoking appears to be associated with the development of cranial autonomic symptoms with migraine headaches.

▶ The relationship between nasal symptoms and migraine is poorly understood. It has been noted that a significant number of migraine patients may also develop autonomic symptoms during their attacks of headache. Why some headache patients activate the trigeminal autonomic reflex (anatomic brainstem connection between the trigeminal cervical complex and cranial parasympathetic outflow system) and thus develop headache and cranial autonomic symptoms while others do not is unknown. Cluster headache, a characteristic trigeminal autonomic cephalalgia, occurs more often in patients with a history of cigarette smoking, suggesting some link between tobacco exposure and cluster headache pathogenesis. This study uses this knowledge and hypothesizes that cigarette smoking leads to activation of the trigeminal autonomic reflex in headache patients. This very interesting study looked at the smoking history of 117 migraine patients to determine if a history of cigarette smoking is associated with the development of cranial autonomic symptoms with migraine headaches. Consecutive patients diagnosed with migraine who were seen over a 7-month time period were asked about the presence of cranial autonomic symptoms (such as eyelid swelling, lacrimation, nasal congestion, rhinorrhea, etc) during headache. Approximately 70% (32/46) of migraineurs with a positive history of cigarette smoking had cranial autonomic symptoms along with their headaches, while only 42% (30/71) of the nonsmoking patients experienced at least 1 autonomic symptom along with headaches.

There was a statistically significant difference between the number of current smokers who had autonomic symptoms with their headaches and the number of patients who never smoked and had autonomic symptoms. Overall, 52% of the studied migraineurs had autonomic symptoms. The study concluded that a history of cigarette smoking appears to be associated with the development of cranial autonomic symptoms with migraine headaches. Cranial autonomic symptoms that occur with headache typically reflect activation of the trigeminal autonomic reflex. This proposed mechanism is interesting and provides some potential explanation for why headache patients get autonomic symptoms such as nasal congestion and rhinorrhea during migraines. It will be exciting to watch how this research progresses.

R. Sindwani, MD

A Systematic Analysis of Septal Deviation Associated With Rhinosinusitis

Orlandi RR (Univ of Utah, Salt Lake City)
Laryngoscope 120:1687-1695, 2010

Objectives/Hypothesis.—Rhinosinusitis might have many etiologies that lead to a common presentation of inflammation and impaired mucociliary clearance. Anatomic factors were once thought to play a large role in the pathogenesis of rhinosinusitis, and septal deviation was examined in multiple studies with conflicting results. With the more recent appreciation that the development of rhinosinusitis is likely multifactorial, it is appropriate to re-examine possible anatomic etiologies. A systematic analysis of septal deviation and rhinosinusitis was therefore performed to better define this association and describe possible etiologic mechanisms. Examination of a large sample, accomplished through systematically identifying and combining previous studies, may compensate for the several shortcomings of these separate analyses. A systematic analysis was therefore performed to answer the question, is septal deviation associated with rhinosinusitis?

Study Design.—Systematic analysis of previously published studies.

Methods.—Following a structured literature search, articles examining the association of septal deviation and rhinosinusitis were analyzed quantitatively and qualitatively. Based on the quantitative results, a septal deviation angle (SDA) cutoff of 10° was chosen for distinguishing positive from negative for septal deviation in the qualitative analysis.

Results.—Of over 300 references initially identified, 13 articles comprised the basis of this review. Increasing angles of septal deviation were associated with increasing prevalence of rhinosinusitis in multiple studies. Combining the results of five previous studies on this subject demonstrated significant association of septal deviation and rhinosinusitis ($P = .0004$, χ^2 analysis). The clinical effect was found, however, to be modest with an odds ratio of 1.47. Interestingly, in all studies that examined the laterality of rhinosinusitis associated with septal deviation, inflammation was found bilaterally. Based on the data from this analysis, it appears that many of the previous analyses were insufficiently powered to detect an association between rhinosinusitis and septal deviation. Others failed to find an association by examining subjects with small SDAs.

Conclusions.—Septal deviation is associated with an increased prevalence of rhinosinusitis, although the impact of this anatomic anomaly is limited. It appears to be one of many possible factors that might lead to the development of rhinosinusitis (Fig 1).

▶ This interesting meta-analysis examines the possible pathophysiological role of septal deviation in chronic rhinosinusitis (CRS). From the outset, anatomic abnormalities have been suspected to play a key role in pathogenesis of rhinosinusitis through obstruction of the ostiomeatal complex or impairment of mucociliary function.

In this analysis, a septal deviation angle (SDA) cutoff of 10° was (arbitrarily) chosen for distinguishing positive from negative for septal deviation. Of over 300 references initially identified, 13 articles comprised the basis of this review. Increasing angles of septal deviation were associated with increasing prevalence of rhinosinusitis in multiple studies. Combining the results of 5 of these studies demonstrated significant association of septal deviation and rhinosinusitis ($P = .0004$, χ^2 analysis). The clinical effect was found, however, to be only modest (odds ratio, 1.47). Noteworthy and I think a major issue that yet needs to be explained is that in all studies that examined the laterality of rhinosinusitis associated with septal deviation inflammation was found bilaterally. The author concluded that septal deviation is associated with an increased prevalence of

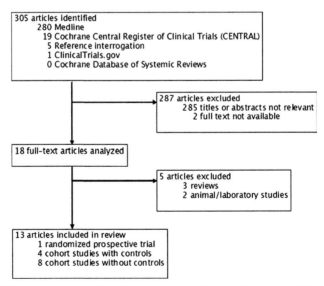

FIGURE 1.—Search strategy and article analysis process. (Reprinted from Orlandi RR. A systematic analysis of septal deviation associated with rhinosinusitis. *Laryngoscope.* 2010;120:1687-1695, with permission The American Laryngological, Rhinological and Otological Society, Inc.)

rhinosinusitis, although the impact of this anatomic finding is limited. Whether a septal deviation plays a role in CRS appears to further depend on the degree of deviation. The study further suggested that the SDA appears to play a significant role, with $>10°$ appearing to be a breakpoint beyond which rhinosinusitis is more reliably seen. Certainly all of us consider the role of anatomic factors including septal deviation in the management of our patients with CRS (if not just for improving access during surgery or postoperatively), but this article takes this 1 step further and suggests a pathophysiologic role for the deviation. The fact that CRS inflammation is and was seen bilaterally in cases of delayed neurological syndrome (DNS) still has not been adequately explained in this article or others in the literature remains a major barrier to the acceptance of this hypothesis. Articles on this topic also do not appropriately take into account the "incidence" of DNS in the general population, which of course could be defined in a large variety of ways ($>10°$ of deflection being just 1), and relate this back to the presence of CRS.

R. Sindwani, MD

Balloon Catheter Technology in Rhinology: Reviewing the Evidence
Batra PS, Ryan MW, Sindwani R, et al (Univ of Texas Southwestern Med Ctr, Dallas; Cleveland Clinic Foundation, OH)
Laryngoscope 121:226-232, 2011

Balloon catheter technology (BCT) for management of paranasal sinus inflammatory disease was introduced to otolaryngology in 2005. Since its introduction, BCT has been a subject of considerable controversy with proponents for and against adoption of the technology. Balloon procedures have been promoted as a less invasive alternative to endoscopic sinus surgery that results in reduced pain and quicker recovery. The technology and its promotion have generated significant press coverage and interest by the lay public looking for new solutions for sinonasal problems. Over time, alternate balloon devices have been advocated for operating room and office-based sinus ostia dilatation. This contemporary review will evaluate the existing evidence on the available balloon devices. The frank strengths and weaknesses of the peer-reviewed literature will be highlighted. The potential complications unique to balloon catheters and radiation exposure from fluoroscopy will also be discussed.

▶ Without a doubt, the use of balloon catheter technology (BCT) has been the most controversial topic to hit the rhinology world for many years. This contemporary review was designed by 4 senior rhinologists who have no vested interest in any balloon manufacturing company and was performed to try and provide a balanced and objective critique of the topic so that otolaryngologists might better be able to decide the role of this new technology (if any) in their practices. It reviews the various BCT available, critically analyzes the published scientific literature, explores special applications, and examines the safety profile of these devices. To date, 3 different devices (Balloon Sinuplasty,

LacriCATH, FinESS) have been reported in the literature that provide alternate strategies for operative suite and office-based sinus ostia dilatation. The Balloon Sinuplasty has been most extensively studied to date. The accrued data attest to its safety, whereas the largest published observational cohort studies have demonstrated the ability to achieve sinus ostia patency for up to 2 years. However, because the selection criteria for these studies were not clearly defined, it is unclear if these data can be extrapolated to the general population with chronic rhinosinusitis (CRS). Furthermore, the apparent benefits of BCT might not extend to those who have moderate or severe paranasal sinus inflammatory disease, especially in the setting of sinonasal polyposis. Historically, recommendations for the use of new technology and procedures within rhinology have admittedly relied on the use of lower levels of evidence. However, as the medical profession has moved to embrace the principles of evidence-based decision making, expectations for minimum standards of evidence have risen. The lack of sufficient comparative outcomes data prevents adequately addressing critical issues, such as the development of appropriate indications or guidelines, assessment of the relative value of a new technology, as well as understanding its impact on the macroeconomics of health care. Further nuances to this evolving saga include new current procedural terminology codes and reimbursement/relative value unit levels for balloon dilatation, a movement afoot to migrate into the clinic from the operating room, and debates over the (central) role of the infundibulum and sanctity of the uncinate process, to name a few. Considering the current body of literature as it relates to BCT, several important issues remain unanswered and need to be addressed. Is BCT equivalent or superior to the existing devices employed in functional endoscopic sinus surgery (FESS) for management of CRS? Equally important, will the use of BCT translate into improvements in patient outcomes, overall health, and/or quality of life to justify any potential increases in cost incurred by the health care system? The many unsettled questions will be best answered by prospective randomized trials that directly compare FESS with BCT or medical with surgical treatment.

R. Sindwani, MD

Clinical value of office-based endoscopic incisional biopsy in diagnosis of nasal cavity masses
Han MW, Lee B-J, Jang YJ, et al (Univ of Ulsan, Songpa-Gu, Seoul, South Korea)
Otolaryngol Head Neck Surg 143:341-347, 2010

Objective.—To evaluate clinical features and the diagnostic accuracy of office-based endoscopic incisional biopsy in patients with nasal cavity masses.

Study Design.—Diagnostic test assessment with chart review.

Setting.—Tertiary referral center.

Subjects and Methods.—From January 1997 to August 2006, preoperative diagnosis was achieved using endoscopic incisional biopsy in 521 patients. Cytopathologic and histologic findings were categorized as malignancy, benign neoplasm, or non-neoplastic lesion. Preoperative imaging was done in 462 patients (computed tomography: 438 cases; magnetic resonance imaging: 24 cases). We investigated the accuracy of endoscopic incisional biopsy and preoperative imaging by comparing it with pathologic results from tumor resection as the "gold standard."

Results.—Most of the patients had unilateral nasal symptoms (e.g., nasal obstruction, unilateral epistaxis, unilateral facial pain), and the clinical symptoms were of little diagnostic value in the differentiation of tumor and inflammatory lesion. The sensitivity and specificity of endoscopic incisional biopsy were 43.7 and 98.9 percent, respectively, for the diagnosis of nasal cavity malignancies, and 78.2 and 96.2 percent, respectively, for the diagnosis of benign neoplasms. The sensitivity and specificity of preoperative imaging were 78.3 and 97.5 percent, respectively, for the diagnosis of nasal cavity malignancies and 66.4 and 86.3 percent, respectively, for the diagnosis of benign neoplasms. Combining the two modalities increased diagnostic accuracy in nasal cavity masses.

Conclusion.—Endoscopic incisional biopsy alone did not ensure accurate diagnosis of nasal cavity tumors, but in combination with preoperative imaging it was helpful for the diagnosis of nasal cavity malignancies (Fig 1, Table 3).

▶ This interesting study aimed to define the roles of endoscopic incisional biopsy and preoperative imaging in the diagnostic workup and management of unilateral nasal cavity masses, comparing them with permanent biopsy achieved by definite resection as the gold standard. The authors point out that incisional biopsies obtained in the clinic can be readily obtained, aid in quickly establishing a tissue diagnosis, and in cases where nonsurgical treatment is the preferred definitive treatment modality, may avoid general anesthesia and possible surgical complications all together. Subjects with unilateral nasal cavity lesions were accrued from 1997 to 2006 with preoperative diagnosis achieved using endoscopic incisional biopsy in 521 patients. Histologic findings were categorized as malignancy, benign neoplasm, or non-neoplastic lesion. Preoperative imaging was done in 462 patients (CT in the large majority, 438 cases and MRI in 24 cases). The accuracy of endoscopic incisional biopsy performed in the clinic setting under local anesthetic using a thru-cutting forceps was investigated by comparing its results with final pathology from definitive tumor resection in the operating room. Most of the patients had unilateral nasal symptoms, and the clinical symptoms were of little diagnostic value with respect to final pathology. The sensitivity and specificity of endoscopic incisional biopsy were 43.7 and 98.9 percent, respectively, for the diagnosis of nasal cavity malignancies, and 78.2 and 96.2 percent, respectively, for the diagnosis of benign neoplasms. Combining results of incisional biopsy and imaging increased diagnostic accuracy in nasal cavity masses. Of note, there were no significant complications (hemorrhage, cerebrospinal fluid leak, etc) encountered during incisional biopsy in the clinic. The study concluded that endoscopic incisional biopsy alone did not ensure accurate

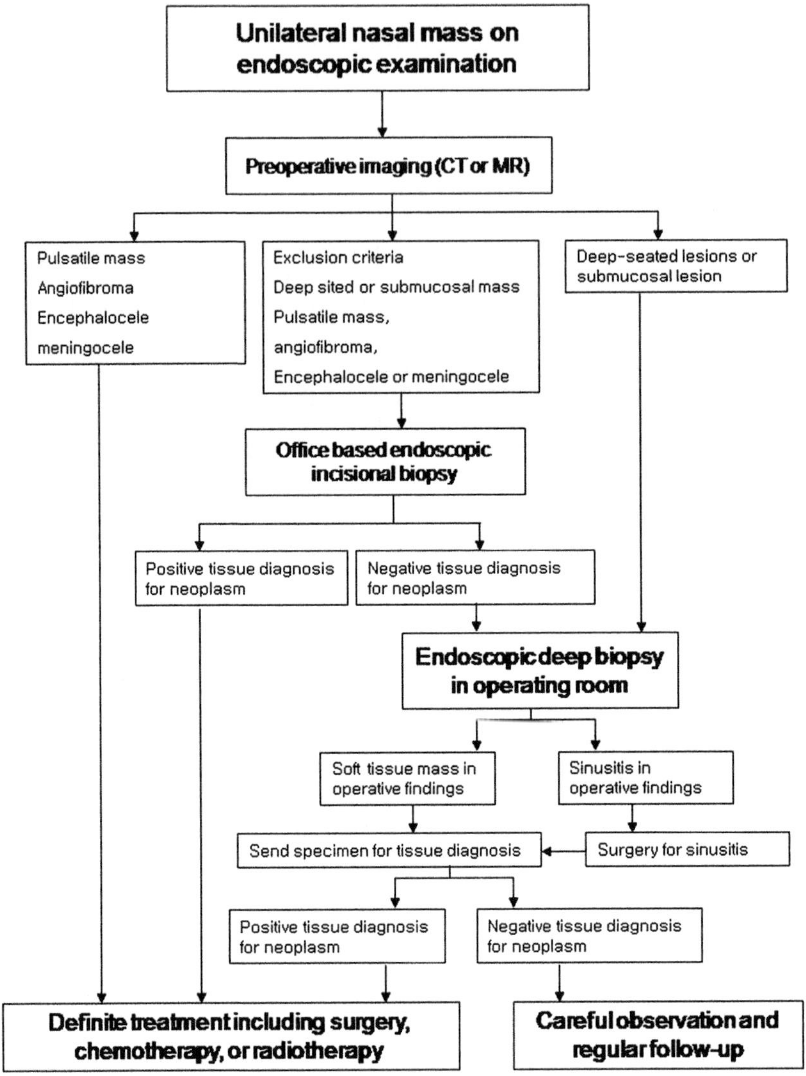

FIGURE 1.—Decision tree for nasal cavity masses. (Reprinted from Han MW, Lee B-J, Jang YJ, et al. Clinical value of office-based endoscopic incisional biopsy in diagnosis of nasal cavity masses. *Otolaryngol Head Neck Surg*. 2010;143:341-347. Copyright 2010, with permission from American Academy of Otolaryngology–Head and Neck Surgery Foundation.)

diagnosis of nasal cavity tumors, but in combination with preoperative imaging, it was helpful for the diagnosis of nasal cavity malignancies. The authors provide a thoughtful analysis of exactly where misdiagnoses (Table 3) were made and provide a decision tree to approach nasal cavity masses (Fig 1). They nicely highlight that presumptive diagnoses of angiofibroma, encephalocele, or meningoceles based on clinical history and imaging studies should skip

TABLE 3.—Misdiagnosis by Office-Based Endoscopic Incisional Biopsy in Malignant Tumors (n = 33)

Histologic Diagnosis	Endoscopic Incisional Biopsy	
Squamous cell carcinoma	Inverted papilloma	4 (15%)
	Inflammatory lesion	11 (40%)
Malignant melanoma	Inflammatory lesion (polyp)	4 (57%)
Undifferentiated carcinoma	Keratinous acellular debris (necrotic tissue)	4 (100%)
Adenoid cystic carcinoma	Inflammatory lesion (granulation)	4 (40%)
NK/T-cell lymphoma	Inflammatory lesion	2 (50%)
Teratocarcinosarcoma	Inflammatory lesion	1 (100%)
Sarcoma	Benign lymphoid hyperplasia	1 (100%)
Malignant myxoid tumor	Spindle cell lesion	1 (100%)
Malignant fibrous histiocytoma	Inflammatory lesion (fibrotic nodule)	1 (100%)

any biopsy steps and move directly to definitive surgical management. Clinicians should be aware that endoscopic incisional biopsy and radiologic evaluation have limitations but when used in combination can be of great assistance in the diagnosis of nasal cavity masses. The article points out, however, that although technically feasible and safe to perform, incisional biopsies obtained in the clinic are fallible, especially for benign lesions, and unless the diagnosis of a frank malignancy is obtained on such a biopsy, more extensive and deeper seated tissue biospsies obtained under general anesthesia should be sought.

R. Sindwani, MD

Correlates of Chemosensory Malingering

Doty RL, Crastnopol B (Univ of Pennsylvania, Philadelphia)
Laryngoscope 120:707-711, 2010

Objectives/Hypothesis.—Smell and taste tests are commonly employed to quantify chemosensory sequelae of head trauma, toxic exposures, and iatrogenesis. Malingering on forced-choice chemosensory tests can be detected by improbable responding. This study determined whether chemosensory test malingerers differ from nonmalingerers in terms of age, sex, education, and a range of self-reported behaviors and symptoms, potentially providing information of value for malingering detection.

Study Design.—Case control.

Methods.—Twenty-two chemosensory malingerers were identified from a large clinical database and matched, randomly, to 66 nonmalingerers on the basis of etiology. Differences in demographics and responses to intake questionnaire items were statistically assessed. Logistic regression was used to identify variables that best predicted malingering behavior.

Results.—Relative to nonmalingerers, malingerers reported significantly fewer allergies, dental problems, cigarettes smoked, surgical operations, nasal sinus problems, and use of medications, and significantly more putative symptom-related psychological duress, interference with daily activities, weight loss, decreased appetite, and taste loss. Litigation involvement was higher in malingerers than nonmalingerers. Age, sex, education, and length of symptom descriptions did not differentiate malingerers from nonmalingerers.

Conclusions.—Malingerers of chemosensory tests exaggerate symptom severity and underreport factors that might be construed as contributing to their dysfunction, such as smoking behavior, medication use, and general health. This contrasts with the behavior of malingerers of psychiatric symptoms, who typically exaggerate their general health problems. These data suggest that careful review of past medical records should be used to verify patient reports to better detect chemosensory malingering in cases where financial or other external incentives are present.

▶ Malingering is "the intentional production of false or grossly exaggerated physical or psychological symptoms motivated by external incentives." Anosmia or hyposmia is frequently misinterpreted as loss of taste function. Although a significant number of people with acquired olfactory dysfunction have total loss, less-than-total dysfunction is actually more common.[1] Importantly, recovery is possible in some cases. Thus, recent longitudinal studies suggest that as many as 8% of those presenting with anosmia and 18% of those with hyposmia may regain normal function over time.[2] This article explored whether chemosensory test malingerers differ from nonmalingerers on a variety of variables and self-reported behaviors and symptoms. Twenty-two chemosensory malingerers were identified from a database and matched randomly to 66 nonmalingerers. Relative to nonmalingerers, malingerers reported significantly fewer allergies, dental problems, cigarettes smoked, surgical operations, nasal sinus problems, and use of medications and significantly more putative symptom-related psychological duress, interference with daily activities, weight loss, decreased appetite, and taste loss. As expected, litigation involvement was higher in malingerers. Interestingly, age, sex, education, and length of symptom descriptions did not differentiate malingerers from nonmalingerers. The authors concluded that malingerers of chemosensory tests exaggerate symptom severity and underreport factors that might be construed as contributing to their dysfunction (such as smoking behavior, medication use, and general health). Malingering on forced-choice chemosensory tests can be detected by improbable responding.

This study suggests that people who feign or overexaggerate the degree to which they cannot smell or taste in a clinical setting differ, on a range of variables, from those with bona fide chemosensory disturbances. This presumably reflects their belief that cigarette smoking and disorders for which medications are used could be viewed as alternative causes for their alleged chemosensory dysfunction. Its findings suggest that careful and detailed review of past medical records is needed to verify patients' reports of their own medical histories when chemosensory dysfunction is claimed and financial or other external incentives are available. Further studies and techniques in reliably identifying malingerers would be of great value.

R. Sindwani, MD

References

1. Deems DA, Doty RL, Settle RG, et al. Smell and taste disorders, a study of 750 patients from the University of Pennsylvania Smell and Taste Center. *Arch Otolaryngol Head Neck Surg.* 1991;117:519-528.
2. London B, Nabet B, Fisher AR, White B, Sammel MD, Doty RL. Predictors of prognosis in patients with olfactory disturbance. *Ann Neurol.* 2008;63:159-166.

Demographical and clinical aspects of sports-related maxillofacial and skull base fractures in hospitalized patients
Elhammali N, Bremerich A, Rustemeyer J (Ctr Hosp, Bremen, Germany)
Int J Oral Maxillofac Surg 39:857-862, 2010

As many as 30% of all maxillofacial fractures (MFFs) and skull base fractures (SBFs) are reported to be sports-related. Participation in sporting activities has grown worldwide and the number of cases of sports-related injuries has also increased. The aim of this study was to evaluate the data of 3596 patients hospitalized by MFF or SBF over a 6-year period; 147 (4%) of these cases were sports-related (mean age 29.7 ± 12.8 years). The highest incidence was found in patients aged 20–29 years (35%), and the fractures resulted mostly from ball sports (74%), especially soccer (59%) and handball (8%). The injuries involved different areas, with a significant prevalence of the midface complex (67%) compared with the mandible region (29%) and the skull base (4%). The commonest diagnoses associated with MFF and SBF were brain concussion (19%), laceration of the skin and soft tissue (16%), and dental injury (8%). Surgery was required for 88% of midface fractures. In cases of mandible fractures 52% were supplied with osteosynthesis. This study identified the significant number of severe sports-related injuries that occur each year, suggesting that changes of rules and safety standards are needed for the prevention of such injuries (Table 1).

▶ The number of sports-related injuries that result in hospitalization is of course relatively small compared with those that are treated in emergency rooms or outpatient clinics, but they represent the more serious end of the spectrum of injuries. The cause of sports-related injuries varies geographically based on cultural preferences for sports (eg, skiing-related injuries in Switzerland vs soccer-related ones in France). The purpose of this study in Germany was to provide an overview of recent sports-related maxillofacial fracture (MFF) and skull base fracture (SBF) with demographic patterns, seasonal differences, type of sports, anatomical sites of MFF, and concomitant injuries. The results are discussed along with findings in comparable studies from several countries. The authors echo concerns raised by similar studies for increased awareness of these injuries and the need for further protective measures in sport. The study evaluated 3596 patients hospitalized by MFF or SBF over a 6-year period; 147 (4%) of these cases were sports related (mean age, 29.7 ± 12.8 years). Interestingly, the highest incidence (35%) was found in patients aged 20 to

TABLE 1.—Distribution of Sports-Related Maxillofacial and Skull Base Fractures and Gender (n = 147)

Sport	%	Male (n)	Female (n)
Ball sports	74	100	9
Soccer	59.2	86	1
Handball	8.2	9	3
Basketball	1.4	1	1
Volleyball	1.4	1	1
Baseball	0.7	1	0
Rugby	0.7	1	0
Squash	0.7	0	1
Hockey	0.7	1	0
Tennis	0.7	0	1
Golf	0.7	0	1
Horse riding	6.8	0	10
Skiing	4.8	6	1
Combat sports	5.5	4	4
Tae-Kwon-Do	1.4	1	1
Karate	2.7	2	2
Boxing	1.4	1	1
Others	8.9	7	6
Biking	0.7	1	0
Jogging	1.4	2	0
Inline-skating	6.8	4	6
Total	100	117	30

29 years, and the fractures resulted mostly from ball sports (74%), especially soccer (59%) and handball (8%) as shown in Table 1. The injuries involved different areas, with a significant prevalence of the midface complex (67%) compared with the mandible region (29%) and the skull base (4%). Surgery was required for 88% of midface fractures. Some authors have suggested that without adequate sports safety measures, sports-related injury and hospitalization will become more frequent. Although participation in sport involves an inherent risk of injury, research has demonstrated that most of these injuries are preventable.[1] The authors conclude that rule changes and augmented protective gear in sports should be considered.

R. Sindwani, MD

Reference

1. Conn JM, Annest JL, Gilchrist J. Sports and recreation related injury episodes in the US population, 1997-99. *Inj Prev.* 2003;9:117-123.

Does reflux have an effect on nasal mucociliary transport?
Durmus R, Naiboglu B, Tek A, et al (Haydarpasa Numune Education and Res Hosp, Istanbul, Turkey)
Acta Otolaryngol 130:1053-1057, 2010

Conclusion.—Gastroesophageal and laryngopharyngeal reflux were found to have no effect on nasal mucociliary transport.

Objective.—Gastroesophageal and laryngopharyngeal reflux have been recognized as causative factors for chronic rhinosinusitis but no definite mechanism has been described yet. We aimed to determine whether gastroesophageal and laryngopharyngeal reflux impair nasal mucociliary transport.

Methods.—This was a prospective cohort study in a tertiary referral center. Fifty patients with both laryngopharyngeal and gastroesophageal reflux comprised the study group. Reflux syndrome index and reflux finding score were calculated for each patient before and after treatment. Antireflux medication was given for 12 weeks. The control group consisted of 30 healthy volunteers. Nasal mucociliary transport was assessed by means of the saccharine test. It was performed before and after the treatment. Statistical analysis was performed using the saccharine test results of the study and control groups.

Results.—No statistical difference was found between the saccharine test results of the study group and control group before treatment. The differences betweeen the pretreatment and post-treatment reflux symptom index and reflux finding scores were statistically significant. The difference between the post-treatment saccharine test results of the patients in whom reflux scores returned to normal and those with remaining high scores was not statistically significant.

▶ This interesting and well-designed prospective study examines the important question of whether gastroesophageal and laryngopharyngeal reflux have an effect on nasal mucociliary clearance. Gastroesophageal reflux (GER) and laryngopharyngeal reflux (LPR) have been purported as causative factors for a variety of otolaryngologic diseases, including chronic sinusitis (CRS), but no definite mechanism has been described. The most common pathophysiologic theory is that the unprotected nasopharynx and nasal cavity mucosa is unable to tolerate a lower pH that results in edema and inflammation and a perturbation in mucociliary function predisposing to CRS. This was a prospective cohort study in a tertiary referral center. Fifty patients with both LPR and GER comprised the study group. Reflux syndrome index and reflux finding score were calculated for each patient. Antireflux medication was given for 12 weeks. The control group comprised 30 healthy volunteers. Nasal mucociliary transport was assessed by means of the saccharine test. It was performed before and after the treatment. Interestingly, no statistical difference was found between the saccharine test results of the study group and control group before treatment. The differences between the pretreatment and posttreatment reflux symptom index and reflux finding scores were statistically significant and supportive of the disease states studied. This study concluded that GER and LPR were found to have no effect on nasal mucociliary transport. Other possible mechanisms, including vagus nerve neuroinflammation and the role of *Helicobacter pylori* among others, need further study.

R. Sindwani, MD

Effect of Head Position and Surgical Dissection on Sinus Irrigant Penetration in Cadavers
Singhal D, Weitzel EK, Lin E, et al (Univ of Adelaide, South Australia; Wilford Hall Med Ctr, San Antonio, TX; et al)
Laryngoscope 120:2528-2531, 2010

Background.—Effective treatment for recalcitrant rhinosinusitis requires unobstructed surgical marsupialization of sinus cavities and use of delivery systems that will topically penetrate the sinuses.

Aims.—To determine the extent of sinus penetration achieved with nasal irrigation by varying the ostial size and head position.

Methods.—Ten thawed fresh-frozen cadaver heads were dissected in a staged manner. After each stage of dissection, sinus squeeze-bottle irrigations were performed in three head positions, and endoscopes placed via external ports into the sinus cavities viewed the sinus ostia. An ordinal scale was developed to grade ostial penetration of irrigations. Three reviewers independently graded the outcomes.

Results.—Irrigant entry into sinuses increased with ostial size ($P < .001$) and the greatest differential of improvement in sinus penetration is obtained at an ostial size of 4.7 mm. Stages 2 and 3 (larger sinus ostia) of maxillary and sphenoid dissections have statistically greater irrigant penetration relative to earlier stages. Frontal sinus irrigation is worse in vertex to ceiling head position. There does not appear to be any significant advantage to head position with maxillary and sphenoid sinuses.

Conclusions.—This study shows that the larger the sinus ostium, the better the penetration of irrigant into the sinus, with an ostium of at least 4.7 mm allowing maximal penetration in the maxillary and sphenoid sinuses. The same benefit was not noted in the frontal sinus. Head position was only relevant to the frontal sinus where less penetration was seen with the head neutral (vertex to ceiling) position when compared to forward angled positions.

▶ A variety of factors are thought to improve irrigant penetration of sinus ostia, including delivery system, particle size, ostial size, irrigant surface tension, and force vector of irrigant relative to ostial position. Nasal delivery experimentation with drops, lavages, sprays, and nebulizers has shown variable degrees of sinus penetration, with recent studies suggesting superiority of squeeze bottles with high volume and high force. Few studies to date have evaluated the penetration of sinuses by varying ostial sizes and head positions. This study evaluated these 2 key concepts by visualizing sinus penetration of irrigant by placing endoscopes into the sinus through external ports in cadavers. Ten fresh-frozen cadaver heads were dissected in a staged manner. After each stage of dissection, sinus squeeze bottle irrigations were performed in 3 head positions and endoscopes placed via external ports into the sinus cavities viewed the sinus ostia. Irrigant entry into sinuses increased with ostial size ($P < .001$), and the greatest differential of improvement in sinus penetration is obtained at an ostial size of 4.7 mm. Larger sinus ostia of maxillary and sphenoid dissections showed statistically greater irrigant penetration relative to earlier stages of dissection (smaller ostia). Frontal sinus irrigation was worse in vertex to ceiling head position. There does not appear to be any significant advantage to head position with maxillary and sphenoid sinuses. The study concluded that the larger the sinus ostium, the better the penetration of irrigant into the sinus, with an ostium of at least 4.7 mm allowing maximal penetration in the maxillary and sphenoid sinuses. Head position was only relevant to the frontal sinus where less penetration was seen with the head neutral (vertex to ceiling) position when compared with forward-angled positions. Irrigant penetration of a sinus requires adequate sinus ostial size. As expected, this study shows the benefits of increasing surgical dissection in the maxillary and sphenoid sinus for increasing irrigant penetration. Interestingly, the same does not hold true for the frontal sinus. Head position was only relevant to the frontal sinus where a disadvantage was seen in the nose to wall position.

R. Sindwani, MD

Effect of nasolacrimal duct obstruction on nasal mucociliary transport
Naiboglu B, Deveci I, Kalaycik C, et al (Haydarpasa Numune Education and Res Hosp, Istanbul, Turkey; et al)
J Laryngol Otol 124:166-170, 2010

Background.—Most patients with nasolacrimal duct obstruction have dry, crusty nasal mucosa. Mucociliary clearance is modulated by the amount and biochemical composition of nasal mucus. Nasolacrimal duct obstruction disturbs the drainage of tears into the nasal cavity.

Objective.—We examined the effect of nasolacrimal duct obstruction on the mucociliary transport of nasal mucosa, by comparing saccharine test results for epiphora patients versus healthy volunteers. Study design: Prospective, randomised, clinical trial.

Methods.—Eight patients with bilateral epiphora and 10 patients with unilateral epiphora were included in the study group. Complete nasolacrimal duct obstruction was demonstrated by studying irrigation of the nasolacrimal system, and by fluorescein dye study. The control group comprised 20 healthy volunteers. Mucociliary transport was assessed by the saccharine test in both the study and control groups. The saccharine transit times of 26 impaired nasal cavities were compared with those of 20 healthy nasal cavities of controls. Also, the saccharine transit times of the healthy nasal cavities of the 10 patients with unilateral epiphora were compared with those of their diseased sides, and also with those of healthy volunteers.

Results.—The saccharine transit times of the epiphora patients were statistically significantly greater than those of the control group. Also, there was a statistically significant difference in saccharine transit times, comparing the healthy and impaired nasal cavities of patients with unilateral epiphora.

Conclusion.—Nasolacrimal duct obstruction has a negative effect on nasal mucociliary clearance. This may be related to changes in the amount and biochemical composition of nasal mucus.

▶ This intriguing study examined the effects of nasolacrimal duct obstruction (NLDO) on mucociliary clearance. This unique study was based on the authors' observations that most patients undergoing dacryocystorhinostomy for epiphora had a dry crusty nasal mucous membrane on the impaired side but normal nasal mucosa on the healthy side. They hypothesized that tears contribute to healthy nasal secretions and effective mucociliary clearance. They examined the effect of the tear film on mucociliary clearance by comparing the mucociliary transport time results (saccharine test) of epiphora patients with those of healthy subjects. This was a randomized study in which 8 patients with bilateral epiphora and 10 patients with unilateral epiphora were included in the study group, while 20 healthy volunteers served as controls. The saccharine transit times of 26 impaired nasal cavities were compared with those of 20 healthy nasal cavities of controls. Also, the saccharine transit times of the healthy nasal cavities of the 10 patients with unilateral epiphora were compared with those of their diseased sides. The saccharine transit times of the epiphora patients were significantly greater than those of the control group. Also, there was a significant difference in saccharine transit times, comparing the healthy and impaired nasal cavities of patients with unilateral epiphora. The authors concluded that NLDO appears to have a negative effect on nasal mucociliary clearance. This is thought to be related to changes in the amount and biochemical composition of nasal mucus, which is negatively influenced by the absence of tear film. This is a very insightful and intriguing topic that deserves further exploration.

R. Sindwani, MD

Improvement in smell and taste dysfunction after repetitive transcranial magnetic stimulation
Henkin RI, Potolicchio SJ Jr, Levy LM (The Taste and Smell Clinic, Washington, DC; George Washington Univ Med Ctr, DC)
Am J Otolaryngol 32:38-46, 2011

Background.—Olfactory and gustatory distortions in the absence of odors or tastants (phantosmia and phantageusia, respectively) with accompanying loss of smell and taste acuity are relatively common symptoms that can occur without other otolaryngologic symptoms. Although treatment of these symptoms has been elusive, repetitive transcranial magnetic stimulation (rTMS) has been suggested as an effective corrective therapy.

Objective.—The objective of the study was to assess the efficacy of rTMS treatment in patients with phantosmia and phantageusia.

Methods.—Seventeen patients with symptoms of persistent phantosmia and phantageusia with accompanying loss of smell and taste acuity were studied. Before and after treatment, patients were monitored by subjective responses and with psychophysical tests of smell function (olfactometry) and taste function (gustometry). Each patient was treated with rTMS that consisted of 2 sham procedures followed by a real rTMS procedure.

Results.—After sham rTMS, no change in measurements of distortions or acuity occurred in any patient; after initial real rTMS, 2 patients received no benefit; but in the other 15, distortions decreased and acuity increased. Two of these 15 exhibited total inhibition of distortions and return of normal sensory acuity that persisted for over 5 years of follow-up. In the other 13, inhibition of distortions and improvement in sensory acuity gradually decreased; but repeated rTMS again inhibited their distortions and improved their acuity. Eighty-eight percent of patients responded to this therapeutic method, although repeated rTMS was necessary to induce these positive changes.

Interpretation.—These results suggest that rTMS is a potential future therapeutic option to treat patients with the relatively common problems of persistent phantosmia and phantageusia with accompanying loss of taste and smell acuity. Additional systematic studies are necessary to confirm these results.

▶ This is a very interesting article evaluating the potential beneficial effects of repetitive transcranial magnetic stimulation (rTMS) on the common otolaryngologic problems of smell and taste dysfunction. Transcranial magnetic stimulation (TMS) has been reported to influence γ-aminobutyric acid and other neurotransmitters, and it was theorized that using it to modify dysfunction in smell and taste may be of value to patients with these sensory disorders. Put simply, this is thought to somehow improve the plasticity of the central nervous system (CNS). rTMS has been reported to modify CNS excitability and enhance sensory function, and its use as a therapeutic treatment for other sensory disturbances is being explored. The study looked specifically at the efficacy of rTMS treatment in 17 patients with phantosmia and phantageusia. Before and after 3 rounds of treatments, 2 rounds of sham rTMS treatment followed by an actual rTMS treatment by design, patients were monitored by subjective responses and with psychophysical tests of smell and taste function. The study found that after sham rTMS, no change in measurements of distortions or acuity occurred in any patient. The rTMS was found to offer significant benefit: after initial (real) rTMS, 15 of 17 patients noted their distortions decreased and acuity increased, and in the majority inhibition of distortions and improvement in sensory acuity gradually decreased but repeated rTMS again inhibited their distortions and improved their acuity. A striking 88% of patients responded to this treatment, although repeated rTMS was needed. The results of this study suggest that rTMS is a potential future therapeutic option to treat patients with persistent phantosmia and phantageusia. The authors have written extensively on this topic for many years and clearly understand this topic very well. The results and implications are impressive and intriguing. However, I felt that this article was written in too factual and conclusive a tone for something clearly in its infancy for clinical applications. There are a lot of data regarding various chemical markers; some of which are modified in a variety of ways by this treatment, giving the sense that the mechanism by which rTMS works (or should work) is all figured out. In truth, a large variety of neurotransmitters are/may be modified by this treatment, and this is still in the experimental phase of development. Furthermore, it is useful to remind oneself that even the disorders we are discussing are highly subjective, variable from patient to patient, and also poorly understood. Further studies are certainly needed to confirm these results and delineate the possible future indications (if any) for this therapeutic modality.

R. Sindwani, MD

Longstanding Giant Frontal Sinus Mucocele Resulting in Extra-Axial Proptosis Orbital Displacement and Loss of Vision
Fernandes R, Pirgousis P (Univ of Florida College of Medicine, Jacksonville)
J Oral Maxillofac Surg 68:3051-3052, 2010

Background.—Frontal mucoceles are the most common of the paranasal sinus mucoceles. These lesions are benign but can severely obstruct the sinus ostium, producing dilatation of the sinus cavity secondary to mucoid material accumulation. The sinus outlet obstruction that causes these masses can result from inflammatory conditions of the frontonasal duct, external trauma to the frontal sinus and/or its drainage system, or growths or tumors in the frontonasal duct area. They characteristically produce progressive enlargement, bony erosion, and intraorbital and intracranial extension. Because they expand in the direction of least resistance, they tend to erode the thin bone of the superior orbital wall and displace the globe inferiorly. Diplopia can result, along with vision loss should the optic nerve be severely compressed by the mucocele's mass effect. A case was described.

Case Report.—Woman, 59, came for assessment of a frontal mass that had been present and enlarging for at least 10 years. On at least two occasions, she experienced spontaneous rupture and drainage of straw-colored fluid. For 4 years she had had progressive displacement of her left eye. Clinical evaluation revealed a large frontal mass with significant frontal bone protuberance and outward displacement of the frontal bone. Extra-axial proptosis of the left eye and displacement of the orbital cavity caudally and laterally were marked. She had lost both vision and light perception in the left eye. A computed tomogram (CT) revealed a large fluid-filled mass emanating from the frontal sinus. No disruption of the sinus' posterior wall or evidence of intracranial communication was found. Significant lateral displacement of the left orbital walls produced a slit effect in the residual cavity, accompanied by lateral displacement of the nasal bone and pressure resorption. As a result there was a large concavity to the left of the central face. Encephalocele was ruled out on the basis of the CT scans. The recommended treatment was surgical removal of the lesion and resultant defect, which is accomplished in a staged reconstructive approach.

Conclusions.—The patient suffered some of the significant sequelae of a giant frontal sinus mucocele. Cases involving paranasal sinus pathology are best explored using CT, although magnetic resonance imaging may be required in complicated cases with intracranial extension or coexisting infection. Treatments for frontal mucoceles vary from functional endoscopic sinus surgery to craniotomy and craniofacial exposure with or without sinus obliteration. With giant lesions, a considerably more aggressive approach is required. The most common method is radical extirpation, cranialization of the sinus, and frontonasal duct obliteration using

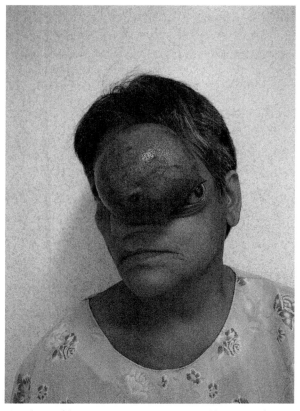

FIGURE 1.—Facial view of the patient at presentation. (Reprinted from Fernandes R, Pirgousis P. Long-standing giant frontal sinus mucocele resulting in extra-axial proptosis orbital displacement and loss of vision. *J Oral Maxillofac Surg.* 2010;68:3051-3052. Copyright 2010, with permission from American Association of Oral and Maxillofacial Surgeons.)

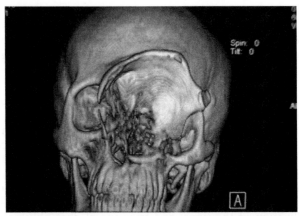

FIGURE 2.—Computed tomographic scan of the frontal mucocele. Note the significant displacement and distortion of the orbital and nasal walls. (Reprinted from Fernandes R, Pirgousis P. Longstanding giant frontal sinus mucocele resulting in extra-axial proptosis orbital displacement and loss of vision. *J Oral Maxillofac Surg.* 2010;68:3051-3052. Copyright 2010, with permission from American Association of Oral and Maxillofacial Surgeons.)

gelfoam, muscle grafts, and fibrin glue via a combined coronal approach; craniotomy may be needed if dural involvement requires resection and duraplasty (Figs 1 and 2).

▶ This is a striking case report of a 59-year-old woman with a remote history of head trauma who presented with a frontal mass that was enlarging over a 10-year period. It ruptured spontaneously a few times in the past. She presented with visual loss and extensive facial deformity (Fig 1). I selected this case report because of the impressive clinical photograph and CT reconstruction (Fig 2) and because it reminds us of (1) the amazing deformity and damage that mucoceles (benign and when discovered early, usually easy to treat lesions) can cause and (2) the power of denial in our patients. Sinus outlet obstruction that results in the formation of frontal sinus mucoceles can include processes such as inflammatory conditions, external trauma, and neoplasia in the region of the frontal outflow tract. Regardless of the etiology, their behavior is similar with progressive enlargement, bony erosion, and intraorbital and intracranial extension.[1] Frontal mucoceles are the most common (65%) among the paranasal sinus mucoceles. As the article discusses, although many mucoceles may be successfully managed endoscopically, massive lesions such as the one presented often require combined and even staged approaches for resection and reconstruction.

R. Sindwani, MD

Reference

1. Stumpe MR, Sindwani R, Chandra RK. Endoscopic management of sinus disease with frontal lobe displacement. *Am J Rhinol.* 2007;21:324-329.

Pharmaceutical Marketing and the New Social Media
Greene JA, Kesselheim AS (Brigham and Women's Hosp and Harvard Med School, Boston, MA)
N Engl J Med 363:2087-2089, 2010

Background.—Control of the Food and Drug Administration (FDA) over drug labels and promotional statements has been a powerful tool used to protect consumer health. The FDA goal is to ensure that any statements are confined to claims about approved indications and do not inflate benefits or minimize risks. Manufacturers have generally waited until the FDA has established explicit codes for acceptable practices before investing in marketing in new media. Regulating drug information on Web-based social media presents some unique challenges.

Problem Areas.—It is not clear how to provide a fair balance between benefit and risk information in the dynamic and expanding matrix of networked media, especially Twitter posts. Static Web sites have used a "one-click rule," with risk information no more than a single keystroke away. However, the access to risk information does not mean that the risks are adequately or realistically presented.

Manufacturers may also lose control over the content of their promotional message on Web-based social media. Even if it is possible to distinguish company media from other online discussions of their products, manufacturers can still support third-party bloggers, posters, and Twitter users whose comments—flattering or negative—are unregulated. Entrepreneurs have effectively blurred the line between a manufacturer's Web site and the general blogosphere.

FDA Alternatives.—The FDA could conclude that achieving a fair balance on Web-based social media is not possible in a manner that protects public health and choose to ban pharmaceutical marketing on these sites. It could also issue new guidelines, which will likely release a flood of marketing in these new media. Certain aspects must be considered by physicians should pharmaceutical promotion be allowed in social media. First, the impact of the media communication about drugs remains to be determined. To address this, an industry-funded, Internet-based social network called #FDASM has an active Twitter feed and is actively soliciting empirical research to support recommendations for Web 2.0 promotional activity that the FDA has sanctioned. Second, it is important to address the disclosure of financial interests. Most Internet users may be able to find data on drugs' risks and benefits, but it is difficult to find information on whether the source is credible and disinterested. Financial disclosure should be as explicit for leading providers of social media content as for authors of articles in peer-reviewed journals. Third, physicians and consumers should hold the FDA and drug manufacturers responsible for maintaining credible information in social media with respect to benefits and risks. It may be time to provide a digital FDA "seal of approval" to identify FDA-reviewed content in posts and discussion threads as well as a hyperlink to pages with content approved by the

FDA. Manufacturers may be in an even better position to monitor online discussions about their products.

Conclusions.—Drug promotion in Web-based social media is as yet unregulated by the FDA. Because of the unique features of these media, both government regulators and manufacturers must share the responsibility for overseeing this marketing so that it benefits and protects consumer health.

▶ This is a thought-provoking article from the *New England Journal of Medicine* on the emerging role of social media and direct-to-consumer pharmaceutical marketing efforts. Outlets such as Facebook and Twitter, the largest social media Web sites, have more than 350 million users worldwide, and surveys indicate that 60% of Americans turn first to the Internet when seeking health-related information.[1] The drug industry allocated less than 4% of the more than $4 billion it spent on direct-to-consumer advertising to Internet outlets in 2008, and only a tiny fraction of that was for social networking sites.[2] In the next year, however, the authors argue that the proportion may change substantially. Since the early 1900s, control by the Food and Drug Administration (FDA) over drug labels has been one of its most powerful tools for protecting the public's health. More recently, the FDA has been putting pressure on companies to ensure the information targeting consumers is fair and balanced, with adequate attention given to information about risks as well as benefits. The FDA may conclude that fair balance in Web-based social media cannot be implemented in a way that is compatible with public health needs, and it may try to ban pharmaceutical promotion entirely from these media. However, the authors point out that analysts predicting the agency will instead issue new guidance, which will result in an explosion of marketing in online social media, as there was in print media in the 1980s and broadcast media in the 1990s. The authors also insightfully highlight 3 aspects of pharmaceutical promotion in new social media to which physicians should pay particular attention. First, there is a dearth of research on the clinical and public health impact of communication about drugs. Second, it is crucial to deal with the problem of disclosure of financial interests in social media. Last, physicians and consumers should hold the FDA and pharmaceutical manufacturers responsible for maintaining credible information in social media. The topic of who will survey and watch-dog information on social media sites with respect to drug/instrument advertisement is of growing concern to both the public and the medical profession. It seems inevitable that this issue will need to be worked out soon, given the pervasiveness of these websites, and industry's zest for accessing them.

R. Sindwani, MD

References

1. Fox S, Jones S. *The Social Life of Health Information: Americans' Pursuit of Health Takes Place Within a Widening Network of Both Online and Offline Sources.* Washington, DC: Pew Internet & American Life Project; June 11, 2009. http://www.pewinternet.org/Reports/2009/8-The-Social-Life-of-Health-Information.aspx. Accessed March 14, 2011.

2. Arnst CA. Why drugmakers don't Twitter. *BusinessWeek*. November 19, 2009. http://www.businessweek.com/magazine/content/09_48/b4157064827269.htm. Accessed April 7, 2011.

Risk stratification of severe acute rhinosinusitis unresponsive to oral antibiotics

Hirshoren N, Hirschenbein A, Eliashar R (Hebrew Univ School of Medicine – Hadassah Med Ctr, Jerusalem, Israel)

Acta Otolaryngol 130:1065-1069, 2010

Conclusions.—C-reactive protein (CRP) levels may predict the extent of acute rhinosinusitis disease in the computed tomography (CT) scans, as well as the specific symptom severity. High levels may direct the physician to change the treatment.

Objective.—To establish tools to define 'high risk' patients suffering from acute rhinosinusitis.

Methods.—Patients suffering from severe unresponsive acute rhinosinusitis filled in health-related quality of life questionnaires and rated their symptoms. Blood tests and CT scans were performed. We examined the value of imaging and inflammatory markers, especially CRP, as predictors of disease severity, defined by subjective and objective means; need for surgery; and occurrence of ocular complications.

Results.—Thirty-two patients were prospectively recruited. A significant association was found between CRP levels, imaging scores, and symptoms severity. Neither ocular complications nor the need for surgery were present in the group with low CRP level.

▶ This study looks at the role of C-reactive protein (CRP) to help risk stratify severe acute rhinosinusitis unresponsive to oral antibiotics. Thirty-two patients with a clinical diagnosis of acute bacterial rhinosinusitis who did not improve after a period of 7 days or more of oral antibiotic treatment (amoxicillin) and a positive CT scan were included. The study found a significant association between CRP levels, imaging scores, and symptoms severity (using the Rhino Sinusitis Disability Index). Neither ocular complications nor the need for surgery was present in the group with low CRP level, while high CRP levels predicted the extent of the disease in the CT scans, as well as the specific symptom severity. The authors proposed a pathway (Fig 1 in the original article) using CRP, a simple and inexpensive blood test, to routinely evaluate severe unresponsive acute bacterial rhinosinusitis (SUABRS). High CRP levels seem to highlight higher risk individuals, and they suggested that this could be used to direct the physician to change the patient's treatment or consider surgical management. Conversely, normal CRP levels indicate a less severe disease process with a milder course, and the physician may reassure the patient and continue first-line antibiotics and symptomatic treatment. The biggest issue that I see with the use of CRP is, of course, that it is a nonspecific marker of inflammation and is in no way specific to sinusitis. Further work is needed on this topic, but I applaud the authors for investigating predictive factors that if established could help decision making in the small but significant group of patients with SUABRS.

R. Sindwani, MD

The Clinical Significance of Nasal Irrigation Bottle Contamination

Keen M, Foreman A, Wormald P-J (Univ of Adelaide, Australia)
Laryngoscope 120:2110-2114, 2010

Objectives/Hypothesis.—This study aimed to assess the clinical relevance of contamination of nasal irrigation bottles in patients with recalcitrant chronic rhinosinusitis (CRS). Secondary investigations to identify the presence of bacterial biofilms on the inner surface of the bottles and to assess different sterilization methods were also undertaken.

Study Design.—Prospective, observational.

Methods.—Eleven patients with recalcitrant CRS who were already using nasal irrigation as part of their treatment regimen were examined every 2 weeks for a period of 6 weeks. At each visit, a culture sample was taken from their irrigation bottle and middle meatus, and they were given a new irrigation bottle. Irrigation bottles from six patients were analyzed with scanning electron microscopy (SEM) to detect biofilm formation. Finally, new bottles were inoculated with different strains of *Staphylococcus aureus* and then cleaned with different methods. The bottles were cultured immediately after cleaning and 48 hours later.

Results.—Overall, 42 of 43 (97%) bottles collected demonstrated bacterial growth. Concurrent sinonasal and bottle infection with *S. aureus* was seen in 51% of patients during the study. Bacterial biofilms were demonstrated on the inner surface of four of the six irrigation bottles tested. Treatment with Milton's solution (1% NaOCl plus 19% NaCl) and microwaving were found to be effective methods for sterilizing the bottles both initially after the cleaning and 48 hours later.

Conclusions.—Patients who irrigate their nose and sinuses commonly contaminate their irrigation bottle, most often with *S. aureus*, which can be in the biofilm form. Simple cleaning methods could reduce contamination of the bottles.

▶ Saline nasal irrigations are now a key component of the medical management of chronic rhinosinusitis (CRS) and routinely used before and after endoscopic sinus surgery. Recent studies have demonstrated that nasal irrigation may be the best method for irrigating the paranasal sinuses and that large-volume low-pressure nasal irrigation is more effective than sprays or nebulizers for sinus penetration.[1,2] Despite their widespread popularity, the potential harm of nasal irrigations has only recently been considered. This simple study evaluated the clinical relevance of contamination of nasal irrigation bottles in patients with CRS by culturing the bottles as well as the patients' noses at the same time. Secondarily, the authors also examined the presence of bacterial biofilms on the inner surface of the bottles and different sterilization methods. Eleven patients with recalcitrant CRS were examined every 2 weeks for a period of 6 weeks. At each visit, a culture sample was taken from their irrigation bottle and from middle meatus, and they were given a new irrigation bottle. The bottles were cultured immediately after cleaning and 48 hours later. The study found that 42 of 43 (97%) bottles collected demonstrated bacterial growth. Interestingly, concurrent sinonasal and bottle infection with *Staphylococcus aureus* was seen in 51% of patients during the study. Bacterial biofilms were demonstrated on the inner surface of 4 of the 6 irrigation bottles tested. Treatment with Milton's solution and microwaving were found to be effective methods for sterilizing. The study concluded that patients who irrigate their nose and sinuses commonly contaminate their irrigation bottle (most often with *S aureus*), which can be clinically relevant. It found a very high rate (81%) of concurrent sinonasal and bottle infection with *S aureus*. The fact that bacteria can form biofilms on the inner surface of the irrigation bottles was also demonstrated. Although nasal irrigation has been shown to be effective in the management of CRS, infection of the bottle with bacteria may actually play a role in potentiating sinonasal infections. *S aureus* and *Pseudomonas* species are frequently found in CRS patients, and interestingly these very species were observed in irrigation bottles, possibly implicating contaminated irrigation fluid in the genesis of these infections. Although this study has a very small number of patients in it, the results do suggest that bacterial contamination of nasal irrigation bottles appears to be a clinically relevant problem. Patients should be counseled about overuse of the same bottles and encouraged to frequently sterilize their bottles.

R. Sindwani, MD

References

1. Pynnonen MA, Mukerji SS, Kim HM, Adams ME, Terrell JE. Nasal saline for chronic sinonasal symptoms: a randomized controlled trial. *Arch Otolaryngol Head Neck Surg.* 2007;133:1115-1120.
2. Wormald PJ, Cain T, Oates L, Hawke L, Wong I. A comparative study of three methods of nasal irrigation. *Laryngoscope.* 2004;114:2224-2227.

Use of Complementary and Alternative Medical Therapies for Chronic Rhinosinusitis: A Canadian Perspective
Rotenberg BW, Bertens KA (Univ of Western Ontario, London, Ontario, Canada)
J Otolaryngol Head Neck Surg 39:586-593, 2010

Background.—Many Canadians use complementary and alternative medicines (CAMs) to treat their chronic diseases. The objective of this study was to report patients' use of CAM for chronic rhinosinusitis (CRS) and to determine factors predictive of CAM use.

Method.—A cross-sectional survey was conducted. Self-report questionnaires were administered to patients with CRS using strict inclusion and exclusion criteria. The questionnaire included demographic information, questions pertaining to disease severity, and CAM use for CRS treatment. Statistical analysis was used to compare gender, age range, symptom duration, pharmacotherapy use, and surgical frequency among CAM users and nonusers. A binomial logistic regression model was developed to predict CAM use. Secondary outcome measures included factors predictive of CAM use, type of CAM used, and reasons for using CAM.

Results.—Data were obtained from 288 patients. Forty-five respondents (15.6%) had used CAM as a treatment for their CRS. CAM users were more likely to be females and more likely to have used each class of pharmacotherapy. On logistic regression, female gender and use of nasal corticosteroids were predictive of CAM use.

Conclusion.—The use of CAM as treatment of CRS is common. Females and those who have used the various classes of pharmacotherapy are more likely to use CAM. Both female gender and nasal corticosteroid use are predictive of CAM use. Physicians should routinely inquire about CAM use from their patients with CRS.

▶ Standard treatment options for chronic rhinosinusitis (CRS), such as pharmacotherapy, immunotherapy, and even endoscopic sinus surgery, result in only modest results for some patients. This may lead some patients to search for alternative treatment options. This article from Canada explored the growing trend of the use of complementary and alternative medicines (CAMs) (including herbal therapies, acupuncture, homeopathy, reflexology, aromatherapy, massage, and chiropractic). The use of alternative treatments has an important and possibly confounding impact on an individual's health status. For example, herbal preparations may potentially improve symptoms but could also lead to significant side effects or drug interactions (that may even be heretofore unrecognized). The use of CAMs has been shown to be more prevalent in patients attempting to self-manage chronic disease processes (like CRS). The authors conducted a cross-sectional survey of 288 consecutive patients with CRS to explore patients' use of CAM and examine factors predictive of CAM use. Self-report questionnaires were administered to patients. Sixteen percent of patients who responded had used CAM as a treatment for their CRS symptoms, with herbal remedies representing the most commonly used alternative. CAM users were more likely to be females and more likely to have used each class of pharmacotherapy. Further analysis with logistic regression demonstrated that female gender and use of nasal corticosteroids were predictive of CAM use in this population. The authors concluded that in Canada, the use of CAM as a treatment of CRS is common and females and those who have used the various classes of pharmacotherapy are more likely to use CAM. Interestingly, the most popular reasons for CAM use indicated by the subjects were desire to improve on existing medical therapy (17%) and frustration with conventional medicine (13%). Although this study has significant limitations (poor response rates to some questions, lack of a validated questionnaire, bias associated with self-reporting design), the results should be of interest to the general otolaryngology community. Although the scientific data supporting the use of CAMs for disease processes, including CRS, is of course quite weak (or nonexistent), this does not seem to be stopping our patients from using these unconventional treatments at an increasing rate.

R. Sindwani, MD

Outcomes

Long-term Results of Radiofrequency Turbinoplasty for Allergic Rhinitis Refractory to Medical Therapy
Lin H-C, Lin P-W, Friedman M, et al (Chang Gung Univ College of Medicine, Kaohsiung, Taiwan; Rush Univ Med Ctr, Chicago, IL; et al)
Arch Otolaryngol Head Neck Surg 136:892-895, 2010

Objective.—To study the long-term outcomes of radiofrequency (RF) turbinate surgery for the treatment of allergic rhinitis refractory to medical therapy.
Design.—A retrospective review of a prospective data set.
Setting.—Tertiary referral center.
Patients.—A total of 146 patients with allergic rhinitis refractory to medical therapy undergoing RF turbinoplasty were included.
Main Outcome Measures.—A standard 0 to 10 visual analog scale (VAS) was used to assess the allergic symptoms including nasal obstruction, rhinorrhea, sneezing, itchy nose, and itchy eyes prior to RF turbinoplasty and at 6 months and 5 years postoperatively. The long-term clinical benefits and complications were reviewed. Statistical analysis was determined by repeated measures of analysis of variance.
Results.—No adverse reactions such as bleeding, infection, adhesions, or olfactory change were encountered. Of the 146 patients, 119 were followed up at least 5 years postoperatively. Five years after treatment, 101 patients had complete data available for analysis. They reported improvement of nasal obstruction, with the mean (SD) VAS score decreasing from 6.65 (1.92) to 4.45 (2.54). The mean (SD) VAS score changed from 5.90 (2.79) to 3.79 (2.97) for rhinorrhea; from 5.15 (2.77) to 3.50 (2.77) for sneezing; from 3.67 (3.03) to 2.41 (2.30) for itchy nose; and from 2.94 (3.02) to 2.02 (2.42) for itchy eyes (all $P < .001$, paired t test with Bonferroni correction).
Conclusion.—This long-term study has demonstrated that the RF turbinoplasty for allergic rhinitis appears to be an effective and safe tool for treating allergic rhinitis refractory to medical therapy.

▶ There are a few very unique things about this study looking at long-term follow-up of radiofrequency (RF) turbinoplasty for allergic rhinitis (AR). First, the follow-up period is an impressive 5 years in duration for most of the cohort studied. Second, and more intriguing, is that unlike most studies on turbinate procedures that evaluate effects of the procedure on nasal obstruction alone, this study uniquely evaluated the effects of the surgery on a host of AR symptoms (in addition to obstruction). A total of 146 patients with AR refractory to medical therapy undergoing RF turbinoplasty were included. Using a 0 to 10 visual analog scale (VAS), allergic symptoms, including nasal obstruction, rhinorrhea, sneezing, itchy nose, and itchy eyes, were measured before RF turbinoplasty and at 6 months and 5 years postoperatively (data available for only 101 patients at this end point). The study found a significant reduction in allergic symptoms at 6 months and although the improvement waned over time, benefits in these symptoms from the turbinate surgery were still evident in many patients at the 5-year mark. The authors concluded that RF turbinoplasty was a safe and effective tool in the treatment of refractory AR. Although this study has its considerable shortcomings (including lack of a control group or randomization, poorly defined medical treatment, use of a nonvalidated VAS scale for outcomes, potentially unaddressed confounders, etc), the finding that all allergic symptoms measured (including ocular symptoms even) significantly improved for any length of time (let alone 5 years postoperatively) is unexpected to say the least. Although not completely convincing, the authors attempt to explain the improvements in general and specifically ocular allergic symptoms on the basis of the inferior turbinate being the site of allergen contact, naso-ocular reflexes, etc. More work is needed to explore these concepts certainly, but the basic notion that manipulation of the inferior turbinate can somehow alter the allergic response and reduce nasal and nonnasal allergic symptoms is intriguing and deserves some attention.

R. Sindwani, MD

Pediatric Acute Sinusitis: Predictors of Increased Resource Utilization
Dugar DR, Lander L, Mahalingam-Dhingra A, et al (George Washington Univ School of Medicine, DC; Univ of Nebraska Med Ctr, Omaha, NE; Yale Univ, New Haven, CT; et al)
Laryngoscope 120:2313-2321, 2010

Objective.—To determine variations in resource utilization in the management of pediatric acute sinusitis.

Study Design.—Retrospective analysis of a publicly available national dataset.

Methods.—The Kids' Inpatient Database 2006 was analyzed using ICD-9codes for acute sinusitis.

Results.—A total of 8,381 patients (55% male, mean age 8.5 years [SE = 0.2]) were admitted with acute sinusitis. Mean total charges was $20,062 (SE = 1,159.1). Mean length of stay was 4.2 days (SE = 0.12), with 4.8 diagnoses (SE = 0.06) and 0.85 procedures (SE = 0.06). Thirty-six percent had concomitant respiratory diseases, 11% otitis media, and 8% orbital symptoms. A total of 703 patients underwent operations on the upper aerodigestive tract (534 were nasal sinusectomies); 582 patients underwent lumbar puncture and 162 underwent orbital surgery. The primary payer was private insurance in 50% and Medicaid in 41%. Predictors of increased total charges were male gender (*P* = .028), being a teaching hospital ($P < .0001$), metropolitan patient location ($P < .0001$), hospitals in the western region ($P < .0001$), admission source from another hospital ($P < .0001$), and discharge status to another inpatient hospital or home healthcare ($P < .0001$). There is a large geographic variation in resource utilization (range = $5,837 [Arkansas] to $48,327 [California]). Race, primary payer, admission type, and urgency were not significant predictors of increased resource utilization.

Conclusions.—Despite being a common diagnosis, there exists a large national variation in management of acute pediatric sinusitis. Predictors of increased resource utilization included male gender, teaching hospital status, metropolitan patient location, western hospital region, admission source, and discharge status. Knowledge of these variables may allow interventions and potentially facilitate benchmarking to reduce the economic burden of this entity while ensuring optimal outcomes.

▶ This is a very revealing article about pediatric sinusitis, which examines many aspects of resource utilization in relation to this disease. Up to 30% of self-limiting viral respiratory syncytial (RS) can progress to bacterial RS in children, compared with less than 2% in adults.[1] Despite the information available on pediatric RS, data do not exist assessing the national demographics of the disorder in the context of variables pertaining to resource utilization. Such data may be used as internal benchmarks within health care systems and potentially to identify variables associated with increased utilization. There is a major trend in US health care to establish and look to such benchmarks. This article reports findings of The Kids' Inpatient Database 2006, a publicly available national data set, which was analyzed using the *International Classification of Diseases, Ninth Revision, Clinical Modification* code for acute sinusitis. A total of over 8300 patients (mean age, 8.5 years) were admitted with acute sinusitis in 2006, which generated mean total charges of $20 062 for care. Mean hospital stay was 4 days. A total of 703 patients underwent surgery (534 were sinus surgeries); 582 patients underwent lumbar puncture, and 162 underwent orbital surgery. The primary payer was private insurance in 50% and Medicaid in 41%. Of interest from a general perspective, significant predictors of increased total charges to the health care system were frontal sinusitis, male gender, being at a teaching hospital, metropolitan patient location, hospitals in the Western region, admission source from another hospital, and discharge status to another inpatient hospital or home health care. The study noted a large geographic variation in resource utilization (range, $5837 [Arkansas] to $48 327 [California]). Somewhat surprisingly, variables including race, admission type, and urgency were not significant predictors of increased resource utilization. This study highlighted that despite being a common diagnosis, large national variations in management of acute pediatric sinusitis exist.

R. Sindwani, MD

Reference

1. Wald ER. Sinusitis in children. *N Engl J Med.* 1992;326:319-323.

Smoker's Nose: Structural and Functional Characteristics
Kjaergaard T, Cvancarova M, Steinsvaag SK (Haukeland Univ Hosp, Bergen, Norway; Norwegian Radium Hosp, Oslo, Norway)
Laryngoscope 120:1475-1480, 2010

Objectives/Hypothesis.—The effects of smoking on endonasal geometry and airflow remain largely unknown. Our study examined the relationship between smoking status and objective measures of nasal cavity dimensions, nasal congestion, and nasal airflow, using acoustic rhinometry (AR) and peak nasal inspiratory flow (PNIF).

Study Design.—Cross-sectional study.

Methods.—Included in the study were 2,523 consecutive patients referred for evaluation of chronic nasal or sleep-related complaints. Smoking history was recorded, and AR and PNIF were measured at baseline and after decongestion of the nasal mucosa. Minimal cross-sectional areas (MCA), nasal cavity volumes (NCV), and PNIF, as well as quantified reversible mucosal congestion based on nasal congestion indexes (NCI) were analyzed to reveal possible associations with smoking status. Linear and logistic regressions were applied adjusting for possible confounders.

Results.—Smokers exhibited lower values of MCA, NCV, and PNIF than nonsmokers, both at baseline and after decongestion. Further, smokers had a lower decongestive capacity of the nasal mucosa, reflected by lower NCI for AR measures. Cigarette consumption, expressed as either pack-years or cigarettes smoked per day, showed a similar inverse relationship with the rhinometric measures even though a linear dose-response relationship could not be established.

Conclusions.—We have clearly demonstrated that smokers exhibit lower MCA and NCV, achieve lower PNIF values, and have a less-compliant nasal mucosa than nonsmokers. Our results are unique, and provide evidence that smoking has adverse effects on the nasal airway, possibly due to mucosal inflammation. This might have further implications because altered nasal function could compromise the lower airways.

▶ The adverse effects of cigarette smoking (CS) on the lower respiratory tract have been extensively studied, but little is known about the effects of CS on nasal structure and function. This study systematically examined the differences between smokers' and nonsmokers' noses using objective measures such as nasal cavity dimensions, congestion, and nasal airflow using acoustic rhinometry (AR) and peak nasal inspiratory flow (PNIF). This is a large cross-sectional study of over 2500 patients referred for chronic nasal or sleep-related complaints. Smoking history was recorded, and AR and PNIF were measured before and after decongestion. The study found that smokers exhibited lower values of minimal cross-sectional area, nasal cavity volume, and PNIF than nonsmokers, before and after decongestion, and that smokers had a lower decongestive capacity. The study concluded that there are significant differences in the noses of smokers versus nonsmokers and smokers have less compliant nasal mucosa. The authors hypothesized that smoking has adverse effects on the nasal airway, possibly because of mucosal inflammation. As discussed in the article, the differences in rhinometric recordings between smokers and nonsmokers were relatively small in absolute numbers, and it is uncertain whether these differences are indeed clinically significant, as the study did not evaluate any subjective outcomes. This is of course a major shortcoming of the study. Nevertheless, the study examined a potentially important and clinically relevant relationship. Further studies including subjective measures and investigations into possible pathophysiologic mechanisms of the effects of CS are warranted.

R. Sindwani, MD

Spontaneous CSF Leaks: Factors Predictive of Additional Interventions
Seth R, Rajasekaran K III, Luong A, et al (Cleveland Clinic Foundation, OH; Univ of Medicine and Science, North Chicago, IL; Univ of Texas Med School at Houston; et al)
Laryngoscope 120:2141-2146, 2010

Objective.—Spontaneous cerebrospinal fluid (CSF) leaks represent a significant challenge due to frequent association with elevated intracranial pressure (ICP) and higher risk of surgical failure. The study objective was to review management strategy and identify factors associated with need for acetazolamide and/or ventriculoperitoneal shunt (VPS) placement.

Study Design.—Retrospective data analysis.

Methods.—Chart review performed from 1999 to 2009 at a tertiary-care medical center.

Results.—A total of 105 patients underwent CSF leak repair; 39 patients (37.1%) were treated for spontaneous CSF leaks. Mean age was 57.7 years and 33 were female (85%). Average body mass index (BMI) was 38.5 kg/m². The most common sites were cribriform plate (51%), sphenoid lateral pterygoid recess (31%), and ethmoid roof (8%). All patients underwent endoscopic repair utilizing image guidance with multilayered closure in most cases. Five patients (12.8%) developed recurrent CSF leak with mean ICP of 27.0 cm H_2O, compared to 25.0 cm H_2O for those without recurrence ($P = .33$). All had successful rerepair at mean follow-up of 2.8 years. Acetazolamide was used in nine patients, whereas six patients underwent VPS placement for elevated ICP management. Diagnosis of benign intracranial hypertension (BIH) was statistically associated with need for acetazolamide or VPS ($P < .001$), whereas elevated ICP reached borderline significance ($P = .049$).

Conclusions.—Management of spontaneous CSF leaks requires a comprehensive strategy after endoscopic repair. Diagnosis of BIH may be associated with requirement of further ICP treatment. Close ICP monitoring, coupled with selective use of acetazolamide and VPS, may decrease risk of failure (Fig 2).

▶ Endoscopic repair of cerebrospinal fluid (CSF) leaks has achieved success rates in excess of 90%,[1,2] but the subgroup of spontaneously occurring CSF leaks have a significantly lower rate of successful closure, ranging from 25% to 87%.[3,4] A suggested reason for this is that spontaneous leaks may have intracranial pressure (ICP) elevation or carry an underlying diagnosis of benign intracranial hypertension (BIH), and successful treatment of spontaneous CSF leaks, therefore, requires repair of the skull base defect and careful assessment and treatment of elevated ICP as well. This single institution study

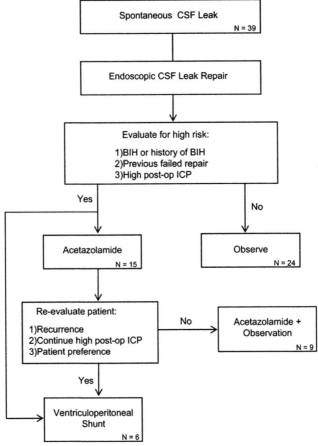

FIGURE 2.—The treatment algorithm utilized in this patient group. Treatment decisions were based on CSF leak recurrence and concern for high risk of recurrence based on ICP elevation and diagnosis of BIH. (Reprinted from Seth R, Rajasekaran K III, Luong A, et al. Spontaneous CSF leaks: factors predictive of additional interventions. *Laryngoscope.* 2010;120:2141-2146, with permission from The American Laryngological, Rhinological and Otological Society, Inc.)

reviewed the management strategy and evaluated factors associated with the need for acetazolamide and/or ventriculoperitoneal shunt (VPS) placement. A total of 105 patients underwent CSF leak repair; with 39 patients (37.1%) treated for spontaneous CSF leaks. Most patients were female (85%), with an average body mass index of 38.5 kg/m². Most of the leaks occurred at the cribriform plate (51%) and the lateral sphenoid sinus (31%). Five patients (13%) with spontaneous leak failed initial endoscopic repair, and these were associated with a mean ICP of 27.0 cm, which was statistically higher than those without recurrence. Acetazolamide was used in 9 patients, whereas 6 patients underwent VPS placement for elevated ICP management. Diagnosis of BIH was statistically associated with need for acetazolamide. The study concluded that the successful management of spontaneous CSF leaks requires concerted postrepair ICP monitoring and aggressive treatment with the selective use of acetazolamide and VPS (Fig 2). This study is consistent with other recent articles in highlighting the importance of establishing the presence of BIH and close ICP monitoring and treatment in spontaneous CSF leaks. Opening pressures (ICP) should be measured routinely at the start of all CSF leak repair operations (not done consistently even in the patients presented in this article), and postoperative management of elevated ICP may decrease surgical failure rates in this higher risk population. A practical consideration worth stressing is that patients who are confirmed at the start of surgery to have elevated ICP (greater than 20 cm of water) and, therefore, at a higher risk for failure should routinely have a lumbar drain placed and left in situ postoperatively. This will help with postoperative healing of the repair site as well as facilitate ICP monitoring.

R. Sindwani, MD

References

1. Hegazy HM, Carrau RL, Snyderman CH, Kassam A, Zweig J. Transnasal endoscopic repair of cerebrospinal fluid rhinorrhea: a meta-analysis. *Laryngoscope.* 2000;110:1166-1172.
2. Senior BA, Jafri K, Benninger M. Safety and efficacy of endoscopic repair of CSF leaks and encephaloceles: a survey of the members of the American Rhinologic Society. *Am J Rhinol.* 2001;15:21-25.
3. Schlosser RJ, Bolger WE. Spontaneous nasal cerebrospinal fluid leaks and empty sella syndrome: a clinical association. *Am J Rhinol.* 2003;17:91-96.
4. Schlosser RJ, Wilensky EM, Grady MS, Bolger WE. Elevated intracranial pressures in spontaneous cerebrospinal fluid leaks. *Am J Rhinol.* 2003;17:191-195.

Surgical Technique

Is Nasal Surgery an Effective Treatment for Obstructive Sleep Apnea?
Rosow DE, Stewart MG (Weill Cornell Med College, NY)
Laryngoscope 120:1496-1497, 2010

Background.—Nasal obstruction is thought to contribute to sleep-disordered breathing and obstructive sleep apnea (OSA), and some have found an association between the presence of nasal obstructive symptoms and OSA. Although considerable research exists in the otolaryngology literature regarding the effectiveness of surgery in OSA, it is unclear to what extent nasal surgery alone benefits these patients.

▶ This article is a focused review examining the literature on whether nasal surgery is an effective treatment option for obstructive sleep apnea (OSA). It has long been held that nasal obstruction can contribute to sleep-disordered breathing and OSA. Although considerable research exists regarding the effectiveness of surgery in OSA, it is unclear to what extent nasal surgery alone benefits these patients. This article evaluated the available literature on the topic. Several prospective trials have been undertaken that examine pre- and postoperative polysomnograms of patients with OSA undergoing corrective nasal surgery. There were 4 case series (level 4 evidence) and only 1 randomized controlled trial (level 1 evidence) cited.

The level 1 study by Koutsourelakis et al in 2008 was a double-blinded randomized controlled trial in which 49 patients with OSA and nasal septal deviation underwent either septoplasty—with or without submucous turbinate resection—or sham surgery. There was no significant reduction of apnea-hypopnea index (AHI) in the surgery group as compared with baseline or with the placebo group. In the surgery group, mean AHI was 31.5 before and after surgery; in the placebo group, mean AHI changed from 30.6 to 32.1 after sham surgery. However, the authors did report a statistically significant improvement in Epworth Sleepiness Scale (ESS) score in the surgical group and not in the placebo group: surgery ESS, 13.4 to 11.7 ($P < .01$); placebo ESS, 13.7 to 12.5 ($P =$ not significant). The analysis concluded that there is no evidence that patients with OSA will experience improvement in the defining measures of OSA (AHI or minimum oxygen saturation) after nasal surgery alone. There is evidence, however, that OSA patients with nasal obstruction will experience subjectively better sleep, less sleepiness, and improved quality of life following corrective nasal surgery. In addition, some have suggested that nasal surgery may improve compliance by making continuous positive airway pressure more tolerable to patients by reducing the pressures necessary for maintaining airway patency. These are important considerations in counseling patients prior to surgery. More well-designed studies are needed.

R. Sindwani, MD

Comparative outcomes of using fibrin glue in septoplasty and its effect on mucociliary activity
Habesoglu TE, Kulekci S, Habesoglu M, et al (Haydarpasa Numune Education and Res Hosp, Istanbul, Turkey)
Otolaryngol Head Neck Surg 142:394-399, 2010

Objective.—Our objective was to determine the efficacy of fibrin glue to prevent complications and nasal mucociliary clearance (MCC) after septoplasty compared with a nonabsorbable packing requiring removal (polyvinyl alcohol [PVA] sponge).

Study Design.—Prospective clinical trial with planned data collection.

Setting.—The study was conducted at Haydarpasa Numune Education and Research Hospital.

Methods.—A total of 44 patients, who had septoplasty operations, were included in the study. We evaluated postoperative pain, sleep disturbance on the night of surgery, bleeding, septal hematoma, synechia, infection, and MCC values in the fibrin glue and PVA sponge groups.

Results.—The pain scores in the fibrin glue group were significantly lower than in the PVA sponge group ($P < 0.01$). A statistically significant difference was noted in the number of patients who had mild bleeding in favor of the fibrin glue group ($P < 0.05$). In the fibrin glue group, 95.7 percent of patients reported that they had normal sleep; in the PVA sponge group, only 23.8 percent of patients reported normal sleep ($P < 0.01$). In the fibrin glue group, a significant decrease was noted in postoperative MCC values compared with preoperative values ($P < 0.01$). However, in the PVA sponge group, a significant increase was noted in postoperative clearance values compared with preoperative values ($P < 0.01$).

Conclusion.—In our series of patients, we have seen no gross complications from fibrin glue usage. Fibrin glue can be readily used in septoplasty; it requires no special treatment, has an adequate hemostatic effect, and appears to promote the regeneration of mucociliary activity of the injured mucosa postoperatively.

▶ This is a randomized controlled study on patients undergoing septoplasty under local anesthesia comparing outcomes of coaptation of septal flaps with fibrin glue versus nonabsorbable nasal packing. There has been a significant trend in sinonasal surgery to avoid the use of uncomfortable and possibly unnecessary nonabsorbable packing.[1] This study evaluated postoperative pain, sleep disturbance on the night of surgery, bleeding, septal hematoma, synechia, infection, and mucociliary clearance (MCC) values in 44 randomized septoplasty patients treated with either fibrin glue or nonabsorbable packing. As one would expect, the pain scores, amount of bleeding, and MCC were significantly better (lower) in the fibrin glue group. Further, the large majority of patients (95%) in the fibrin glue group reported that they had normal sleep after surgery versus only 24% of patients who were packed. No obvious complications from fibrin glue usage were noted. The authors concluded that fibrin glue can be readily and effectively used in septoplasty and suggested (based on improvement in MCC) that the use of this substance in septoplasty appears to promote the regeneration of mucociliary activity of the injured mucosa postoperatively. Many have shifted from using removable nasal packing after sinonasal surgery including septoplasty, which I think is well founded and good practice. For most routine septoplasties, packing is unnecessary and adds to the recovery of our patients. This well-designed study nicely demonstrates this and even highlights impairment in sleep that can come from having nasal packing in place. However, suggesting that the use of fibrin glue actually improves mucosal healing is really beyond the purview of this study and cannot be addressed by this article. In fact, several studies on healing sinonasal mucosa suggest that compounds containing active clotting factors such as fibrin may actually interfere with mucosal regeneration and lead to synechia formation and granulation tissue as they also stimulate the inflammatory cascade.[2] Placing the glue within the septal flaps may potentially protect somewhat from some of these deleterious effects. In addition to additional costs, animal-based products, such as fibrin glue, also carry the risk of disease transmission and hypersensitivity reactions, which must be acknowledged.[3] Lastly, another simple (and more cost-effective) alternative to the placement of nasal packing or fibrin glue after septoplasty is endoscopically suturing the flaps together using either mattress or interrupted dissolvable sutures.

R. Sindwani, MD

References

1. Orlandi RR, Lanza DC. Is nasal packing necessary following endoscopic sinus surgery? *Laryngoscope.* 2004;114:1541-1544.
2. Valentine R, Wormald PJ, Sindwani R. Advances in absorbable biomaterials and nasal packing. *Otolaryngol Clin North Am.* 2009;42:813-828.
3. Dorion RP, Hamati HF, Landis B, Frey C, Heydt D, Carey D. Risk and clinical significance of developing antibodies induced by topical thrombin preparations. *Arch Pathol Lab Med.* 1998;122:887-894.

Endoscopic Coblator™-Assisted Management of Encephaloceles
Smith N, Riley KO, Woodworth BA (Univ of Alabama at Birmingham)
Laryngoscope 120:2535-2539, 2010

Objectives.—Numerous studies have demonstrated the efficacy and safety of endoscopic management of cerebral spinal fluid (CSF) rhinorrhea, encephaloceles, and anterior skull base defects. Techniques have evolved as new instrumentation has developed, but typically involve meticulous bipolar cautery to decrease the potential for intracranial bleeding. The present study evaluated the Coblator™ as a novel tool in transnasal endoscopic management of encephaloceles.

Study Design.—Outcomes study.

Methods.—A prospective cohort involving 19 patients with 22 encephaloceles (19 spontaneous, 3 traumatic) reduced with the Coblator™ (radiofrequency coblation plus bipolar modality) was compared to a retrospective cohort of six encephaloceles (five spontaneous, one traumatic) removed with endoscopic bipolar cautery. Main outcome measures included duration of encephalocele removal and bleeding events. Bleeding encountered during removal was considered a minor event unless more than one attempt at cauterization was required. Other data collected included standard demographics, encephalocele size, and complications.

Results.—Average duration of coblation-assisted encephalocele removal was 15.8 minutes compared to 46 minutes with standard bipolar cautery ($P = .0003$). Average number of bleeding episodes did not significantly differ between groups (Coblator™, 1.0 ± 1.57 vs. bipolar, 1.17 ± 0.98; $P = .80$). One episode of major bleeding occurred in the coblation group

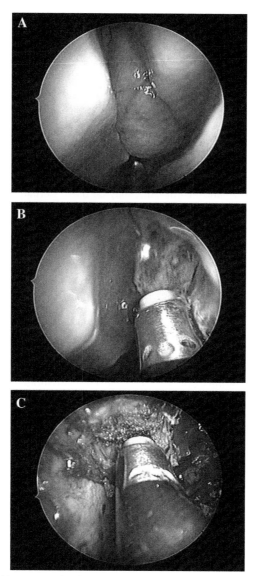

FIGURE 1.—Coblation-assisted endoscopic encephalocele removal. Transnasal endoscopic view of a left sided cribriform encephalocele. (A) The inferior portion of the encephalocele is removed with radio-frequency coblation. (B) The encephalocele has been completely removed/reduced and the circular defect in the cribriform plate identified. (C) Bipolar coagulation function is primarily utilized during this portion of the procedure. [Color figure can be viewed in the online issue, which is available at wileyonlinelibrary.com.] (Reprinted from Smith N, Riley KO, Woodworth BA. Endoscopic Coblator™-assisted management of encephaloceles. *Laryngoscope.* 2010;120:2535-2539, with permission from The American Laryngological, Rhinological and Otological Society, Inc.)

when an anterior ethmoid artery was encountered during removal. Encephalocele size was similar between groups (Coblator™, 17.4 mm vs. bipolar, 16.6 mm; $P = .65$).

Conclusions.—Radiofrequency coblation significantly increased intraoperative speed during encephalocele removal with similar hemostatic properties when compared to bipolar cautery alone and represents a useful instrument in the management of encephaloceles (Fig 1).

▶ Successful endoscopic repair of encephaloceles includes removal of the encephalocele to the skull base and repair of the bony defect. The techniques used to remove the encephalocele itself are actually not very well described in the literature, although a variety of devices, including powered instruments, bipolar cautery, and hand instruments, may be used. Certainly, most surgeons prefer the use of some form of cautery to decrease the potential for a blood vessel within the substance of an encephalocele bleeding into the intracranial space during reduction.[1] My experience has been that the currently available bipolar instruments are cumbersome to use and not very ergonomic when accessing the varying geometries of the skull base, so I read this article with interest. This study evaluated the use of the Coblator as a novel tool in transnasal endoscopic management of encephaloceles. This prospective study of 22 encephaloceles (19 spontaneous and 3 traumatic) reduced with the Coblator (radiofrequency coblation plus bipolar modality) was compared with a retrospective cohort of 6 encephaloceles (5 spontaneous and 1 traumatic) removed with more conventional endoscopic bipolar cautery. Main outcome measures included duration of encephalocele removal and bleeding events. The study found that the use of the Coblator was associated with more efficient encephalocele resection; there was no difference in bleeding episodes. The authors concluded that radiofrequency coblation significantly increased intraoperative speed during encephalocele removal with similar hemostatic properties when compared with bipolar cautery alone and represents a useful instrument in the management of encephaloceles. Coblation has been used for procedures such as tonsillectomy, turbinectomy, removal of respiratory papillomas, and nasal polypectomy. Coblation works by using an oscillating electrical current to disrupt surrounding tissue through radiofrequency energy that is produced by electrodes at the tip of the wand. A conductive medium (normal saline) is used to deliver the electrical energy instead of direct contact keeping tissue temperatures low (40°C-70°C) compared with standard electrosurgery (400°C-600°C).[2,3] Given the exposure/proximity to neurovital structures, the fact that bipolar energy is delivered is important. The use of the Coblator for encephalocele resection appears to be a promising application of this technology.

R. Sindwani, MD

References

1. Woodworth BA, Palmer JN. Spontaneous cerebrospinal fluid leaks. *Curr Opin Otolaryngol Head Neck Surg.* 2009;17:59-65.

2. Woloszko J, Stalder KR, Brown IG. Plasma characteristics of repetitively-pulsed electrical discharges in saline solutions used for surgical procedures. *IEEE Trans Plasma Sci.* 2002;30:1376-1383.
3. ArthoCare ENT: Coblation Web site. http://www.arthrocareent.com/wt/page/coblation_explained. Accessed April 6, 2011.

Endoscopic Endonasal Surgery for Petrous Apex Lesions
Zanation AM, Snyderman CH, Carrau RL, et al (Univ of North Carolina Memorial Hosps, Chapel Hill; Univ of Pittsburgh Med Ctr, PA)
Laryngoscope 119:19-25, 2009

Background.—Endoscopic endonasal approaches to the ventral skull base are categorized based on their orientation in coronal and sagittal planes. For all of these approaches, the sphenoid sinus is the starting point, and provides orientation to important vascular and neural structures. Surgical approaches to the petrous apex include 1) a medial approach, 2) a medial approach with internal carotid artery (ICA) lateralization, and 3) a transpterygoid infrapetrous approach (inferior to the petrous internal carotid artery). The choice of a surgical approach depends on the relationship of the lesion to the internal carotid artery (medial or inferior), degree of medial expansion, and pathology. The purpose of this paper is to discuss the anatomic and technical features of endoscopic surgical approaches to the petrous apex, provide a new classification for approaches that focuses on the relationship of the lesion to the petrous internal carotid artery, and provide outcomes data on our first 20 endoscopic petrous apex approaches.

Methods.—A retrospective clinical outcome study of endoscopic petrous apex surgeries was performed at the University of Pittsburgh Medical Center. The medical records from patients with endoscopic endonasal approaches to isolated petrous apex lesions were reviewed for demographics, diagnoses, presentation, endoscopic approach, and clinical outcomes. Patients with lesions that extended into the petrous apex but were not isolated to the petrous apex were excluded (e.g., clival chordoma with extension into the petrous apex).

Results.—Twenty patients were included in the analysis: 13 inflammatory cystic lesions (9 cholesterol granulomas and four petrous apicitis) and 7 solid lesions. Chondrosarcoma was the most common solid petrous apex lesion in our series. Twelve of 13 cystic lesions were drained endoscopically (one surgery was aborted early in the series). All drained patients had resolution of presenting symptoms. One patient had closure of the outflow tract without return of symptoms and one patient had revision endoscopic drainage due to scarring and neo-osteogenesis and return of unilateral headache. No carotid injuries and no new cranial neuropathies occurred perioperatively. The advantages and limitations of the medial transsphenoidal approaches (with and without carotid mobilization) and the transpterygoid infrapetrous approach are discussed.

Conclusions.—The endoscopic endonasal approach to petrous apex lesions is safe and effective for appropriately selected patients in the hands of experienced endoscopic skull base surgeons. If offers advantages of removing the hearing and facial nerve risks from the transtemporal/transcranial approaches and allows for a larger and more natural drainage pathway into the sinuses (Figs 1 and 2).

▶ There has been a large proliferation of endoscopic techniques and approaches to the skull base over the past several years. In this article, the authors describe surgical approaches to the petrous apex that include (1) a medial approach, (2) a medial approach with internal carotid artery (ICA) lateralization, and (3) a transpterygoid infrapetrous approach (inferior to the petrous ICA) (Fig 1). The approach preferred depends upon the relationship to the ICA (medial or inferior), degree of medial expansion, and pathology. The article reviews the anatomic and technical features of endoscopic surgical approaches to the petrous apex and provides a classification scheme for approaches that focuses on the relationship of the lesion to the petrous ICA. Outcomes data on the center's first 20 endoscopic petrous apex cases are also presented. Most lesions managed were inflammatory cystic lesions (9 cholesterol granulomas and 4 petrous apicitis), with 7 solid lesions. Twelve of 13 cystic lesions were drained endoscopically into the sphenoid sinus, and all drained patients had resolution of symptoms. No carotid injuries and no new cranial neuropathies were noted (Fig 2). The advantages and limitations of the medial transsphenoidal approaches (with and without carotid mobilization) and the transpterygoid infrapetrous approach are reviewed. The authors conclude that endoscopic endonasal approaches to petrous apex lesions are safe and effective. They acknowledge that this is highly technical and demanding surgery and caution that it should be reserved for experienced endoscopic skull base surgeons. Endonasal approaches are particularly attractive for inflammatory petrous apex lesions (the large majority encountered in this series) because they do not risk injury to hearing or the facial

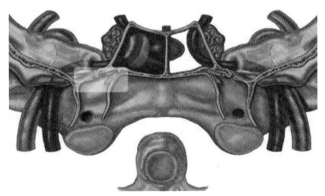

FIGURE 1.—Schematic of petrous apex approaches. Shaded oval represents the medial transsphenoid approaches. Shaded rectangle represents the transpterygoid infrapetrous approach. (Reprinted from Zanation AM, Snyderman CH, Carrau RL, et al. Endoscopic endonasal surgery for petrous apex lesions. *Laryngoscope.* 2009;119:19-25, with permission from The American Laryngological, Rhinological and Otological Society, Inc.)

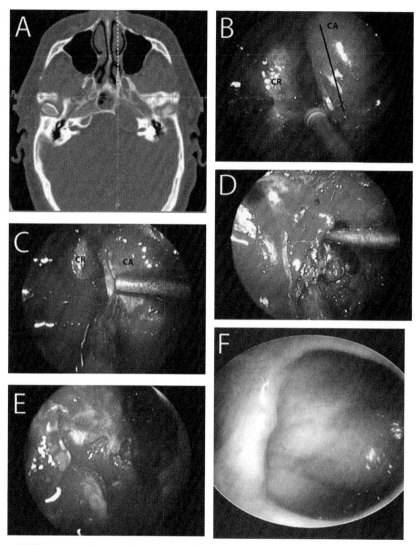

FIGURE 2.—Medial transsphenoid approach with internal carotid artery lateralization. (A) Image guidance screenshot showing left petrous apex lesion. (B) Thinning of the bone of the paraclival carotid canal with a high-speed drill. (C) Lateralization of the carotid artery exposing the medial canal wall. (D) Petrous apex granuloma opened showing removal of the cholesterol content. (E) Evacuated petrous apex cavity with wide communication into the sphenoid sinus. (F) Postoperative month 3 picture showing wide opening into the petrous cavity. CR = clival recess of the sphenoid; CA = carotid artery, the line represents the vertical portion of the paraclival carotid artery. (Reprinted from Zanation AM, Snyderman CH, Carrau RL, et al. Endoscopic endonasal surgery for petrous apex lesions. *Laryngoscope.* 2009;119:19-25, with permission from The American Laryngological, Rhinological and Otological Society, Inc.)

nerve associated with external approaches, offer far less morbidity and shorter hospital stays, and, importantly, allow for a larger and more natural drainage pathway of the lesions into the sinuses thereby decreasing recurrences. Even if one is not interested in mobilizing the ICA, many lesions of the petrous apex can be accessed through the posterior sphenoid sinus wall and when large and inflammatory in nature, the ICA may not need to be retracted. Often large lesions of the petrous apex may produce a bulge into the posterior aspect of the sphenoid, which, augmented by surgical navigation, may greatly assist the surgeon in localization and drainage. This technique of course takes exquisite advantage of the anatomic relationship between the posterior sphenoid and the petrous apex. The trend toward minimally invasive endoscopic neurorhinologic procedures on the skull base and adjacent regions is sure to continue.

R. Sindwani, MD

Endoscopic sphenoid nasalization for the treatment of advanced sphenoid disease
Soler ZM, Sindwani R, Metson R (Harvard Med School, Boston, MA; Saint Louis Univ School of Medicine, MO)
Otolaryngol Head Neck Surg 143:456-458, 2010

Background.—Usually, enlarging a blocked sinus ostium will allow the retained secretions to drain out and permit mucociliary clearance to be reestablished. In patients who have failed previous sphenoidotomy or who have advanced disease, conventional sphenoidotomy may be insufficient to give relief. Sphenoid nasalization may be able to open the sphenoid sinus, allow intraoperative exposure, facilitate postoperative drainage, and permit long-term monitoring.

Patients and Technique.—Twenty-two patients were managed using sphenoid nasalization between 2000 and 2009. Seven men and 15 women (mean age 54.7 years) were included, all with indications for sphenoid nasalization surgery as a primary or revision procedure.

First, the sphenoid ostium is exposed between the superior turbinate and the septum in the sphenoethmoid recess. To permit better access to the sphenoid face, the inferior part of the superior turbinate is removed. A small spoon curette is used to enlarge the sphenoid ostium inferiorly and laterally. The surgeon carefully notes the positions of the optic nerve and carotid artery while removing the remaining bone of the sphenoid face laterally to the lamina papyracea and superiorly to the ethmoid roof. The sphenoid sinus floor is then removed posteriorly and laterally toward the clivus. The relatively thick bone of this area is removed using a high-speed drill. If the sphenoid nasalization is to be bilateral, the 1 to 2 cm of the nasal septum located posteriorly must be resected. This improves surgical exposure and bone removal efforts. The endocope is passed through one side of the nose and the drill through the other. It is then quite easy to take down the midline sphenoid face and most of the intersphenoidal septum. The result is a wide common aperture extending between the two laminae papyraceae. Both sphenoid sinuses are marsupialized to the nasal cavity anteriorly and to the nasopharynx inferiorly.

Results.—Bilateral sphenoid nasalization was done in 17 cases and unilateral nasalizatioan in 5 cases. None of the patients suffered intraoperative or postoperative complications. Blood loss averaged 90 mL, with a range of 20 to 250 mL. After a mean follow-up of 13.5 months, nasal endoscopy revealed all patients had a widely spaced sphenoid sinus. Recurrent inverted papilloma along the lateral wall of the sphenoid sinus required revision surgery after 30.1 months in a single patient, but none of the other patients required surgery up to a mean of 46.7 months postoperatively.

Conclusions.—Sphenoid nasalization is performed only after conventional sinusotomy has failed or when the pathologic condition cannot be addressed otherwise. Removing the sphenoid floor permits drainage by

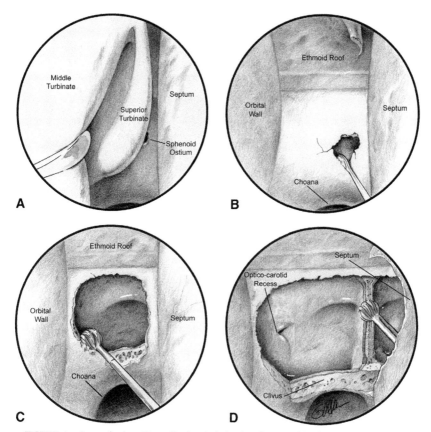

FIGURE 1.—Steps of sphenoid nasalization include identification of landmarks along the anterior sphenoid wall (**A**), enlargement of the sphenoid ostium (**B**), removal of the anterior wall and floor of the sphenoid sinus (**C**), and resection of the posterior nasal septum with drilling of the intersphenoidal septum when bilateral sphenoid nasalization is performed (**D**). (Reprinted from Soler ZM. Sindwani R, Metson R. Endoscopic sphenoid nasalization for the treatment of advanced sphenoid disease. *Otolaryngol Head Neck Surg.* 2010;143:456-458. Copyright 2010, with permission from American Academy of Otolaryngology–Head and Neck Surgery Foundation.)

gravity into the nasopharynx. The wide opening allows access for postoperative debridement of the interior of the sphenoid, either manually or using saline irrigations. Neoplastic disease treatments and monitoring are more readily carried out as well. However, sphenoid nasalization may be associated with an increased risk for surgical complications such as injury to the carotid artery and optic nerve. Sphenoid anatomy must be clearly understood to avoid these situations. In experienced hands, sphenoid nasalization offers a safe procedure for patients with refractory inflammatory disease for whom conventional sphenoidotomy has failed or for patients whose advanced disease requires maximal access to the sphenoid interior (Figs 1 and 2).

▶ In most cases of chronic sphenoid sinusitis, widening of the obstructed sinus ostium is sufficient to provide drainage and ventilation. However, in the setting of failed prior sphenoidotomy or advanced disease, a standard sphenoidotomy technique may prove inadequate. In such instances, sphenoid nasalization may be of value to widely open the sinus, providing enhanced intraoperative exposure, postoperative drainage, and long-term surveillance in the case of neoplasia. This article describes a novel procedure on the sphenoid sinus

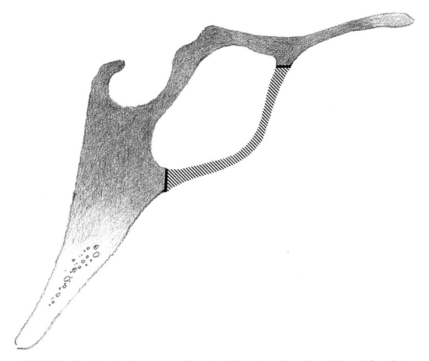

FIGURE 2.—Sagittal view demonstrates the region of bone along the sphenoid face and floor that are removed during the nasalization procedure. (Reprinted from Soler ZM. Sindwani R, Metson R. Endoscopic sphenoid nasalization for the treatment of advanced sphenoid disease. *Otolaryngol Head Neck Surg.* 2010;143:456-458. Copyright 2010, with permission from American Academy of Otolaryngology–Head and Neck Surgery Foundation.)

whereby the sinus interior is marsupialized and widely opened into the naso-pharynx through resection of the anterior face, intersphenoidal septum, and floor via a posterior septectomy approach (Fig 1). As shown, with the endo-scope passed through one side of the nose and the drill through the other, the midline sphenoid face and most of the intersphenoidal septum can be readily taken down (Fig 1D). This results in a wide common aperture (spanning from lamina papyracea to lamina papyracea) with both sphenoid sinuses mar-supialized to the nasal cavity anteriorly and the nasopharynx inferiorly (Fig 2). This is of course similar conceptually to the frontal drillout procedure (or Draf III procedure) advocated for advanced exposure of the frontal sinus. The authors describe their rationale for this procedure and outline indications and the tech-nique in detail. There were no complications in this series of 22 patients. Sphe-noid nasalization provides the surgeon with maximal exposure for controlled tumor resection and enhanced postoperative tumor surveillance.

R. Sindwani, MD

Middle Turbinectomy for Exposure in Endoscopic Endonasal Transsphenoidal Surgery: When is it Necessary?
Guthikonda B, Nourbakhsh A, Notarianni C, et al (Louisiana State Univ Health Sciences Ctr, Shreveport)
Laryngoscope 120:2360-2366, 2010

Objectives.—To evaluate the benefits of middle turbinectomy on the exposure of the skull base structures.
Design.—An anatomical study on 20 fresh cadaver heads.
Methods.—The extent of the exposure of the skull base structures during endoscopic endonasal approach has not been addressed specifically in respect to the whether or not the middle turbinectomy is performed. We compared the extent of exposure obtained by endonasal transsphenoidal approaches without middle turbinectomy (NMT), with unilateral turbi-nectomy (UMT), and with bilateral turbinectomy (BMT). Our preselected target points in the skull base consisted of sella turcica, tuberculum sella, planum sphenoidale, clivus (upper and middle third), and ipsilateral sphe-nopalatine artery (SPA).
Results.—Of our preselected anatomic target points, only the middle third of the clivus and ipsilateral SPA had enhanced exposure in UMT (100% for both structures) compared to NMT (45% and 20%, respec-tively). The addition of a BMT did not provide added exposure to any target compared with a UMT.
Conclusions.—Middle turbinectomy may not be necessary for endo-nasal transsphenoidal approach to the lesions of the sella, planum sphenoi-dale, and upper third of the clivus. However, gaining access to the middle clival region is facilitated by resection of middle turbinate.

▶ This is a systematic study in 20 cadavers performed to evaluate when a middle turbinectomy is and is not necessary during endonasal transsphenoidal surgery. The study reviewed the extent of exposure of skull base structures obtained without middle turbinectomy, with unilateral turbinectomy (UMT), and with bilateral turbinectomy (BMT) while performing approaches to targets, including the sella, planum sphenoidale, clivus, and sphenopalatine artery. Generally, the authors found that taking the ipsilateral middle turbinate (MT) did not offer a significant improvement in exposure to the skull base in the large majority of approaches. The 2 scenarios in which ipsilateral MT resection improved exposure were in access to the inferior portion of the clivus and more lateral exposure of the sphenopalatine artery/fractional pulse pressure. BMT resection did not provide added exposure to any target compared with a UMT. The authors concluded that turbinectomy may not be necessary for the majority of endonasal transsphenoidal approaches. This cadaver study, in which the authors unblindedly gauged exposure to skull base structures during transsphenoidal surgery, has significant limitations and, I think, makes too much of the goal of sparing the MT, but I do appreciate the sentiment of structural preservation. Transsphenoid approaches can be quite complex and even a small improvement in exposure afforded by resection of a MT, if the surgeon feels is helpful, should be performed. I would also underscore that merely lateralizing the MT during the procedure, as the authors recommend, must also be followed by a purposeful remedialization of this structure at the conclusion of the procedure to ensure that postoperative sinusitis related to turbinate lateralization is avoided. I do agree that a BMT for transsphenoidal surgery is rarely needed (if ever). In my view, the authors' list of potential concerns and complications related to MT resection (in this setting), such as derangements in nasal function, frontal sinusitis, ethmoid scarring, postoperative epistaxis, anosmia, loss of a landmark, although real, are somewhat overstated. In summary, I would not routinely take the MT during any procedure and would try and preserve it (along with all normal structures), but I would not hesitate to resect it, if during the course of a more complex procedure I felt that in so doing, the procedure would be significantly facilitated in any way (ease of completion, better exposure, improved outcomes, etc).

R. Sindwani, MD

Midterm outcomes of outfracture of the inferior turbinate
Aksoy F, Yildirim YS, Veyseller B, et al (Haseki Res and Training Hosp, Istanbul, Turkey)
Otolaryngol Head Neck Surg 143:579-584, 2010

Objective.—A variety of medical and surgical treatment alternatives exists for the management of inferior turbinate hypertrophy, indicating a lack of consensus on the optimal technique. The purpose of the present study was to evaluate the inferior turbinate objectively by means of radiologic methodology during the early and late periods in patients treated with inferior turbinate outfracture.

Study Design.—Case series with planned data collection.

Setting.—Tertiary referral center.

Subjects and Methods.—Eighty inferior turbinates of 40 patients (28 males, 12 females) who underwent surgery because of septum deviation and inferior turbinate hypertrophy were included in this prospective clinical study. All patients were evaluated by paranasal sinus computed tomography preoperatively and at one and six months postsurgery. The angle and the distance between the inferior turbinate and the lateral wall of the nasal fossa and the area lateral to the inferior turbinate bone were measured on the coronal plane anterior posteriorly at five different anatomic levels.

Results.—Statistically significant reductions were noted in the angle and distances in all sections one and six months postoperatively when compared with the preoperative measurements ($P < 0.005$).

Conclusion.—Compared with the preoperative status, those patients who underwent turbinate outfracture procedures displayed a reduction in the angle and the distance between the inferior turbinate bone and the lateral wall of the nasal fossa and the area lateral to the inferior turbinate bone one month following surgery. Ongoing outcomes of this treatment method have been objectively shown.

▶ The main objective of inferior turbinate surgery is to provide more comfortable nasal breathing while minimally disturbing normal physiology through a procedure with the fewest possible complications. There are many procedures, of course, that have been advocated to achieve this, but certainly the best side effect profile is associated with the simple turbinate outfracture procedure. Described in 1904 by Killian as a means to avoid the complications associated with turbinate resection, there is a real paucity of data on this technique, which largely fell out of favor over concerns that over time the turbinate medializes.[1-3]

This study evaluated the position of the inferior turbinates after outfracture by means of CT imaging at 1 and 6 month postoperatively. Eighty inferior turbinates of 40 patients (28 males and 12 females) who underwent surgery because of septum deviation and inferior turbinate hypertrophy were included. The angle and the distance between the inferior turbinate and the lateral wall of the nasal fossa and the area lateral to the inferior turbinate bone were measured on the coronal plane anterior posteriorly at 5 different anatomic levels (Figs 1 and 2 in the original article). There were statistically significant reductions noted in the angle and distances in all sections 1 and 6 months postoperatively when compared with the preoperative measurements ($P < .005$), suggesting that patients who undergo turbinate outfracture procedures do get some lasting displacement with respect to the final position of the inferior turbinate after surgery. Whether this translates to a significant improvement in symptoms and whether this technique is more or less efficacious than the many other techniques available deserves further study.

R. Sindwani, MD

References

1. O'Flynn PE, Milford CA, Mackay IS. Multiple submucosal out-fractures of interior turbinates. *J Laryngol Otol.* 1990;104:239-240.

2. Thomas PL, John DG, Carlin WV. The effect of inferior turbinate outfracture on nasal resistance to airflow in vasomotor rhinitis assessed by rhinomanometry. *J Laryngol Otol.* 1988;102:144-145.

3. Fradis M, Goldz A, Danino J, et al. Inferior turbinectomy versus submucosal diathermy for inferior turbinate hypertrophy. *Ann Otol Rhinol Laryngol.* 2000; 109:1040-1045.

Minimally Invasive Endoscopic Pericranial Flap: A New Method for Endonasal Skull Base Reconstruction

Zanation AM, Snyderman CH, Carrau RL, et al (Univ of North Carolina Memorial Hosps, Chapel Hill; Univ of Pittsburgh Med Ctr, PA)
Laryngoscope 119:13-18, 2009

Objectives.—One of the major challenges of cranial base surgery is reconstruction of the dural defect. Following a craniofacial resection, the standard reconstructive technique is direct suture repair of the dural defect with a fascial graft and rotation of an anteriorly based pericranial scalp flap to cover the dura. The introduction of endoscopic techniques and an endonasal approach to the ventral skull base has created new challenges for reconstruction. The nasoseptal flap has become the workhorse for vascularized endoscopic skull base reconstruction; however at times, the septal mucosal flap may be unavailable for reconstruction. This can be due to prior surgical resection or involvement of the nasal septum by sinonasal cancer. We have developed a minimally invasive endoscopic pericranial flap for endoscopic skull base reconstruction. The use of a pericranial scalp flap for reconstruction during endonasal skull base surgery using minimally invasive techniques has not been previously reported.

Methods.—We performed cadaveric studies to illustrate feasibility of an endoscopic pericranial flap for endonasal skull base reconstruction, then applied this novel technique to an elderly patient after endonasal skull base and dural resection of an esthesioneuroblastoma.

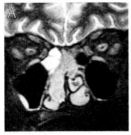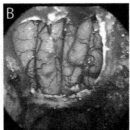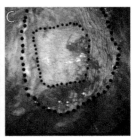

FIGURE 1.—(A) T1 MRI with contrast showing tumor involving both posterior ethmoid sinuses, skull base and posterior septum. (B) Endoscopic cranial base defect after resection and negative frozen margins. (C) Endoscopic reconstruction with the pericranial flap. The small dots outline the defect shown in B and the large dots outline the pericranial flap margins. (Reprinted from Zanation AM, Snyderman CH, Carrau RL, et al. Minimally invasive endoscopic pericranial flap: a new method for endonasal skull base reconstruction. *Laryngoscope.* 2009;119:13-18, with permission from The American Laryngological, Rhinological and Otological Society, Inc.)

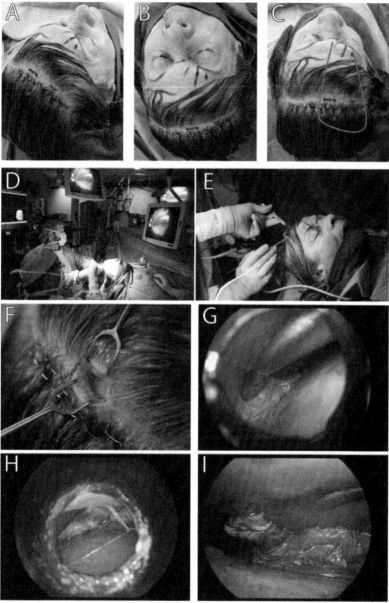

FIGURE 2.—(A) Minimally invasive pericranial flap setup. The pedicle is marked along the right supraorbital rim (3 cm wide) and 2-cm and 1-cm scalp incisions are also marked in the coronal plane. (B) Minimally invasive pericranial flap setup. The 1-cm glabellar incision is marked in a natural skin crease. (C) The area of the pericranial flap is outlined in red. (D) Operative setup. The surgeon works from the apex of the patient's head. (E) Endoscopic scalp dissection technique. (F) An incision (2 cm) taken down to the subgaleal plane only. (G) Endoscopic subgaleal dissection. (H) Guarded and bent extended needle-tip cautery is used to incise the pericranial flap from the underlying bone. (I) A periosteal dissector is used to elevated the flap from the skull. (Reprinted from Zanation AM, Snyderman CH, Carrau RL, et al. Minimally invasive endoscopic pericranial flap: a new method for endonasal skull base reconstruction. *Laryngoscope.* 2009;119:13-18, with permission from The American Laryngological, Rhinological and Otological Society, Inc.)

Results.—The technical report of the minimally invasive pericranial flap is outlined and the advantages and limitations during endonasal skull base reconstruction are discussed. The patient had excellent healing of her skull base and had no evidence of any postoperative cerebrospinal fluid leak.

Conclusions.—The minimally invasive endoscopic pericranial flap provides another option for endonasal reconstruction of cranial base defects. There is minimal donor site morbidity, and it provides a large flap that can cover the entire ventral skull base. The issues of intranasal tissue tumor involvement and the need for radiotherapy make the endoscopic pericranial flap an ideal reconstruction for anterior cranial base defects resulting from endonasal sinonasal and skull base cancer resections (Figs 1-3).

▶ The pedicled pericranial scalp flap (PCF) has been the workhorse of anterior cranial base reconstruction for decades. This pedicled flap is based on the supraorbital and supratrochlear vessels and can extend from the superior orbital rim to the occiput. Following an anterior craniofacial resection with a subfrontal approach, traditionally the flap has been passed inferior to the supraorbital bone segment through a bone defect at the nasion to cover the dura. One of the major challenges of cranial base surgery is reconstruction of the dural defect, a hurdle that has been extenuated with endoscopic techniques, which are further limited by availability of local vascularized tissue that can be used for reconstruction.

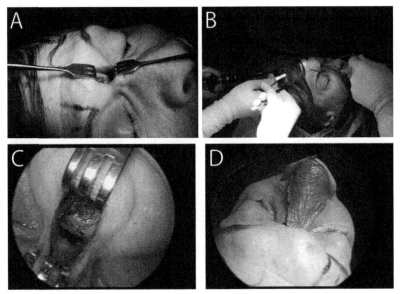

FIGURE 3.—(A) A 1-cm glabellar incision taken down to the nasion. (B) A subperiosteal pocket is raised from the nasion up to the flap dissection site. (C) The nasionectomy visualized through the glabellar incision. (D) The pericranial flap transposed through the glabellar incision. (Reprinted from Zanation AM, Snyderman CH, Carrau RL, et al. Minimally invasive endoscopic pericranial flap: a new method for endonasal skull base reconstruction. *Laryngoscope.* 2009;119:13-18, with permission from The American Laryngological, Rhinological and Otological Society, Inc.)

Intranasally, a variety of free mucosal and pedicled flaps off of the sphenopalatine artery have been described, each with limitations, most notably limited size and proximity to the field of resection. This is a case report and description of an innovative technique used to harvest and place a PCF endoscopically through a bony defect in the nasion into the nose for anterior skull base reconstruction in an elderly patient with an esthesioblastoma (Fig 1). The technical description of the minimally invasive pericranial flap is outlined (Figs 2 and 3 and Fig 4 in the original article), and its advantages and limitations during endonasal skull base reconstruction are discussed. The PCF was harvested using minimally invasive surgical techniques: small scalp incisions, endoscopic dissection, and a minimal cosmetic bone defect. The only visible scar was a 1-cm incision at the level of the nasion in a glabellar skin crease. This flap provides another option for endonasal reconstruction of cranial base defects and recruits vascularized tissue from a remote site, away from the tumor being treated. This technique has minimal donor site morbidity and provides a large flap that can cover the entire ventral skull base. The minimally invasive endoscopic pericranial flap provides another option for endonasal reconstruction of cranial base defects. There is minimal donor site morbidity, and it provides a large flap that can cover the entire ventral skull base. The authors advocate consideration of this flap when reconstruction with a septal mucosal flap is not feasible. Further experience with this method of harvesting the PCF is needed, but the technique appears very promising.

R. Sindwani, MD

Outcomes After Middle Turbinate Resection: Revisiting a Controversial Topic

Soler ZM, Hwang PH, Mace J, et al (Oregon Health and Science Univ, Portland; Stanford Univ Med Ctr, Palo Alto, CA)
Laryngoscope 120:832-837, 2010

Objectives/Hypothesis.—To evaluate differences in endoscopy exam, olfactory function, and quality-of-life (QOL) status after endoscopic sinus surgery (ESS) for patients with and without bilateral middle turbinate (BMT) resection.

Study Design.—Open, prospective, multi-institutional cohort.

Methods.—Subjects completing enrollment interviews, computed tomography (CT), and endoscopy exam were asked to provide pre- and postoperative responses to the Smell Identification Test (SIT), Rhinosinusitis Disability Index (RSDI), Chronic Sinusitis Survey (CSS), and the Medical Outcomes Study Short Form-36 Health Survey (SF-36). Bivariate and multivariate analyses were performed at the .05 alpha level.

Results.—Forty-seven subjects with BMT resection were compared to 195 subjects without BMT resection with a mean follow-up of 17.4 months postoperatively. Patients with BMT resection were more likely to have asthma $(P=.001)$, aspirin intolerance $(P=.022)$, nasal polyposis $(P=.025)$, and prior sinus surgery $(P=.002)$. Patients with BMT resection had significantly higher baseline disease burden measured by endoscopy,

CT, and SIT scores $(P < .001)$. No significant differences in improvement were found in RSDI, CSS, or SF-36 scores between patients with BMT resection and those with BMT preservation $(P > .05)$. Patients undergoing BMT resection were more likely to show improvements in mean endoscopy $(-4.5 \pm 5.2$ vs. -1.9 ± 4.3; $P = .005)$ and olfaction $(5.3 \pm 10.8$ vs. 1.3 ± 7.6, $P = .045)$ compared to those with BMT preservation.

Conclusions.—This investigation found no difference in QOL outcomes in patients with BMT preservation vs. resection. Patients undergoing BMT resection did, however, show greater improvements in endoscopy and SIT scores, which persisted after controlling for confounding factors.

▶ Resection of the middle turbinate (MT) during the course of sinus surgery has been a controversial practice since throughout the history of sinus surgery. Some early teachings advocated routine MT resection, whereas the era of functional endoscopic sinus surgery found thought leaders strongly discouraging MT resection, almost at any cost. Those in favor of resection touted improved visualization (intra- and post-op), decreased synechiae formation, and improved sinus ostial patency as advantages. Preservationists described risks of atrophic rhinitis, anosmia, postoperative epistaxis, destruction of intraoperative landmarks, and iatrogenic frontal sinusitis as reasons against the practice. This well-constructed controlled study examined this issue by comparing subjective and objective outcomes of patients with and without bilateral middle turbinate (BMT) resections. Forty-seven subjects with BMT resection were compared with 195 subjects without BMT resection, with a mean follow-up of 17 months. Not surprisingly, patients with BMT resection were more likely to have asthma, acetylsalicylic acid intolerance, nasal polyposis, and prior sinus surgery. Patients with BMT resection showed no significant differences in quality-of-life (QOL), and improvements were found in patients with BMT preservation versus resection. It should be noted that this study does not directly address the question of whether the MT should be routinely resected or routinely preserved. Rather, it shows that thoughtful resection of the MT can be done with no apparent consequence to long-term disease-specific or general QOL outcomes. As this study showed, most patients who end up having MT resections have advanced disease, a history of prior surgery, and nasal polyps. Presumably the decision to resect the MT was made at the time of surgery because the surgeon felt that the turbinate was in some way a factor in the disease process/prior surgical failure or there was significant concern that sparing this structure might in some contribute to failure or a worse surgical outcome (eg, lateralization). As a general rule, surgeons should plan on preserving the MT (and any other nondiseased nasal structure for that matter), which is such a reliable landmark in sinus surgery, but as this study shows there are plenty of scenarios that may serve as exceptions to this rule. Importantly, sacrificing the MT in such an instance is not associated with any significant sequelae and may actually prevent further surgical failures.

R. Sindwani, MD

Reverse Rotation Flap for Reconstruction of Donor Site After Vascular Pedicled Nasoseptal Flap in Skull Base Surgery

Caicedo-Granados E, Carrau R, Snyderman CH, et al (Univ of Minnesota, Minneapolis; Univ of Pittsburgh, PA)
Laryngoscope 120:1550-1552, 2010

Endonasal skull base surgery is growing exponentially as a subspecialty. In recent years, advances in endoscopic techniques and intraoperative navigation systems have allowed us to expand the indications of endoscopic skull base surgery. Major skull base centers worldwide are addressing larger and more complex lesions using endoscopic techniques. As a consequence, the skull base defects are more challenging to reconstruct. In this report, we present a novel technique to reconstruct the denuded septum remaining after the use of the vascular pedicled nasoseptal flap (Figs 1 and 2).

▶ There has been a major proliferation in expanded endonasal approaches and endoscopic skull base surgery in recent years. As larger and larger lesions are

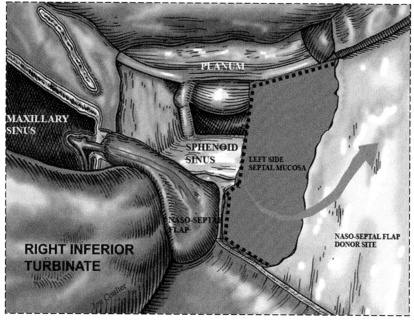

FIGURE 1.—Illustration of right nasal cavity after endoscopic endonasal approach shows right maxillary antrostomy, vascular pedicled nasoseptal flap placed in the nasopharynx, and posterior septectomy with preservation of opposite nasal septal mucosa (reverse rotation flap). Black dotted line shows incisions (superior, posterior, and inferior) on opposite nasal septal mucosa. Big gray arrow depicts the direction of flap transposition. (Reprinted from Caicedo-Granados E, Carrau R, Snyderman CH, et al. Reverse rotation flap for reconstruction of donor site after vascular pedicled nasoseptal flap in skull base surgery. *Laryngoscope.* 2010;120:1550-1552, with permission The American Laryngological, Rhinological and Otological Society, Inc.)

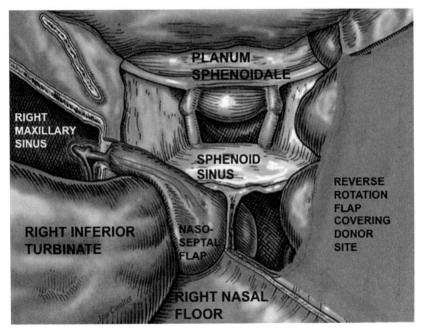

FIGURE 2.—Illustration of right nasal cavity after reverse rotation flap is in place and right maxillary antrostomy. The vascular pedicled nasoseptal flap and reverse rotation flap in position covering the denuded nasal septum are depicted. (Reprinted from Caicedo-Granados E, Carrau R, Snyderman CH, et al. Reverse rotation flap for reconstruction of donor site after vascular pedicled nasoseptal flap in skull base surgery. *Laryngoscope.* 2010;120:1550-1552, with permission The American Laryngological, Rhinological and Otological Society, Inc.)

addressed endoscopically, the requirement to repair skull base defects with pedicled regional flaps, including those involving the posterior nasal septum, has emerged. Although only a short communication, this report presents a novel technique to reconstruct/cover the denuded septum remaining after the use of the pedicled nasoseptal flap. This is illustrated in Figs 1 and 2. The technique described is a clever method of providing extended exposure to the sphenoid and skull base through a septectomy approach with coverage using a pedicled nasoseptal flap and then using the contralateral posterior mucoperiosteum to rotate 180° from posterior to anterior to cover the denuded site of the ipsilateral flap. Usually, these septal flap sites are left to heal in by secondary intention (or perhaps covered with some synthetic material), which contributes to postoperative crusting, the need for extensive irrigations, etc.

Because the contralateral mucoperiosteum is used for coverage, there is no increased morbidity with this technique, and it seems like an effective method of augmenting remucosalization of the septum and possibly improving postoperative quality of life (QOL) in patients after expanded endonasal approaches. However, data on the subjective impact of this technique (less crusting, more or less pain, and improvement in QOL) are not presented in this article and would be of interest to review in a systematic and objective way.

R. Sindwani, MD

Revision Frontal Sinusotomy Using Stepwise Balloon Dilation and Powered Instrumentation

Bhandarkar ND, Smith TL (Oregon Health and Science Univ, Portland)
Laryngoscope 120:2015-2017, 2010

Objectives/Hypothesis.—To report a novel approach toward revision frontal sinusotomy using a technique of balloon dilation followed by the use of powered instrumentation.

Study Design.—Case report.

Methods.—The frontal sinus outflow tract location was first confirmed with image guidance and then dilated with a balloon to address the soft tissue stenosis. Subsequently, the drill was introduced to accomplish a Draf 2B frontal sinusotomy.

Results.—An advantage of initial balloon dilation of the frontal sinus outflow tract was to quickly address the soft tissue stenosis with minimal tissue trauma and therefore less bleeding. This subsequently enabled insertion and clear visualization of the entire drill bit within the inferior aspect of the frontal outflow tract. The increased visualization makes other instrumentation safer as well, and avoids relatively blind removal of scar tissue that could result in inadvertent entry into the orbit or skull base.

Conclusions.—We describe the utility of the balloon as a tool for revision frontal sinusotomy to efficiently and safely allow subsequent instrumentation of the frontal outflow tract with larger more aggressive instruments, such as the drill. We have found this to be a safe and effective technique provided proper preoperative patient selection and assessment for limiting factors (Figs 2-4).

▶ The introduction of balloon catheter technology (BCT) for the dilatation of the sinuses has been one of the most novel (and perhaps contentious)

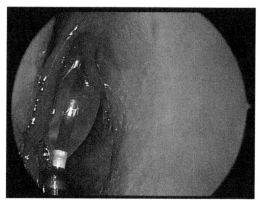

FIGURE 2.—Intraoperative endoscopic view of balloon dilation of left frontal sinus outflow tract. [Color figure can be viewed in the online issue, which is available at wileyonlinelibrary.com.] (Reprinted from Bhandarkar ND, Smith TL. Revision frontal sinusotomy using stepwise balloon dilation and powered instrumentation. *Laryngoscope.* 2010;120:2015-2017, with permission from The American Laryngological, Rhinological and Otological Society, Inc.)

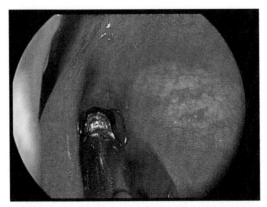

FIGURE 3.—Intraoperative endoscopic view of left frontal sinus outflow tract following balloon dila-tion. Note that the entire drill bit is visible in the dilated area. [Color figure can be viewed in the online issue, which is available at wileyonlinelibrary.com.] (Reprinted from Bhandarkar ND, Smith TL. Revision frontal sinusotomy using stepwise balloon dilation and powered instrumentation. *Laryngoscope.* 2010;120:2015-2017, with permission from The American Laryngological, Rhinological and Otological Society, Inc.)

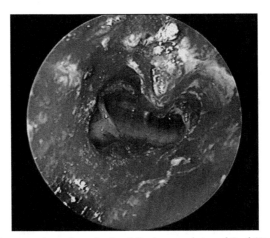

FIGURE 4.—Intraoperative endoscopic view following completion of Draf 2B procedure. [Color figure can be viewed in the online issue, which is available at wileyonlinelibrary.com.] (Reprinted from Bhandarkar ND, Smith TL. Revision frontal sinusotomy using stepwise balloon dilation and powered instrumentation. *Laryngoscope.* 2010;120:2015-2017, with permission from The American Laryngo-logical, Rhinological and Otological Society, Inc.)

technologies to impact the world of rhinology in the recent past. The exact role of the balloon in the management of chronic rhinosinusitis has yet to be estab-lished,[1] and there are many other layers to its use including financial implica-tions (such as correct billing codes, charges, ascribed relative value units, and high cost of the technology, to name a few). This "How I do it" article is included for a few simple reasons. First, it demonstrates a novel common sense application to the use of BCT to a focused indication (revision frontal sinusotomy). Second, the authors have no conflicts of interest or biases toward the technology. This article reports a novel technique to revision frontal sinusotomy incorporating the use of balloon dilation to initially enlarge the frontal recess area, followed by the use of powered instrumentation to more definitively widen it (illustrated by Figs 2-4). The authors prefer to localize the frontal sinus outflow tract and ostium with image guidance and then dilated with a balloon to address the soft tissue stenosis and make more room for powered instruments that are used next. The drill is then introduced to accomplish a Draf 2B frontal sinusotomy. They suggest that the advantage of initial balloon dilation of the frontal sinus outflow tract was to quickly address the soft tissue stenosis with minimal tissue trauma and possibly less bleeding, which further enables their ability to drill and open up the outflow tract. Although this may be the case, it should be noted that there are no data presented (or available in the literature) to support these and other claims mentioned as some of the advantages of this technique (such as shorter operating room time and reflected cost savings, improved visualization, safer drilling, etc). As the authors admit, these practical implications as well as the potential impact of this technique on outcomes of course need to be explored in an objective manner. On the note of outcomes, it could be successfully argued that although the use of BCT in rhinology is gaining popularity, it has not yet been shown that dilating a sinus ostium is superior (or even equivalent) to enlarge it using conventional instrumentation. This of course is the 800-pound gorilla in the room that has still curiously managed to be avoided...

R. Sindwani, MD

Reference

1. Batra PS, Ryan MW, Sindwani R, Marple BF. Balloon catheter technology in rhinology: reviewing the evidence. *Laryngoscope.* 2011;121:226-232.

The utility of intrathecal fluorescein in cerebrospinal fluid leak repair

Seth R, Rajasekaran K, Benninger MS, et al (Cleveland Clinic, OH; Chicago Med School at Rosalind Franklin Univ of Medicine and Science, North Chicago, IL; et al)
Otolaryngol Head Neck Surg 143:626-632, 2010

Objective.—To evaluate the utility of intrathecal fluorescein (IF) for intraoperative localization and successful repair of cerebrospinal fluid (CSF) leaks.

Study Design.—Case series with chart review.

Setting.—Tertiary-care medical center.

Subjects and Methods.—Subjects included those undergoing endoscopic CSF leak repair with or without the use of IF. Informed consent was obtained from all patients undergoing the administration of IF (total dose 10 mg).

Results.—A total of 103 patients underwent CSF leak repair, and in 47 cases (45.6%), IF was used. Patients who were administered IF were more likely to have spontaneous CSF leak etiology (61.7% vs 16.1%; $P < 0.001$). Of the 47 cases with IF use, fluorescein was visualized at the skull base in 31 cases (66.0%), 11 (23.4%) had visible CSF leak without fluorescein coloration, and five (10.6%) had neither clear nor fluorescein-colored CSF visualized. Sensitivity and specificity for fluorescein detection was 73.8 percent (95% confidence interval [CI] 57.7%-85.6%) and 100 percent (95% CI 46.3%-100%), respectively. The false-negative rate was 26.2 percent (95% CI 15.8%-43.5%). Localization of the leak site was greater when fluorescein-colored CSF was visualized (100% vs 81.3%; $P = 0.035$). When fluorescein-colored CSF was not visualized intraoperatively, recurrence rates were 31.3 percent versus 9.7 percent when fluorescein coloration was seen, although this finding was not statistically significant ($P = 0.10$).

Conclusion.—The use of IF facilitates the accurate localization of CSF leaks and may assist the surgeon in confirming a watertight closure. The lack of intraoperative fluorescein visualization should not rule out the presence of CSF leak, as evidenced by a false-negative rate of 26.2 percent (Fig 1).

▶ Despite large safety studies, there are relatively few articles in the literature examining the diagnostic use of intrathecal fluorescein (IF) intraoperatively.

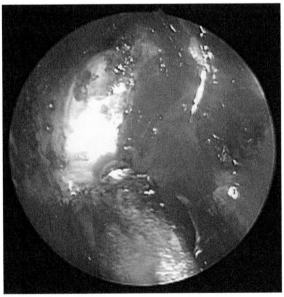

FIGURE 1.—View with 30° endoscope illustrates CSF admixed with fluorescein emanating from left cribriform plate defect in patient with spontaneous leak. (Reprinted from Seth R, Rajasekaran K, Benninger MS, et al. The utility of intrathecal fluorescein in cerebrospinal fluid leak repair. *Otolaryngol Head Neck Surg.* 2010;143:626-632. Copyright 2010, with permission from American Academy of Otolaryngology–Head and Neck Surgery Foundation.)

Most rhinologists have occasionally experienced successfully administered IF that was not present at a skull base defect site even after sufficient transfusion time (false negative). This single institution study sought to evaluate the use of IF for intraoperative localization and successful repair of cerebrospinal fluid (CSF) leaks. A total of 47 cases of IF use were examined. Fluorescein was visualized at the skull base in 31 cases (66.0%), 11 (23.4%) had visible CSF leak without fluorescein (FL) coloration, and 5 (10.6%) had neither clear nor FL-colored CSF visualized. Sensitivity and specificity for FL detection was 73.8% and 100%, respectively. The false-negative rate was a surprising 26.2%. However, the visualization of IF did not appear to impact the success rate of CSF leak repair. The authors concluded that the use of IF facilitates the accurate localization of CSF leaks but cautioned that the lack of intraoperative FL visualization should not rule out the presence of a CSF leak. In such cases, the surgeon must continue to thoroughly examine the skull base and look for the presence of clear CSF. The article discusses possible explanations for false-negative IF visualization, including a transient lack of CSF (which may occur with CSF loss during lumbar subarachnoid drain placement or during CSF reinjection with FL) hindering diffusion of FL to site, interference with FL getting to the fistula site (secondary to postmeningitis arachnoid or dural adhesions restricting flow), or possibly increased clearance of FL in some patients by either replacement of CSF volume or metabolism of the dye.

R. Sindwani, MD

Trans-blepharoplasty orbitofrontal craniotomy for repair of lateral and posterior frontal sinus cerebrospinal fluid leak
Chu EA, Quinones-Hinojosa A, Boahene KDO (Univ of California, Irvine; Johns Hopkins School of Medicine, Baltimore, MD)
Otolaryngol Head Neck Surg 142:906-908, 2010

The majority of anterior cranial base defects and associated cerebral spinal fluid (CSF) leaks are currently repaired by the endoscopic transnasal approach. Nevertheless, frontal sinus CSF leaks, especially far lateral, posterior, and superiorly located leaks, remain difficult to access with transnasal endoscopic techniques. These frontal sinus–related CSF leaks are traditionally approached through a bicoronal incision and variations of frontotemporal craniotomies. With the increasing push for minimally invasive procedures, the supraorbital keyhole craniotomy approach through an eyebrow incision has increased in popularity as a minimal access modification of the traditional orbitofrontal craniotomy to access anterior cranial base tumors and aneurysms. We present a novel direct and minimally invasive approach to frontal sinus defects for CSF repair through an eyelid incision and a mini-fronto-orbital craniotomy. We illustrate this approach with a representative case.

▶ Although most cerebrospinal fluid (CSF) leaks can be successfully managed with endoscopic techniques, defects involving the lateral, posterior, and superior

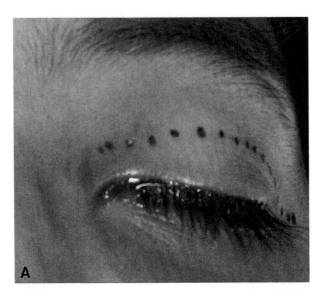

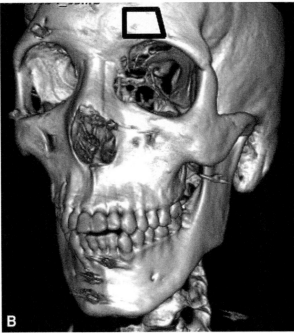

FIGURE 1.—(A) Upper eyelid crease incision for the trans-blepharoplasty approach. The incision is outlined with the patient sitting upright and may extend lateral to the lateral canthus within a natural crease. (B) Osteotomy sites marked out on a three-dimensional reconstruction of CT scan of the head. (Reprinted from Chu EA, Quinones-Hinojosa A, Boahene KDO. Trans-blepharoplasty orbitofrontal craniotomy for repair of lateral and posterior frontal sinus cerebrospinal fluid leak. *Otolaryngol Head Neck Surg.* 2010;142:906-908, with permission from the American Academy of Otolaryngology–Head and Neck Surgery Foundation.)

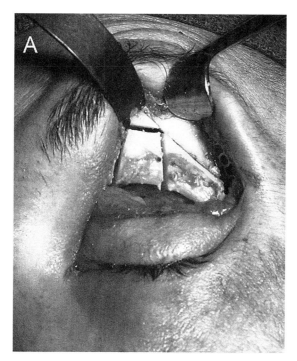

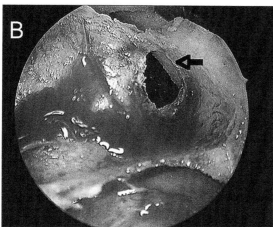

FIGURE 2.—Anterior cranial base dural defect with cerebral spinal fluid rhinorrhea following aneurysm clipping. (A) Supraorbital craniotomy has been completed and incorporates a small portion of the orbital roof. The bone cut seen laterally was from the original orbitotemporal craniotomy for access to the aneurysm. (B) Endoscopic view (4 mm, 0° rigid endoscope) of the frontal sinus and posterior frontal sinus wall. The defect in the posterior wall of the frontal sinus is identified (*black arrow*). (Reprinted from Chu EA, Quinones-Hinojosa A, Boahene KDO. Trans-blepharoplasty orbitofrontal craniotomy for repair of lateral and posterior frontal sinus cerebrospinal fluid leak. *Otolaryngol Head Neck Surg.* 2010;142:906-908, with permission from the American Academy of Otolaryngology–Head and Neck Surgery Foundation.)

frontal sinus are usually accessed through a bicoronal approach and a frontal or frontotemporal craniotomy. More recently, the supraorbital keyhole craniotomy approach through an eyebrow incision has increased in popularity as a minimal access modification of the traditional orbitofrontal craniotomy to access the anterior cranial base. This well-written article describes a novel direct and minimally invasive approach to frontal sinus defects for CSF repair through an eyelid incision and a mini-fronto-orbital craniotomy. This trans-blepharoplasty approach allows wide access to the posterior and superolateral frontal sinus interior and anterior cranial vault through a mini-craniotomy. This elegant technique also employs the adjunctive use of the endoscope and surgical navigation to maximally enhance localization and minimize morbidity. Through this technique, the entire posterior frontal sinus wall can be directly accessed. The upper eyelid incision is placed in the natural crease and as expected heals with excellent cosmesis (Figs 1 and 2). This is a distinct advantage over the previously reported supraorbital approaches, which may afford similar exposure but are accessed though a brow incision, which could interrupt the supraorbital or supratrochlear neurovascular bundle, resulting in prolonged numbness and a more conspicuous scar near the brow. As the authors highlight, great care must be taken not to disrupt the frontal sinus outflow, and a mucosal sparing technique is important to decrease the risk of postoperative mucocele formation. A larger series of this type of procedure with long-term follow-up is needed to better elucidate the indications and possible contraindications to this type of approach.

R. Sindwani, MD

7 Thyroid and Parathyroid

Basic and Clinical Research

Central Neck Lymph Node Dissection for Papillary Thyroid Cancer: Comparison of Complication and Recurrence Rates in 295 Initial Dissections and Reoperations
Shen WT, Ogawa L, Ruan D, et al (Univ of California, San Francisco)
Arch Surg 145:272-275, 2010

Background.—The American Thyroid Association recently changed its management guidelines for papillary thyroid cancer (PTC) to include routine central neck lymph node dissection (CLND) during thyroidectomy. We currently perform CLND during thyroidectomy only if enlarged central nodes are detected by palpation or ultrasonography; we perform CLND in the reoperative setting for recurrence in previously normal-appearing or incompletely resected nodes. Critics of this approach argue that reoperative CLND has higher complication and recurrence rates than initial CLND. We sought to test this argument, using it as our hypothesis.

Design.—Retrospective review.

Setting.—University hospital.

Patients.—All patients undergoing CLND for PTC between January 1, 1998, and December 31, 2007.

Interventions.—Thyroidectomy and CLND.

Main Outcome Measures.—Complications (neck hematoma, recurrent laryngeal nerve injury, and hypoparathyroidism) and recurrence of PTC.

Results.—Altogether, 295 CLNDs were performed: 189 were initial operations and 106 were reoperations. The rate of transient hypocalcemia (41.8% vs 23.6%) was significantly higher in patients undergoing initial CLND compared with those undergoing reoperative CLND. Rates of neck hematoma (1.1% vs 0.9%), transient hoarseness (4.8% vs 4.7%), permanent hoarseness (2.6% vs 1.9%), and permanent hypoparathyroidism (0.5% vs 0.9%) were not different between initial and reoperative CLND. In addition, recurrence rates in the central (11.6% vs 14.1%) and lateral (21.7% vs 17.0%) compartments were not different between the 2 groups.

Conclusions.—Reoperative CLND for PTC has a lower rate of temporary hypocalcemia, the same rate of other complications, and the same rate of recurrence compared with initial CLND. Choosing to observe nonenlarged central neck lymph nodes for PTC does not result in increased complications or recurrence if reoperation is required.

▶ It is generally accepted that in papillary thyroid carcinoma cervical lymph node metastases do not affect overall survival. However, presence of cervical lymph node metastases is associated with increased incidence of locoregional recurrence, justifying intraoperative removal of clinically or radiographically positive cervical lymph nodes in both lateral and central compartments. On the other hand, the issue of prophylactic cervical lymphadenectomy in clinically and radiographically negative cases remains subject to significant controversy. This holds particularly true for the prophylactic central compartment lymphadenectomy, which is associated with increased risk for recurrent laryngeal nerve injury and permanent hypoparathyroidism. The high incidence of central compartment micrometastases in clinically negative cases (50%-60%) is often used by proponents of prophylactic neck dissection to justify their approach, while the detractors cite increased incidence of complications without proven benefit of survival or even change in the course of the disease to justify their objection. To make things even more confusing, the American Thyroid Association recently came out with a recommendation to consider lymph node dissection (basically leaving the decision to individual surgeon) in all patients undergoing thyroidectomy for papillary thyroid carcinoma, regardless of whether the nodes are enlarged. In the backdrop of this confusion, I found this selected article, coming from a highly respected group of thyroid surgeons, very balanced and logical. First, the authors showed in their retrospective case analysis that central compartment neck dissection is indeed associated with increased incidence of recurrent laryngeal nerve and parathyroid gland injury as compared with total thyroidectomy alone. Second, they found that reoperation for central compartment lymphadenopathy is not associated with increased risk of complications or locoregional recurrence as compared with central compartment lymphadenectomy performed at the time of thyroidectomy. Based on their findings as well as on their overall philosophy, the authors recommend observation for clinically negative central compartment and surgery only for clinically or radiographically positive nodes. In my practice, in addition to outlined philosophy, I use risk stratification to guide my surgical approach: prophylactic central compartment lymphadenectomy in high-risk patients, and no lymphadenectomy in patients with low-risk scores.

M. Gapany, MD

The Effectiveness of Radioactive Iodine for Treatment of Low-Risk Thyroid Cancer: A Systematic Analysis of the Peer-Reviewed Literature from 1966 to April 2008

Sacks W, Fung CH, Chang JT, et al (Cedars-Sinai Med Ctr, Los Angeles, CA; Univ of California-Los Angeles; Zynx Health Incorporated, Los Angeles, CA)
Thyroid 20:1235-1245, 2010

Background.—Radioactive iodine (RAI) remnant ablation has been used to eliminate normal thyroid tissue and may also facilitate monitoring for persistent or recurrent thyroid carcinoma. The use of RAI for low-risk patients who we define as those under age 45 with stage I disease or over age 45 with stage I or II disease based on American Joint Committee on Cancer (AJCC) 6th edition, or low risk under the metastases, age, completeness of resection, invasion, size (MACIS) staging system (value <6) is controversial. In this extensive literature review, we sought to analyze the evidence for use of RAI treatment to improve mortality and survival and to reduce recurrence in patients of various stages and disease risk, particularly for those patients who are at low risk for recurrence and death from thyroid cancer.

Methods.—A MEDLINE search was conducted for studies published between January 1966 and April 2008 that compared the effectiveness of administering versus not administering RAI for treatment of differentiated thyroid cancer (DTC). Studies were grouped A through D based on their methodological rigor (best to worst). An analysis, focused on group A studies, was performed to determine whether treatment with RAI for DTC results in decreased recurrences and improved survival rates.

Results.—The majority of studies did not find a statistically significant improvement in mortality or disease-specific survival in those low-risk patients treated with RAI, whereas improved survival was confirmed for high-risk (AJCC stages III and IV) patients. Evidence for RAI decreasing recurrence was mixed with half of the studies showing a significant relationship and half showing no relationship.

Conclusions.—We propose a management guideline based on a patient's risk—very low, low, moderate, and high—for clinicians to use when delineating those patients who should undergo RAI treatment for initial postoperative management of DTC. A majority of very low-risk and low-risk patients, as well as select cases of patients with moderate risk do not demonstrate survival or disease-free survival benefit from postoperative RAI treatment, and therefore we recommend against postoperative RAI in these cases.

▶ The use of radioiodine for well-differentiated thyroid cancer in the United States is standard. It is routinely used in conjunction with aggressive thyroid resection (total and/or near-total thyroidectomy) even in the vast majority of patients who fall into the low-risk category. In another reviewed article, Japanese authors present outstanding long-term outcomes in low-risk, early-stage well-differentiated thyroid cancers without the use of radioactive iodine and with less aggressive partial thyroidectomy.[1] This thorough analysis of English language literature confirms what our Japanese colleagues have been claiming, that is, that radioiodine therapy in patients with low-risk well-differentiated cancer offers no disease-specific survival advantage and this type of cancer can be safely managed with surgery only. Improved survival with radioiodine therapy appears to be evident in high-risk patients and should be used in conjunction with total thyroidectomy and central compartment as well as lateral cervical lymphadenectomy, when indicated. It appears to me that most low-risk well-differentiated thyroid cancers in this country are being overtreated.

M. Gapany, MD

Reference

1. Ito Y, Masuoka H, Fukushima M, et al. Excellent prognosis of patients with solitary T1N0M0 papillary thyroid carcinoma who underwent thyroidectomy and elective lymph node dissection without radioiodine therapy. *World J Surg.* 2010; 34:1285-1290.

Diagnostics

Clinical Usefulness of Positron Emission Tomography–Computed Tomography in Recurrent Thyroid Carcinoma
Razfar A, Branstetter BF IV, Christopoulos A, et al (Univ of Pittsburgh, PA; et al)
Arch Otolaryngol Head Neck Surg 136:120-125, 2010

Objectives.—To determine the efficacy of combined positron emission tomography–computed tomography (PET-CT) in identifying recurrent thyroid cancer and to elucidate its role in the clinical management of thyroid carcinoma.

Design.—Retrospective study.

Setting.—Tertiary care referral academic center.

Patients.—One hundred twenty-four patients with previously treated thyroid carcinoma who underwent PET-CT.

Main Outcome Measures.—PET-CT images were correlated with clinicopathologic information. The influence of PET-CT findings on disease status determination and the treatment plan was evaluated.

Results.—Among 121 patients undergoing iodine I 131 (^{131}I) imaging (an ^{131}I image was unavailable for 3 patients), 80.6% had negative findings on ^{131}I imaging before undergoing PET-CT. Among 75 patients who had positive findings on PET-CT, 71 were true positive results. Among 49 patients who had negative findings on PET-CT, 32 were true negative results. Therefore, PET-CT demonstrated a sensitivity of 80.7%, specificity of 88.9%, positive predictive value of 94.7%, and negative predictive value of 65.3%. A significant difference was noted in the mean serum thyroglobulin levels between patients with positive vs negative PET-CT findings (192.1 vs 15.0 ng/mL, P=.01) (to convert thyroglobulin level to micrograms per liter, multiply by 1.0). Overall, distant metastases were detected in 20.2% of patients using PET-CT. There was an alteration of the treatment plan in 28.2% of patients as a result of added PET-CT information, and 21.0% of patients underwent additional surgery.

Conclusions.—PET-CT is usually performed in patients with thyroid cancer having elevated thyroglobulin levels but non-^{131}I–avid tumors and has high diagnostic accuracy for identifying local, regional, and distant metastases. Additional information from PET-CT in patients with ^{131}I-negative and thyroglobulin-positive tumors frequently guides the clinical management of recurrent thyroid carcinoma.

▶ This is yet another study in the series of recently published articles lending very substantial support to the use of positron emission tomography-computed tomography (PET-CT) for detection of thyroglobulin-positive/iodine-negative patients with suspected recurrent well-differentiated thyroid cancer. PET-CT offers excellent sensitivity and specificity (80.7% and 88.9%, respectively, in the present study), which appears to be better than with PET alone or CT alone. It also helps with specific anatomic localization of recurrence, which is important when planning surgical removal of metastatic cervical lymph nodes or external beam radiotherapy for recurrence in the thyroid bed. There are now enough data in the literature to recommend PET-CT as the imaging study of choice in cases of thyroglobulin-positive/iodine-negative well-differentiated thyroid cancer patients. Based on their experience, the authors of this reviewed study proposed an algorithm (Fig 3 in the original article) for the use of PET-CT in surveillance of recurrent thyroid carcinoma.

M. Gapany, MD

Diagnostic Value and Cost Considerations of Routine Fine-Needle Aspirations in the Follow-up of Thyroid Nodules with Benign Readings
van Roosmalen J, van Hemel B, Suurmeijer A, et al (Univ of Groningen, The Netherlands)
Thyroid 20:1359-1365, 2010

Background.—Fine-needle aspiration (FNA) is the most accurate tool to identify malignancy in solitary thyroid nodules. Although some recommend routinely repeating FNA for nodules that are initially read as benign, there is no consensus. We evaluated clinical relevancy and considered costs of routine follow-up FNA in nodules initially read as benign.

Methods.—We reviewed the records of all 739 patients who underwent FNA of solitary thyroid nodules at our institution from 1988 to 2004. A total of 815 aspirations were required to obtain satisfactory specimens. According to their physicians practice, some patients had a "follow-up biopsy" after an initially benign FNA reading as a matter of routine (Group I approach) or if their clinical status changed (Group II approach). The outcome information for at least 4 years after the initial FNA in these two groups was compared. In addition, hypothetical costs relating to both methods for deciding whether to do a follow-up FNA were considered.

Results.—The initial FNA was benign in 576 (78%), suspicious for follicular neoplasms in 106 (14.4%), and malignant in 57 patients (7.7%). Follow-up FNA was performed in 292 patients with initially benign lesions, 235 in Group I approach and 57 in Group II approach. The FNA diagnosis according to Group I approach remained benign on follow-up biopsy in 96.2% (226/235), was altered to follicular neoplasm in 3% (7/235), and was suspicious for malignancy in 0.8% (2/235). When following Group II approach, the follow-up FNA was benign in 93% (53/57), undetermined in 1.7% (1/57), and showed follicular neoplasm in 5.3% (3/57). Combining Groups I and II methods, 5 of 292 patients had a malignant nodule on histological examination, a false-negative rate of 1.7% for the initial FNA, but without a difference in prevalence of thyroid malignancy between the groups. Cost-consequence analysis showed no benefit in routine follow-up FNA after initially benign FNA readings.

Conclusions.—Routine follow-up FNA in patients whose initial FNA is benign has a low diagnostic upgrading value and is relatively costly. In patients whose initial FNA is benign, we recommend the FNA be repeated only if clinically suspicious signs or complaints develop.

▶ Fine-needle aspirate (FNA) is the most important diagnostic test used for the workup of thyroid nodules. Albeit very accurate, it is, nevertheless, primarily a screening test. The accuracy of FNA significantly reduces in large nodules, measuring 3 cm or more, and most clinicians believe that such nodules should be removed even when cytologic test results are negative for cancer. For smaller nodules, a "negative for malignancy" FNA result does not rule out cancer by 100%, and therefore, a strategy for subsequent follow-up has to be adopted by the managing clinician. To me, repeating screening tests never made much sense, and once the negative-for-malignancy result was obtained, I chose to follow up patients with serial thyroid ultrasounds, repeating them every 6 months for the first year and then once a year for another few years. Any increase in size of the nodule triggered excision (I never repeated FNA, neither on stable nor on growing nodules). I was, therefore, very pleased to read the results of this selected article, which in a retrospective single-institutional study assessed the diagnostic value and cost-effectiveness of repeated FNA for nodules initially diagnosed as benign on original FNA. This study confirmed the low yield and excessive cost of routine repeated FNA in this particular clinical setting.

M. Gapany, MD

General

Approach to the Patient with Incidental Papillary Microcarcinoma
Bernet V (Uniformed Services Univ of Health Sciences, Washington, DC)
J Clin Endocrinol Metab 95:3586-3592, 2010

Analysis of the Surveillance Epidemiology and End Results database reveals that since 1995 a 2.4-fold increase in thyroid cancer has occurred. A concomitant rise in cases of thyroid microcarcinoma has also been noted, with the frequency rising by approximately 50% as well. Increased detection of thyroid nodules, many of them below 1 cm in size, is at least partly responsible for this trend. The wide use of sensitive imaging modalities for various indications leads to the incidental discovery of thyroid nodules, some of which contain thyroid cancer, including cases of microcarcinoma. Although the vast majority of patients with thyroid cancer foci smaller than 1 cm will do exceedingly well long term, exceptions do occur, with some patients experiencing recurrence either locally or less frequently with distant metastasis. There has been some debate on the optimal management for these patients to include: extent of surgery required, the usefulness of ablation with radioactive iodine, as well as the optimal level for TSH suppression. In this article, we will review the available data and recommendations surrounding the management of patients with incidental thyroid microcarcinoma.

▶ Incidental thyroid microcarcinomas are on the rise, mainly because of wide use of sensitive radiographic studies such as CT and MRI scans and, recently, positron emission tomography scans. Data from large retrospective studies show that microcarcinomas of the thyroid gland (defined as tumors smaller than 1 cm in diameter) carry an excellent long-term prognosis, with disease-specific mortality significantly less than 1%. Nevertheless, the management of this incidental cancer is subject to some controversy, with many authors recommending quite aggressive surgery, including total thyroidectomy and central-compartment neck dissection. The argument for more aggressive surgery by the authors, who advocate it, is the reduced incidence of local-regional recurrence, which, by the way, does not translate into improved survival. This selected case report and review of the literature succinctly summarize the current recommendations for management of this early form of well-differentiated thyroid cancer. In my opinion, it is important not to overtreat a disease that has an outstanding long-term outcome and when morbidity of the aggressive surgical therapy might exceed the morbidity of the disease itself, including recurrence.

M. Gapany, MD

Clinical Presentation, Staging and Long-Term Evolution of Parathyroid Cancer

Talat N, Schulte K-M (King's College Hosp, London, UK)
Ann Surg Oncol 17:2156-2174, 2010

Background.—Parathyroid cancer is rare and often fatal. This review provides an in-depth analysis of 330 clinical cases reported in detail. These data are used to inform a proposal for a hitherto lacking TNM staging system.

Materials and Methods.—All case reports or series with sufficient case details of parathyroid cancer were identified from PubMed, and data were analyzed using SPSS.

Results.—Of 330 patients, 117 (35%) died of disease and 207 (63%) experienced recurrence in a total of 2007 follow-up years and a mean length of follow-up of 6.1 years. Histopathology findings rather than biochemical or clinical features predict outcome. In univariate analysis, survival and recurrence rates are significantly influenced by gender (male relative risk [RR] 1.7, 95% confidence interval [95% CI] 1.0–2.7, $P < .01$), and presence of vascular invasion (RR 4.3, 95% CI 1.1–17.7, $P < .01$), or lymph node metastases (RR 6.2, 95% CI 0.9–42.9, $P < .001$). Failure to perform onco-logical surgery carries a high risk for recurrence and death (local versus *en bloc* resection RR 2.0, CI 1.2–3.2, $P < .01$) as for redo surgery. Staging by a novel anatomy-based TNM system identifies significant outcome varia-tion as to recurrence and death. Separation of patients into low and high risk identifies a 3.5–7.0 fold higher risk of recurrence and death ($P < .01$) for the high-risk group. Distant metastases predominantly target medias-tinum and lung.

Conclusion.—Understaging and undertreatment are shown to contribute to high recurrence rates and death toll. To improve outcome, *en bloc* resec-tion including central lymph node dissection should be the minimal surgical approach in any patient with suspected parathyroid cancer.

▶ This is an outstanding study of parathyroid cancer based on a review of 330 published cases. Parathyroid carcinoma is a very rare cancer, and the biology and clinical course of this malignant tumor is not well understood. As a result, there is no agreed-upon staging system or an oncologic approach to managing parathyroid carcinoma, and this cancer is frequently underdiagnosed, under-stated, and undertreated. This selected study sheds some new light on the impact of gender, age, calcium levels, and lymph node metastases on the clin-ical course and long-term outcome of parathyroid carcinoma. The authors also propose a classification of this cancer into low- and high-risk groups to opti-mize prognostication and therapy. Based on their findings in this study, the authors have proposed a modification to currently existing Classification of Malignant Tumors (TNM) staging system, which they have found to be inade-quate. Taking into account the fact that collecting data on this cancer is partic-ularly difficult, I find this study very helpful in widening our insight into this rare malignancy.

M. Gapany, MD

Outcomes

Clinical Outcomes of Patients with Papillary Thyroid Carcinoma after the Detection of Distant Recurrence
Ito Y, Higashiyama T, Takamura Y, et al (Kuma Hosp, Kobe City, Japan)
World J Surg 34:2333-2337, 2010

Purpose.—Papillary thyroid carcinoma generally has an excellent prognosis but can have recurrence to the distant organs that is often life-threatening. To date, prognosis and prognostic factors of papillary carcinoma have been intensively investigated, but our knowledge regarding prognosis after the detection of distant recurrence remains inadequate.

Methods.—We investigated the prognosis and prognostic factors of papillary carcinoma after distant recurrence was detected during follow-up in a series of 105 patients who underwent locally curative surgery between 1987 and 2004.

Results.—To date, 30 patients (29%) have died of carcinoma, and the 5-year and 10-year cause-specific survival (CSS) rates after the detection of distant recurrence were 71 and 50%, respectively. Patients aged 55 years or older at recurrence or with massive extrathyroid extension of primary lesions demonstrated a significantly worse CSS. On multivariate analysis, these two parameters were recognized as independent prognostic factors. Gender, tumor size, and lymph node metastasis did not affect patient prognosis. Uptake of radioactive iodine (RAI) to distant metastasis was not significantly linked to CSS, but none of the patients younger than aged 55 years showing RAI uptake died of carcinoma. Appearance of distant recurrence to organs other than lung also predicted a dire prognosis.

Conclusions.—Age at recurrence and extrathyroid extension of primary lesions were significantly related to patient prognosis after the detection of distant recurrence. RAI therapy is effective, especially for younger patients, if metastatic lesions show RAI uptake.

▶ This selected article is interesting because it focuses on clinical outcomes in a very specific cohort of patients with well-differentiated thyroid carcinoma, namely patients who develop distant metastases later in the course of their disease, following the initial therapy for their tumor. While prognostic criteria for well-differentiated thyroid carcinoma are well established and widely used in prognostication and guidance of therapy, the clinical course of patients who develop distant metastases has not been well researched. In general, we know that distant metastases are associated with poor outcome, but little is known about the prognostic criteria in this specific group of patients. This retrospective study was designed to gain more insight into the clinical course of well-differentiated thyroid cancer in this specific group of patients. The authors found that lymph node metastasis had no prognostic implication on the clinical course of the disease, but patient's age at the time of recurrence and extrathyroidal extension at the time of the initial operation did have a negative impact.

M. Gapany, MD

Excellent Prognosis of Patients with Solitary T1N0M0 Papillary Thyroid Carcinoma Who Underwent Thyroidectomy and Elective Lymph Node Dissection Without Radioiodine Therapy

Ito Y, Masuoka H, Fukushima M, et al (Kuma Hosp, Chuo-ku, Kobe City, Japan)
World J Surg 34:1285-1290, 2010

Background.—The extent of surgery for papillary carcinoma significantly differs between western countries and Japan. Almost routine total thyroidectomy with radioiodine ablation therapy has been performed in western countries, whereas limited thyroidectomy has been adopted in Japan, especially for low-risk cases. In this study, the prognosis of patients with solitary papillary carcinoma measuring 2 cm or less without massive extrathyroid extension, clinically apparent lymph node metastasis or distant metastasis at diagnosis (T1N0M0 in the UICC TNM classification) was investigated to elucidate the appropriate extent of surgery for these patients.

Methods.—We investigated the prognosis of 2,638 patients with solitary T1N0M0 papillary carcinoma who underwent initial surgery between 1987 and 2004. Total or near total thyroidectomy was performed for 1,037 patients and the remaining 1,601 patients underwent more limited thyroidectomy. Elective central node dissection was performed for 2,511 patients, accounting for 96%, and 1,545 (59%) also underwent prophylactic lateral node dissection. Radioiodine ablation therapy was performed only for three patients.

Results.—The 10-year disease-free survival (DFS) rate of our series was 97%. To date, recurrence was observed in 62 patients (2%) and 41 showed recurrence to the regional lymph nodes. Seventeen of 1,601 patients who received limited thyroidectomy (1%) showed recurrence to the remnant thyroid. Pathological nodal-positive patients showed a worse DFS, but the 10-year DFS rate was still high at 96%. Patients with total or near total thyroidectomy had a better DFS, but the difference disappeared if recurrence to the remnant thyroid was excluded. A number needed to treat (NNT) for total or near total thyroidectomy over hemithyroidectomy was 83 to prevent 1 recurrence.

Conclusions.—These findings suggest that solitary T1N0M0 patients have an excellent prognosis when they undergo thyroidectomy and elective lymph node dissection without radioiodine therapy. Regarding the extent of thyroidectomy, hemithyroidectomy is adequate for these patients, if a 1% risk of recurrence to the remnant thyroid is accepted.

▶ Management of well-differentiated thyroid cancer in low-risk patients remains controversial. The guideline adopted by the American Thyroid Association calls for total thyroidectomy followed by radioiodine ablation in all cases of well-differentiated thyroid carcinoma with the exception of well-differentiated thyroid cancers that are less than 1 cm in diameter. There are other data, however, from well-respected centers in the United States, that do not support the use of radioiodine ablation in patients with low-risk thyroid cancers (review articles published by Dr Hay et al, from the Mayo Clinic). While use of radioiodine for well-differentiated thyroid cancer in the United States is standard, in Japan, it is restricted by law, reflecting the national attitude toward use of radioactive materials for medical purposes in Japan. The data on therapy of well-differentiated thyroid cancer coming from Japan are therefore very interesting to review. First, the Japanese surgeons are more conservative when it comes to resecting thyroid gland in tumors that are 2 cm or less in diameter and fall into the good prognostic category (ie, T1N0M0). Second, cervical lymph node sampling in Japan is routinely performed as part of the operation for well-differentiated thyroid cancer. This selected article exemplifies those trends. In this large series, the authors show that excellent outcomes can be achieved in T1N0M0 thyroid cancer without routine use of radioiodine ablation and with less aggressive partial thyroidectomy. Are we overtreating patients with low-risk well-differentiated thyroid cancer?

M. Gapany, MD

Five-Year Follow-up of a Randomized Clinical Trial of Unilateral Thyroid Lobectomy with or Without Postoperative Levothyroxine Treatment
Barczyński M, Konturek A, Gołkowski F, et al (Jagiellonian Univ College of Medicine, Krakow, Poland)
World J Surg 34:1232-1238, 2010

Background.—The aim of this study was to compare the prevalence of recurrent nodular goiter in the contralateral thyroid lobe among patients after unilateral thyroid lobectomy for unilateral multinodular goiter (MNG) receiving versus not receiving postoperative prophylactic levothyroxine (LT4) treatment.

Methods.—From January 2000 through December 2003, 150 consenting patients underwent a unilateral thyroid lobectomy for unilateral MNG at our institution. They were randomized to two groups with 75 patients in each group. Patients in group A received prophylactic LT4 treatment postoperatively (dose range 75–125 µg/day to maintain thyroid-stimulating hormone values below 1.0 mU/L), whereas patients in group B received no postoperative LT4 treatment. All the patients underwent ultrasonographic, cytologic, and biochemical follow-up for at least 60 months postoperatively. The primary outcome was the prevalence of recurrent goiter in the contralateral thyroid lobe. The secondary outcome was the reoperation rate for recurrent goiter. The outcomes were stratified according to individual iodine metabolism status assessed by urinary iodine excretion.

Results.—During the 5-year follow-up, among patients receiving vs. not receiving LT4, recurrent goiter within the contralateral thyroid lobe was found in 1.4% vs. 16.7% of patients, respectively ($p = 0.001$). Moreover, 1.4% vs. 8.3%, respectively, of patients receiving vs. not receiving LT4 required contralateral thyroid lobe surgery ($p = 0.05$). LT4 decreased the recurrence rate among iodine-deficient patients (3.4% vs. 36%, respectively; $p = 0.002$) but not among iodine-sufficient patients (0% vs. 6.4%, respectively; $p = 0.09$).

Conclusions.—Prophylactic LT4 treatment significantly decreased the recurrence rate of nodular goiter in the contralateral thyroid lobe and the need for completion thyroidectomy, mostly among patients with iodine deficiency.

▶ This selected study is very important to review for otolaryngologists who perform thyroid surgery. It is a randomized open-label study that evaluated the efficacy of levothyroxine therapy on recurrence rates of multinodular goiter in patients who underwent thyroid lobectomy for this disease and had no clinical evidence of contralateral goiter. The authors have confirmed in this well-designed and well-conducted study that over a 5-year follow-up period, levothyroxine therapy is primarily effective in preventing recurrence of the goiter in iodine-deficient patients. While iodine deficiency is common worldwide, it was considered almost nonexistent in the United States. However, it is again on the rise here as well. The first National Health and Nutrition Examination Survey (NHANES I), which took place between 1971 and 1974, found that just 2.6% of US citizens had iodine deficiency. The follow-up NHANES III survey, conducted between 1988 and 1994, found that 11.7% are iodine deficient. The October 1998 issue of the *Journal of Clinical Endocrinology & Metabolism* reported that over the previous 20 years, the percentage of Americans with low intake of iodine has more than quadrupled. Of particular concern is the fact that the percentage of iodine-deficient pregnant women has increased from 1% in 1974 to 7% in 1994. It is therefore wise to assess iodine status in patients who undergo partial thyroid surgery for multinodular goiter, prior to deciding on levothyroxine suppression therapy.

M. Gapany, MD

High Recurrent Rate of Multicentric Papillary Thyroid Carcinoma
Lin J-D, Chao T-C, Hsueh C, et al (Chang Gung Univ, Taoyuan Hsien, Taiwan ROC)
Ann Surg Oncol 16:2609-2616, 2009

Background.—Multicentric papillary thyroid carcinoma (PTC) is not unusual in patients with PTC. However, its clinical features concerning cancer recurrence and mortality are not well described.

Methods.—A total of 1682 PTC patients at a single institution who underwent total thyroidectomy were retrospectively reviewed; the mean follow-up period was 7.7 ± 0.1 years. Postoperative radioactive iodide ablation for thyroid remnant was performed after surgery for most patients.

Results.—Of all the PTC cases reviewed, 337 cases (20.0%) were categorized as multicentric PTC. Compared with patients with unifocal PTC, multicentric PTC patients demonstrated older age, advanced TNM staging, and higher recurrence. A higher recurrence rate for multicentric PTC (20.2%) was observed compared with that for unifocal PTC; 45.8% of multicentric PTC cases with ≥ 5 foci experienced cancer recurrence. Mean tumor size of the largest nodule in patients with multicentric PTC was significantly smaller than that found in unifocal PTC. Patients with multicentric papillary microcarcinoma (≤1 cm) had higher recurrence rate and cancer mortality than those with unifocal papillary microcarcinoma. Of the recurrent multicentric PTC cases, 52.9% were persistent or diagnosed within the first year of thyroidectomy and had a cancer-related mortality of 27.8%. The 5-, 10-, and 20-year survival rates of multicentric PTC patients were 97.7%, 94.4%, and 84.7%, respectively, which were not statistically different from those of unifocal PTC patients.

Conclusions.—Multicentric PTC warrant postoperative adjuvant therapy and close surveillance within the first year. Patients with multicentric papillary thyroid microcarcinoma need to be treated as high-risk patients.

▶ Papillary thyroid carcinoma is often multifocal; as a matter of fact, as many as one-third of all patients with papillary thyroid cancer can harbor more than 1 focus of disease in their thyroid glands. The true clinical significance of this finding as well as its prognostic impact is not well understood. For example, it is known that up to 30% of normal thyroid glands examined postmortem may harbor thyroid microcarcinomas. Accepted prognostic criteria, widely used in clinical practice to determine the risk for poor outcome, do not as a rule include multifocality. However, there is an increasing chorus of voices calling for more aggressive management of multifocal papillary thyroid carcinoma. This selected retrospective study finds an association between multicentricity of papillary thyroid carcinoma and the risk for recurrence of the disease. In this study, as it frequently is with well-differentiated thyroid cancer, the increased rate of recurrence did not, however, translate into worse long-term disease-specific survival. Thus, in the absence of other poor prognostic criteria, multicentricity of papillary thyroid carcinoma alone might not be of such great prognostic importance after all. The authors' call for treating all patients with multicentricity as high-risk patients should be taken with some caution.

M. Gapany, MD

Impact of Pregnancy on Outcome and Prognosis of Survivors of Papillary Thyroid Cancer

Hirsch D, Levy S, Tsvetov G, et al (Beilinson Hosp, Petach Tikva, Israel; Academic College of Tel Aviv-Yaffo, Israel)
Thyroid 20:1179-1185, 2010

Background.—Papillary thyroid cancer (PTC) commonly affects women of child-bearing age. During normal pregnancy, several factors may have a stimulatory effect on normal and nodular thyroid growth. The aim of the study was to determine whether pregnancy in thyroid-cancer survivors poses a risk of progression or recurrence of the disease.

Methods.—The files of 63 consecutive women who were followed at the Endocrine Institute for PTC in 1992–2009 and had given birth at least once after receiving treatment were reviewed for clinical, biochemical, and imaging data. Thyroglobulin levels and neck ultrasound findings were compared before and after pregnancy. Demographic and disease-related characteristics and levels of thyroid-stimulating hormone (TSH) during pregnancy were correlated with disease persistence before conception and disease progression during pregnancy using Pearson's analysis.

Results.—Mean time to the first delivery after completion of thyroid-cancer treatment was 5.08 ± 4.39 years; mean duration of follow up after the first delivery was 4.84 ± 3.80 years. Twenty-three women had more than one pregnancy, for a total of 90 births. Six women had evidence of thyroid cancer progression during the first pregnancy; one of them also showed disease progression during a second pregnancy. Another two patients had evidence of disease progression only during their second pregnancy. Mean TSH level during pregnancy was 2.65 ± 4.14 mIU/L. There was no correlation of disease progression during pregnancy with pathological staging, interval from diagnosis to pregnancy, TSH level during pregnancy, or thyroglobulin level before conception. There was a positive correlation of cancer progression with persistence of thyroid cancer before pregnancy and before total I-131 dose was administered.

Conclusions.—Pregnancy does not cause thyroid cancer recurrence in PTC survivors who have no structural or biochemical evidence of disease persistence at the time of conception. However, in the presence of such evidence, disease progression may occur during pregnancy, yet not necessarily as a consequence of pregnancy. The finding that a nonsuppressed TSH level during pregnancy does not stimulate disease progression suggests that it may be an acceptable therapeutic goal in this setting.

▶ This study is an important contribution to a relatively small body of existing literature that addresses the potentially detrimental effect of pregnancy on thyroid cancer recurrence and/or progression. Since well-differentiated thyroid cancer is prevalent in women of childbearing age, a question frequently arises in thyroid cancer survivors whether it is safe to conceive and whether the pregnancy itself poses a risk for recurrence or progression of the disease. While this dilemma is most commonly tackled by endocrinologists and obstetricians/gynecologists, the otolaryngologist who performed the original thyroid cancer operation might also be part of the decision-making team. It is therefore very important for otolaryngologists who treat thyroid cancer to be up to date on this topic. In a way, this study is good news for women who have no evidence of persistent disease (as evidenced by negative ultrasonography and undetectable thyroglobulin levels) and wish to conceive. It confirms the data from some previously published studies that pregnancy in itself does not constitute a risk for recurrence of well-differentiated thyroid cancer.

M. Gapany, MD

No survival difference after successful ^{131}I ablation between patients with initially low-risk and high-risk differentiated thyroid cancer
Verburg FA, Stokkel MPM, Düren C, et al (Univ of Würzburg, Germany; Leiden Univ Med Ctr, The Netherlands; et al)
Eur J Nucl Med Mol Imaging 37:276-283, 2010

Purpose.—To compare disease-specific survival and recurrence-free survival (RFS) after successful ^{131}I ablation in patients with differentiated thyroid carcinoma (DTC) between those defined before ablation as low-risk and those defined as high-risk according to the European Thyroid Association 2006 consensus statement.

Methods.—Retrospective data from three university hospitals were pooled. Of 2009 consecutive patients receiving ablation, 509 were identified as successfully ablated based on both undetectable stimulated serum thyroglobulin in the absence of antithyroglobulin antibodies and a negative diagnostic whole-body scan in a follow-up examination conducted 8.1 ± 4.6 months after ablation. Of these 509 patients, 169 were defined as high-risk.

Results.—After a mean follow-up of 81 ± 64 months (range 4–306 months), only three patients had died of DTC, rendering assessment of disease-specific survival differences impossible. Of the 509 patients, 12 (2.4%) developed a recurrence a mean 35 months (range 12–59 months) after ablation. RFS for the duration of follow-up was 96.6% according to the Kaplan-Meier method. RFS did not differ between high-risk and low-risk patients ($p=0.68$). RFS differed slightly but significantly between those with papillary and those with follicular thyroid carcinoma ($p=0.03$) and between those aged ≤ 45 years those aged >45 years at diagnosis ($p=0.018$).

Conclusion.—After (near) total thyroidectomy and successful ^{131}I ablation, RFS does not differ between patients classified as high-risk and those classified as low-risk based on TNM stage at diagnosis. Consequently, the follow-up protocol should be determined on the basis of the result of initial treatment rather than on the initial tumour classification.

▶ American Thyroid association guidelines and several other recent consensus statements recommend total thyroidectomy followed by adjuvant radioiodine ablation for well-differentiated thyroid carcinomas (with the exception of microcarcinomas). While very few endocrinologists nowadays disagree with the recommendation for a total thyroidectomy for well-differentiated thyroid cancer, the role of radioiodine ablation has been a subject of controversy. Some experts in the field believe that patients with low-risk differentiated thyroid cancer do not benefit from adjuvant radioiodine therapy and advocate iodine ablation only for high-risk thyroid cancers. This large multicenter study has demonstrated (confirming some previously published data) that successful radioiodine ablation as an adjuvant therapy to total thyroidectomy is associated with equally good recurrence-free survival in both low-risk and high-risk tumors. Furthermore, successful radioiodine ablation (negative thyroid-stimulating hormone-stimulated serum thyroglobulin levels) can serve as a good prognostic indicator for excellent recurrence-free survival even in patients with tumors classified as falling into the poor prognostic category.

M. Gapany, MD

Article Index

Chapter 1: Allergy and Immunology

Chapter 2: Head and Neck Surgery and Tumors

Chapter 3: Laryngology

Chapter 4: Otology

Chapter 5: Pediatric Otolaryngology

Chapter 6: Rhinology and Skull Base Surgery

Chapter 7: Thyroid and Parathyroid

Author Index

Printed and bound by CPI Group (UK) Ltd, Croydon, CR0 4YY

08/05/2025

01864677-0002